An Atlas of CORNEAL TOPOGRAPHY

An Atlas of

Corneal Topography

Edited by

Donald R. Sanders, MD, PhD
Associate Professor of Ophthalmology
University of Illinois
at Chicago Eye Center
Center for Clinical Research
Chicago, Illinois

Douglas D. Koch, MD
Associate Professor of Ophthalmology
Cullen Eye Institute
Baylor College of Medicine
Houston, Texas

Project Coordinator
Michelle Van Der Karr

SLACK Incorporated, 6900 Grove Road, Thorofare, NJ 08086-9447

SLACK International Book Distributors

In Japan
Igaku-Shoin, Ltd.
Tokyo International P.O. Box 5063
1-28-36 Hongo, Bunkyo-Ku
Tokyo 113
Japan

In Canada
McGraw-Hill Ryerson Limited
300 Water Street
Whitby, Ontario
L1N 9B6
Canada

In all other regions throughout the world, SLACK professional reference books are available through offices and affiliates of McGraw-Hill, Inc. For the name and address of the office serving your area, please correspond to

McGraw-Hill, Inc.
Medical Publishing Group
Attn: International Marketing Director
1221 Avenue of the Americas —28th Floor
New York, NY 10020
(212)-512-3955 (phone)
(212)-512-4717 (fax)

Editorial Director: Cheryl D. Willoughby
Publisher: Harry C. Benson

An Atlas of corneal topography / edited by Donald R. Sanders, Douglas D. Koch,
p. cm.
Includes biobliographical references and index.
ISBN 1-55642-218-0 (hard)
1. Corneal topography--Atlases. 2. Computer-assisted videokeratography--Atlases. 3. Cornea--Diseases--Diagnosis--Atlases. I. Sanders, Donald R. II. Koch, Douglas D.
[DNLM: 1. Cornea--anatomy & physiology--atlases. 2. Corena--surgery--atlases. 3. Corneal Diseases--radiography--atlases. 4. Image Processing, Computer-Assisted--Atlases. WW 17 A88037
RE336.A84 1993
617.7'1907656--DC20
DNLM/DLC

for Library of Congress 92-49273

Printed in the United States of America

Published by: SLACK Incorporated
6900 Grove Road
Thorofare, NJ 08086-9447

Last digit is print number: 10 9 8 7 6 5 4 3 2 1

To Wanda
My Wife
My Love
My Friend
DRS

Contents

Contributing Authors

Timothy B. Cavanaugh, MD
Hunkeler Eye Clinic
Kansas City, Missouri

David Dulaney, MD
Dulaney Eye Clinic
Phoenix, Arizona

Daniel S. Durrie, MD
Hunkeler Eye Clinic
Kansas City, Missouri

James P. Gills, MD
Clinical Professor
University of South Florida
Tampa, Florida

Elizabeth A. Haft, BS
Cullen Eye Institute
Baylor College of Medicine
Houston, Texas

Douglas Horner, OD, PhD
School of Optometry
Indiana University
Bloomington, Indiana

Douglas D. Koch, MD
Associate Professor of Ophthalmology
Cullen Eye Institute
Baylor College of Medicine
Houston, Texas

Robert B. Mandell, OD, PhD
School of Optometry
University of California
Berkeley, California

Robert G. Martin, MD
Director, Medical Care International
Ophthalmic Research and Training
Institute
Founder, Carolina Eye Associates
Southern Pines, North Carolina

Ellen Kelley McHale, COT
Center for Eye Research
Boston, Massachusetts

Linda J. Rhodes, FCLSA, NCLE
Cullen Eye Institute
Baylor College of Medicine
Instructor, Baylor College of Medicine
Houston, Texas

Donald R. Sanders, MD, PhD
Associate Professor of Ophthalmology
University of Illinois at Chicago Eye Center
Director, Center for Clinical Research
Chicago, Illinois

Roger F. Steinert, MD
Harvard Medical School
Tufts University School of Medicine
Center for Eye Research
Boston, Massachusetts

Spencer P. Thornton, MD
Director, Cataract and Corneal Service
Baptist Hospital
Director, Thornton Eye Surgery Center
Nashville, Tennessee

Michael Vrabec, MD
Assistant Professor of Ophthalmology
University of Vermont
College of Medicine
Burlington, Vermont

Preface

There have been few truly innovative and revolutionary products that have changed the practice of ophthalmology. In the surgical arena, the development of intraocular lenses, Nd:YAG lasers, and phacoemulsifiers fundamentally changed the methodology and dramatically improved the results of cataract surgery. In the refractive area, lasers have the potential to provide predictable methods of correcting refractive errors. In the area of diagnostic equipment, major advances have been truly rare. One of the most notable of these has been A-scan biometry with implant power calculation, which evolved from a new innovation to a necessity in remarkably little time. Computer-assisted videokeratography represents a major technological breakthrough that promises to change the way the cornea is evaluated. The scope and breadth of this book document the changes that have already occurred, from the way pathological conditions such as keratoconus and keratoglobus are diagnosed and followed, to the way surgical and laser procedures such as cataract surgery, astigmatic keratotomy, penetrating keratoplasty, and photorefractive keratectomy are planned, evaluated, and followed, and including also the way contact lenses are fitted. The applications of this new technology as discussed in this book truly represent only the "tip of the iceberg". We hope this atlas serves both as an educational tool and as a stimulus to further innovations in this exciting field.

Acknowledgments

The editors wish to acknowledge the kind assistance of:

Carol Ballew, PhD
Mark Findahl
Barbara Ellen Lowe

1

DOUGLAS D. KOCH, MD
ELIZABETH A. HAFT, BS

Introduction to Corneal Topography

The Importance of the Cornea in Refractive Surgery

In refractive surgery the surgeon must be able to measure precisely and modify predictably. The cornea, lens, and axial length are the key refractive elements of the eye. Of these three factors, only the cornea is clinically accessible for both measurement and modification. Measurement of lens power is problematic, and lens power can only be modified by lens extraction, intraocular lens implantation, or both. Axial length can be measured, but refractive surgical modification is not possible. At this time, the cornea offers the greatest opportunities for surgical correction of refractive errors.

Evaluating Topographical Maps

Since we will be illustrating a number of the points in this chapter with examples of corneal topographic maps, it may be appropriate to discuss how to interpret them. Figure 1.1 is a typical color contour map of a normal, essentially non-astigmatic cornea. In interpreting these maps, it is important to recognize that the so-called "hot" colors—red, orange, and yellow—are steeper portions of the cornea. Green is intermediate and cool colors—light and dark blue—are flatter portions. It is extremely important when looking at these maps to look at the color scale to the left to see which colors correspond to which dioptric powers and to determine the dioptric interval between color changes. In this case the color changes are in half-diopter increments, and since there are 15 distinct colors represented on the scale to the right, the entire range represents 7.5 D. In this case the central cornea is in the 46.5 to 47 D power range. The white circle in the center of the image represents the pupil outline.

The cursor represented by a "+" is initially located at the point which represents the center of the corneoscopic rings. This

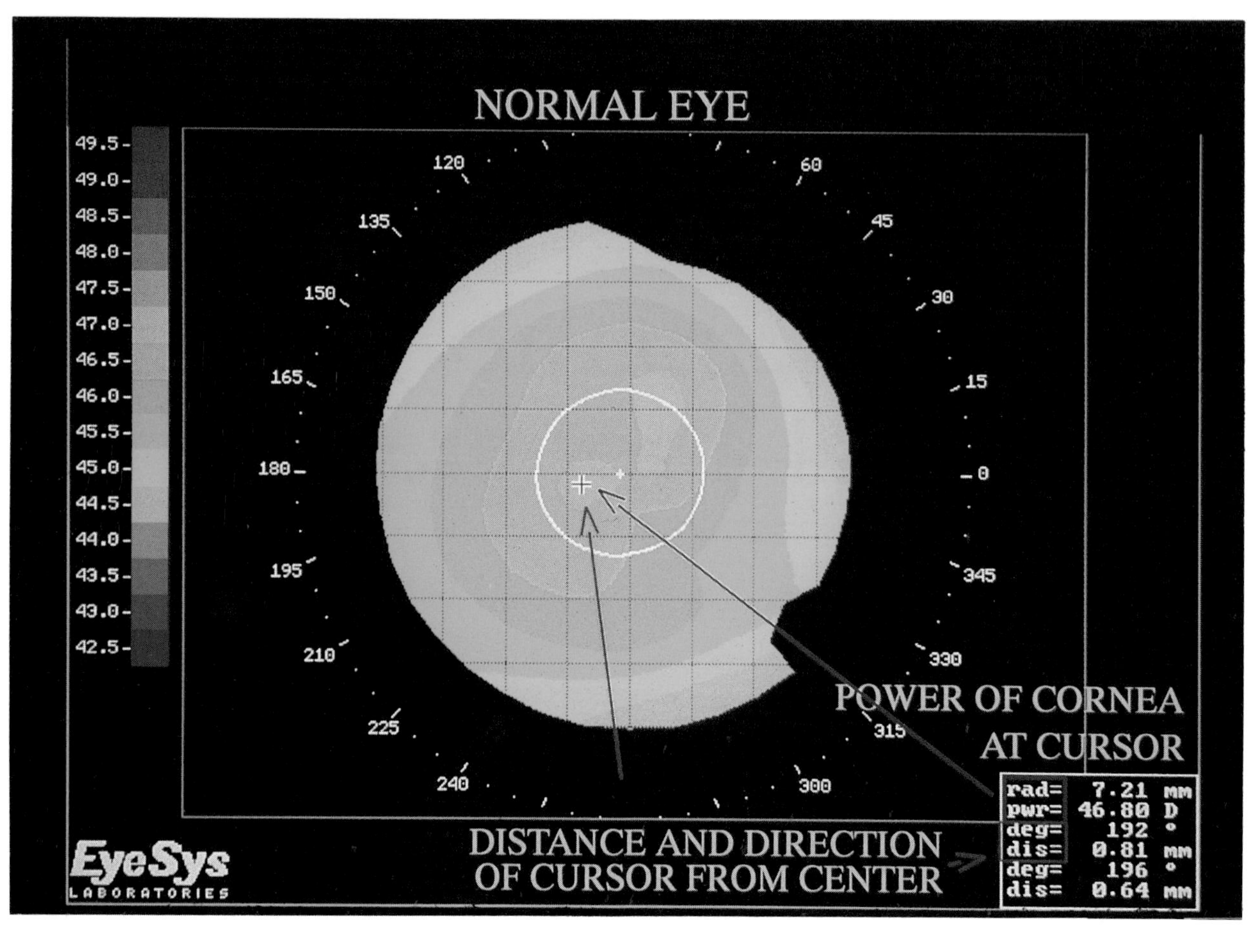

Figure 1.1: Corneal topographic map of an essentially normal aspheric right cornea. The cornea is steepest centrally with progressive flattening peripherally, especially in the nasal area.

center point is referred to as the videokeratographic (or VK) axis or as the vertex normal. When viewing the topographical map on the color monitor of the system, the cursor can be moved around the color map with the computer mouse. The information box in the lower right corner reports the radius of curvature (mm) and dioptric power at the location of the mouse cursor (Figure 1.1). The position with respect to the center of the rings is displayed in radial degrees and millimeters. This and most of the other maps shown have a grid pattern superimposed upon the image. Each square is 1 mm by 1 mm, which allows one to quickly determine how far from the corneal center an abnormality occurs. Also note the peripheral circle which marks the meridians for 360°, which is especially helpful in astigmatism cases.

One can decrease the sensitivity by using larger increments on the dioptric scaling to screen for gross pathology. One can also increase the sensitivity for detecting much smaller and more subtle corneal topographic changes by decreasing the increments between color changes. Figures 1.2A-D demonstrate the same eye displayed with four different dioptric intervals or sensitivities. Keep in mind that when you "zoom in" for a closer look at the corneal curvature it is essential to be aware of the magnification (that is, the dioptric power scale) or you may become confused by clinically insignificant corneal changes. The color changes in the central pupillary area in Figure 1.2D are clinically insignificant in this essentially spherical central cornea.

In addition to the highly flexible "normalized" scale where the dioptric intervals and colors can be individualized, the system also generates an absolute scale ranging from 35 D to 52 D in 0.5 D steps, effectively producing a 17 D range and 34 separable intervals (Figure 1.3). While not as dramatic in appearance as the normalized scale, the value of an absolute scale is that the same color and pattern always represent a specific dioptric range, and once learned avoids confusion that may occur if the user fails to pay attention to the color scale. Its value, especially in pathological corneas, will be demonstrated.

Normal Corneal Curvature and Power

The normal cornea is aspheric and is typically steepest centrally with progressive flattening towards the periphery (Figures 1.1 through 1.3). The nasal cornea is often flatter than the temporal cornea. This aspheric curvature is similar to the curvature of the long end of an ellipse.

A wide variety of different corneal shape patterns can be seen in some virgin corneas and in great frequency in corneas that have been extrinsically modified. For example, following radial keratotomy, the cornea typically flattens centrally and steepens toward the periphery.

Corneal refractive power is determined by both its anterior and posterior curvatures. The power of the anterior surface of normal corneas is approximately 49 D, and that of the posterior surface is approximately −6 D. Since we can presently measure only the anterior curvature of the cornea, and since clinically we wish to know the true corneal refractive power, a modified value for corneal refractive index is used for calculating corneal power. For most corneal measuring devices, instead of 1.376, which is the true refractive index (n) of the cornea, the value 1.3375 is used. For example, for a radius of curvature of 8.00 mm, the actual anterior corneal curvature is 47.00 (using $n = 1.376$), but from a clinical device we would obtain the value of 42.19 for net corneal power (using $n = 1.3375$).

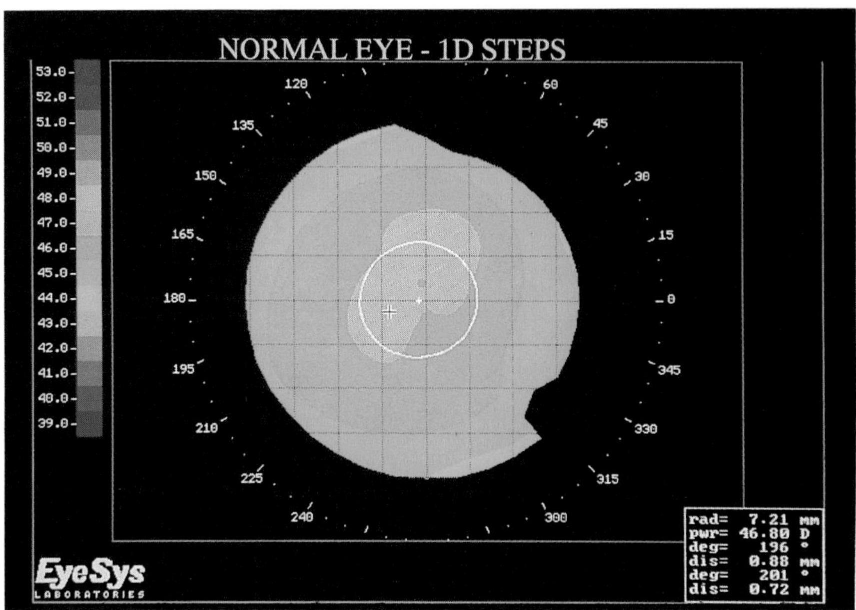

Figure 1.2A.

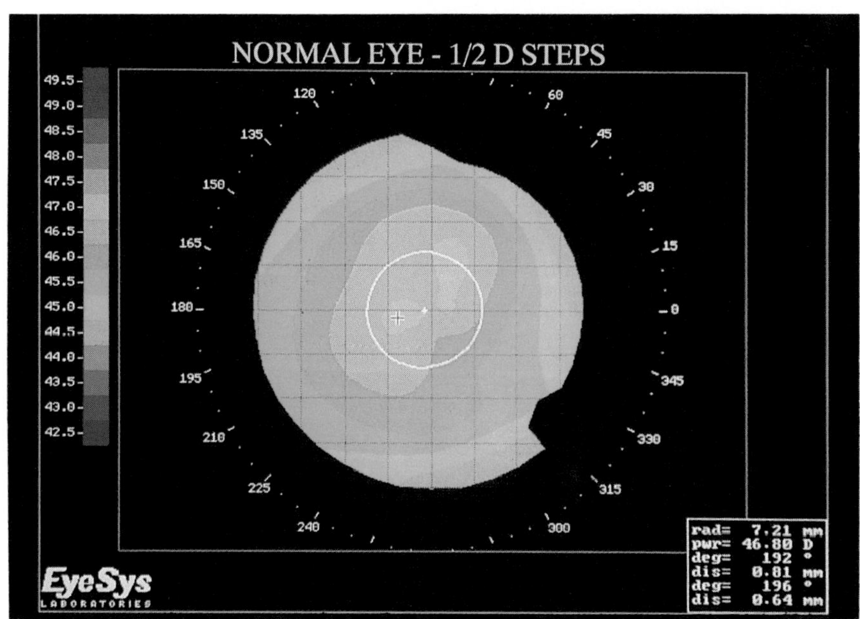

Figure 1.2B.

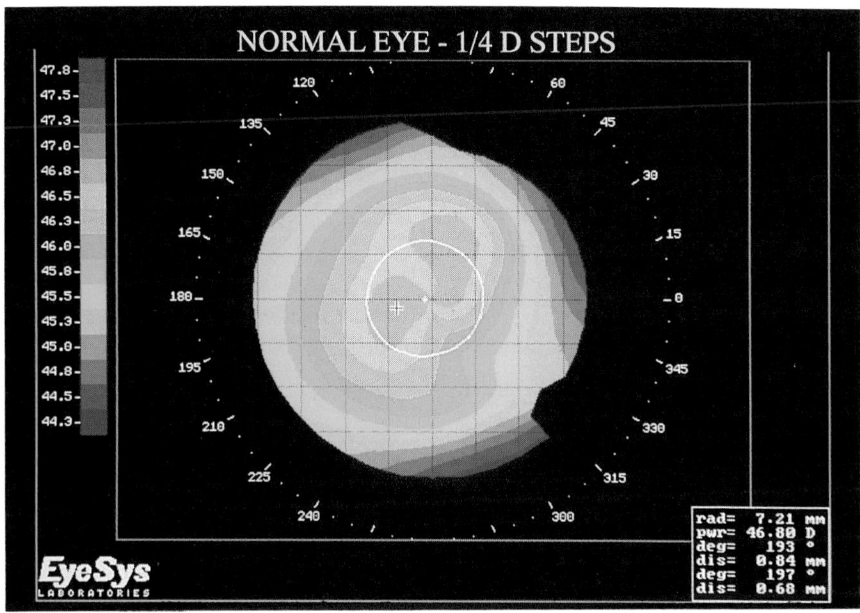

Figure 1.2C.

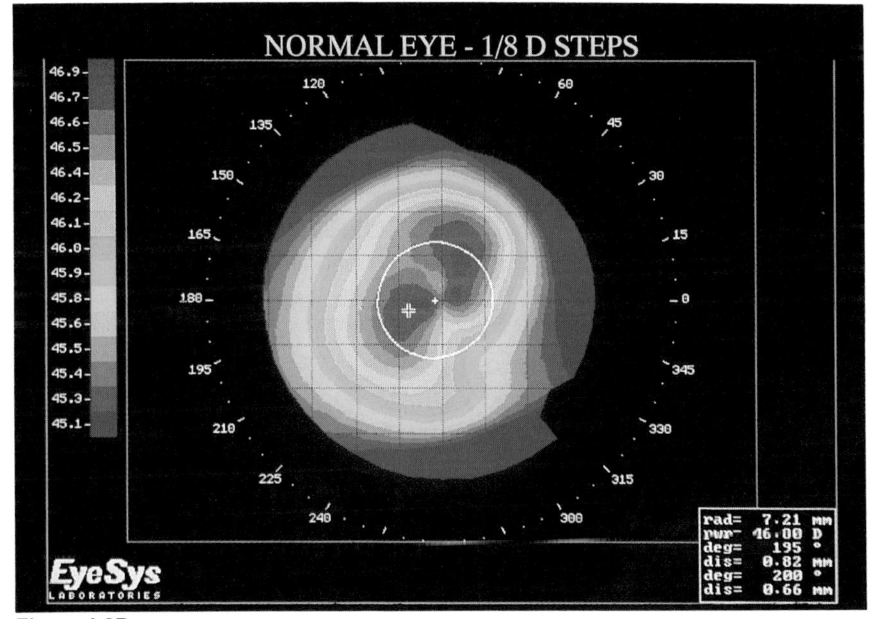

Figure 1.2D.

Figure 1.2: Same cornea as Figure 1.1 showing the effect of changing the dioptric intervals of the scale on the appearance of the topographic map. (A) 1 diopter intervals, (B) 1/2 diopter intervals, (C) 1/4 diopter intervals, (D) 1/8 diopter intervals.

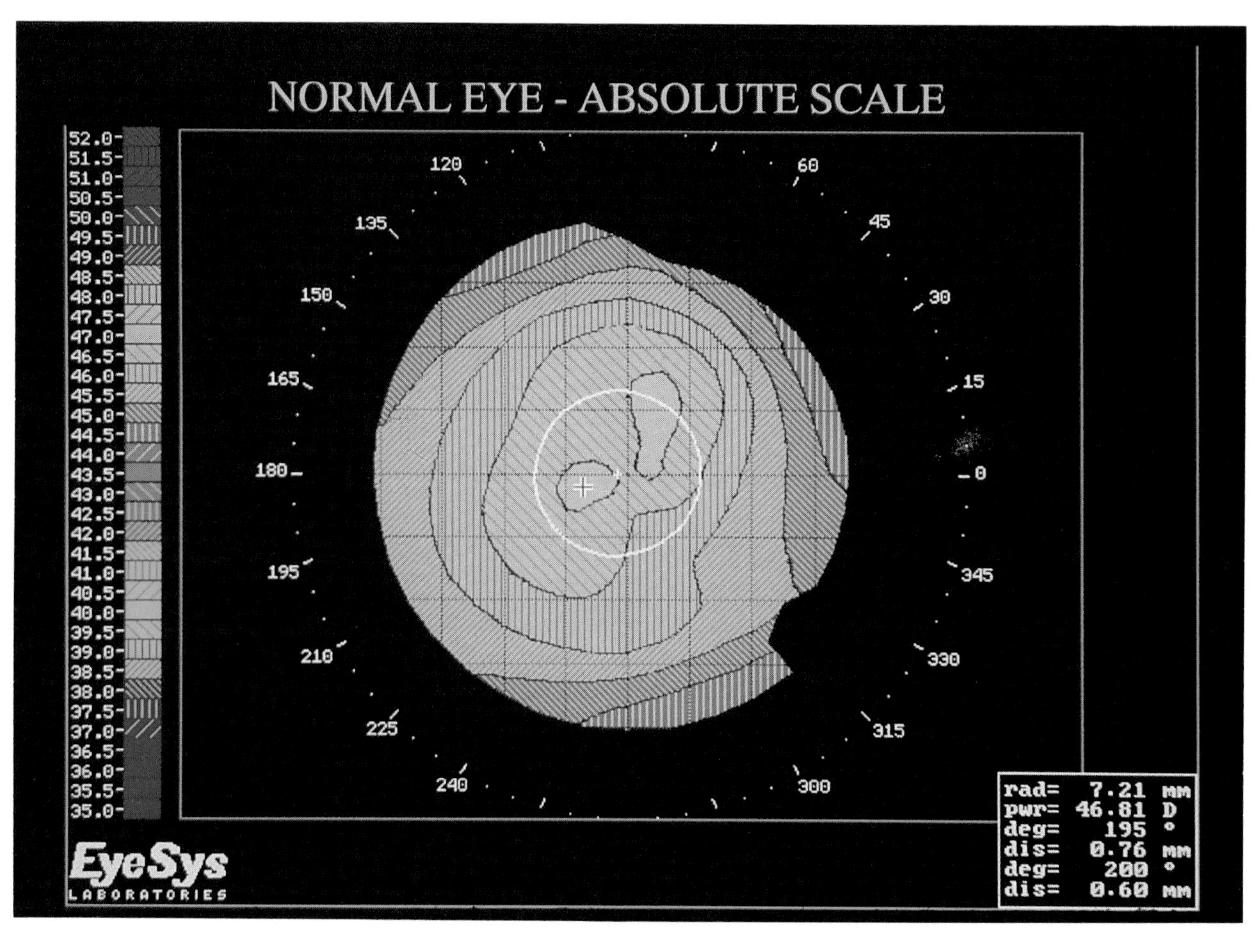

Figure 1.3: Same cornea as Figures 1.1 and 1.2 using the absolute scale.

Limitations of the Keratometer

For decades, the keratometer was the standard for measuring corneal curvature, and, until recently, keratometric data were sufficient for most clinical situations. The keratometer projects a single mire on the cornea, and the separation of two points on the mire is used to determine corneal curvature. The zone measured depends upon corneal curvature; the steeper the cornea, the smaller the zone. For a 36 D cornea, the keratometer measures a 4 mm zone; for a 50 D cornea, the size of this zone is 2.88 mm.

The keratometer has several positive features:

1) accuracy and reproducibility for measuring regular corneas within the normal range of curvatures (40-46 D),
2) speed,
3) ease of use,
4) low cost, and
5) minimal maintenance requirements.

Unfortunately, however, the keratometer has several major inherent limitations:

1) The keratometer measures only a small region of the cornea; central and peripheral regions are ignored.
2) The keratometer assumes that the cornea is symmetrical; it therefore averages the two semimeridians of any given meridian.
3) For corneas of different powers, the keratometer measures different regions.
4) The keratometer loses accuracy when measuring very flat or very steep corneas, particularly those in excess of 50 D.

With these limitations in mind, the keratometer gives a reasonable estimate of central corneal curvature for normal regular corneas. However, many cases with undetected pathology (Figure 1.4) and virgin corneas (i.e., no previous surgery or contact lens wear) are not regular, and corneas that have sustained some form of trauma typically demonstrate some degree of topographical irregularity. As a result, keratometric readings are subject to at least four types of clinically important errors:

1) Inaccurate reading for central corneal curvature (Figure 1.5),
2) Incorrect or misleading dioptric assessment of 3 mm zone (Figure 1.6),
3) Incorrect reading for orientation of steep and flat meridians (Figure 1.7), and
4) Omission of critical information regarding the topography of the corneal periphery (Figure 1.8).

As these and numerous additional examples in this book will illustrate, to understand corneal topography, one must be able to evaluate central and peripheral corneal curvature. The central 3 to 5 mm region of the cornea refracts the light that provides central vision; the precise regions of the cornea responsible for this refraction are determined by pupil size and the Stiles-Crawford effect.[1] The corneal periphery also has an important refractive function, since its refraction of off-axis light affects contrast sensitivity and glare, again as a function of pupil size; more importantly, the topography of the corneal periphery determines central corneal curvature. With the need for this information in mind, it is apparent that the keratometer has become outmoded as the primary means of evaluating corneal curvature.

Qualitative Measurement of Corneal Topography

Several devices have been developed for qualitative measurement of corneal topography. These include the von Loehnan keratoscope (JedMed) (Figure 1.9), the Klein keratoscope (Keeler Instruments), and the Placido image that Rowsey and colleagues provided in their

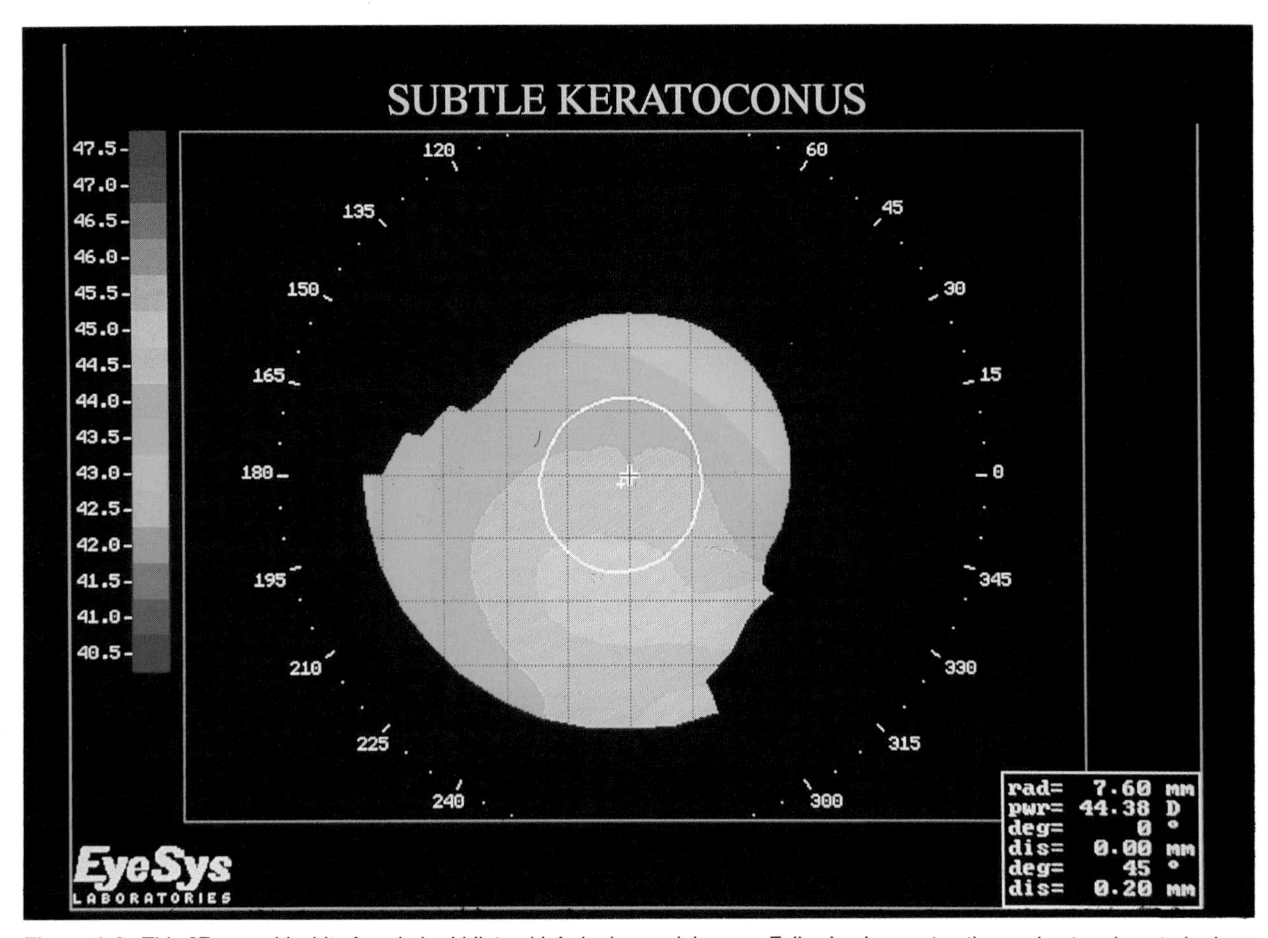

Figure 1.4: This 37-year-old white female had bilateral inferior lens colobomas. Following lens extraction and sutured posterior lens implantation, best-corrected vision was only 20/30. Computerized videokeratography revealed subtle keratoconus bilaterally (seen here in the right eye preoperatively). Vision was 20/20 with a contact lens. Note the subtle asymmetric inferior steepening.

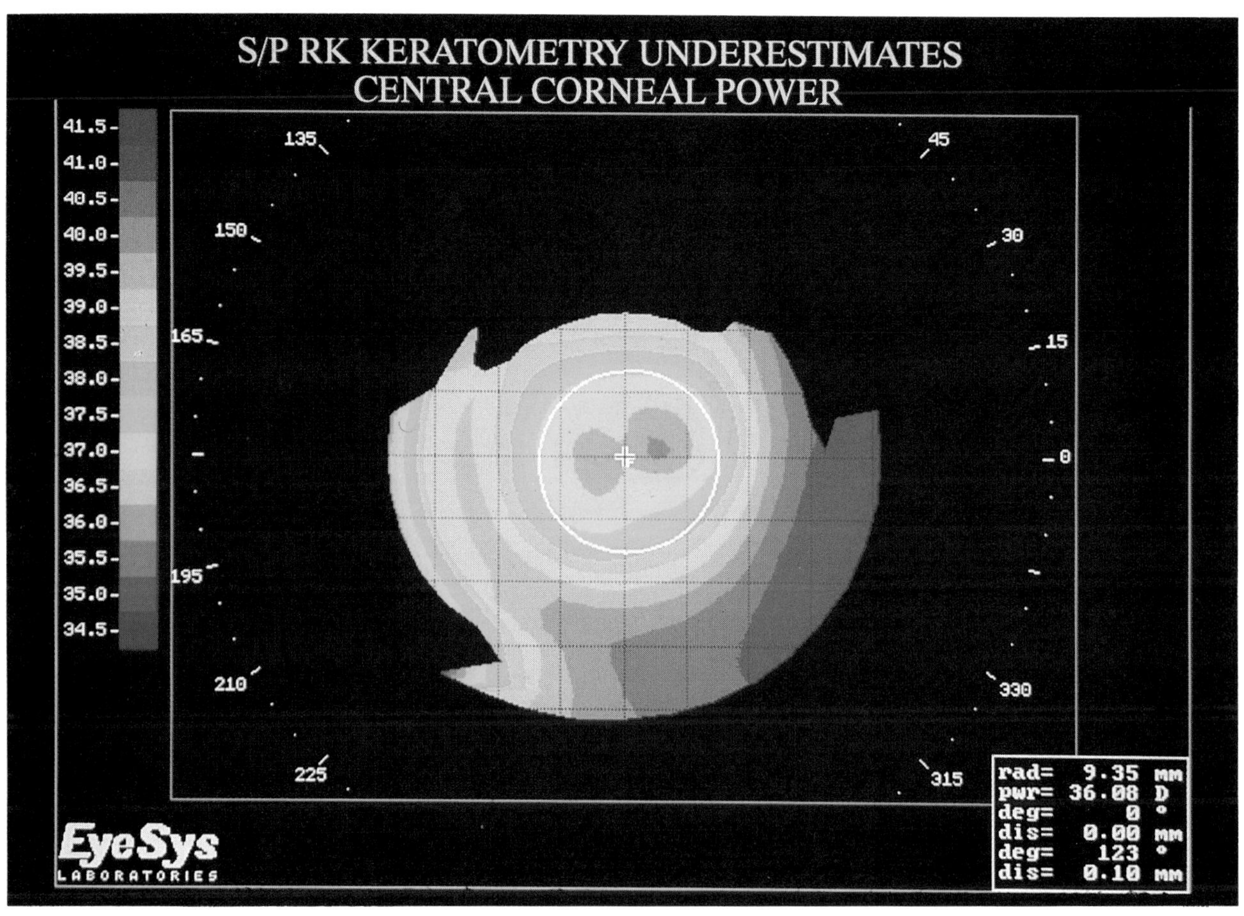

Figure 1.5: Marked central corneal flattening 2 weeks following 8-incision radial keratotomy. Keratometry was 37/37.5 at 80°, but central corneal power by CVK is 36.08 D, consistent with +2.00 D refraction.

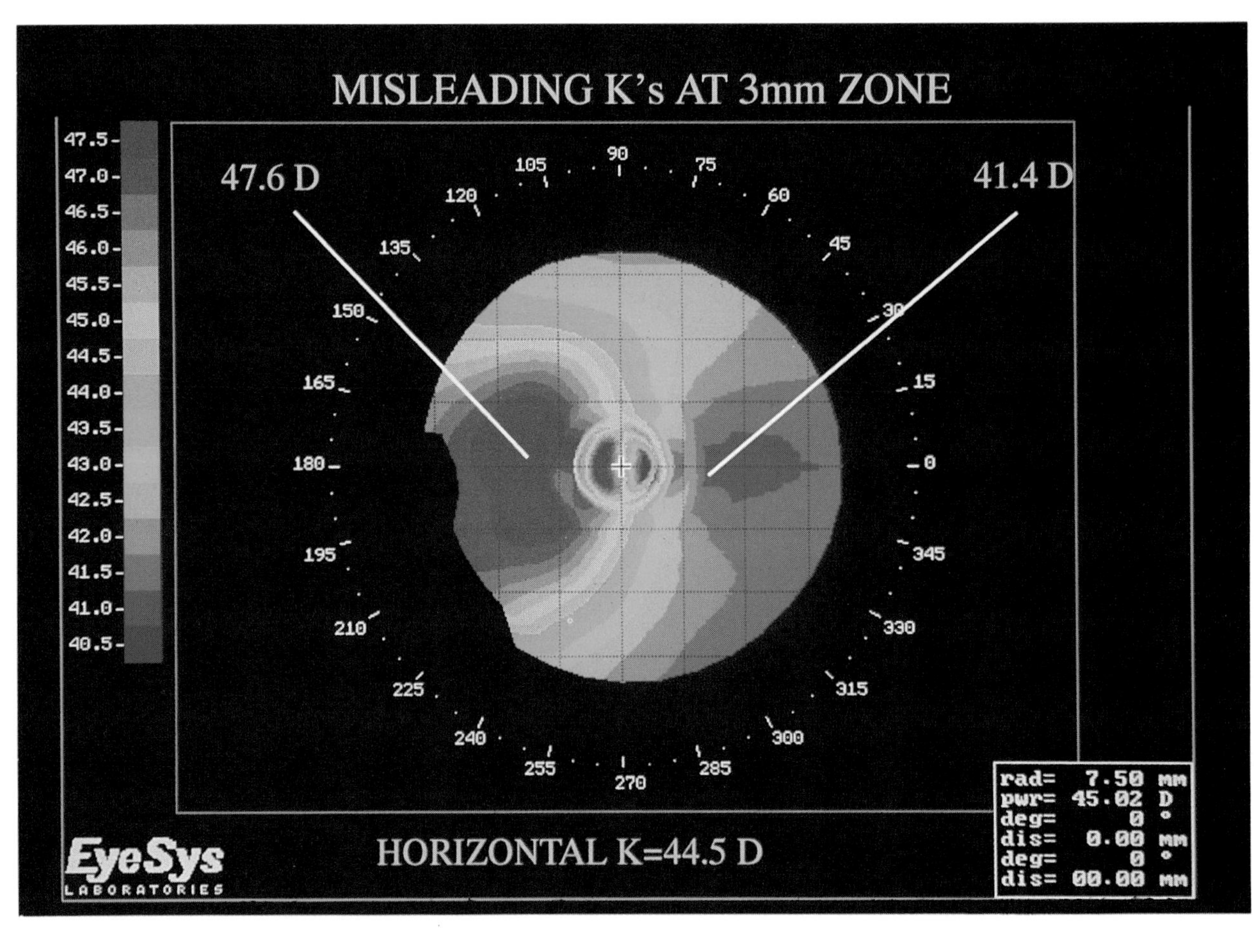

Figure 1.6: Postoperative astigmatic keratotomy case (OS) with steep nasal area and flat temporal area. Temporal measurement was 41.4 D and nasal was 47.6 D. The keratometer averaged these values and gave a value of 44.5 D for the horizontal meridian (0-180° axis).

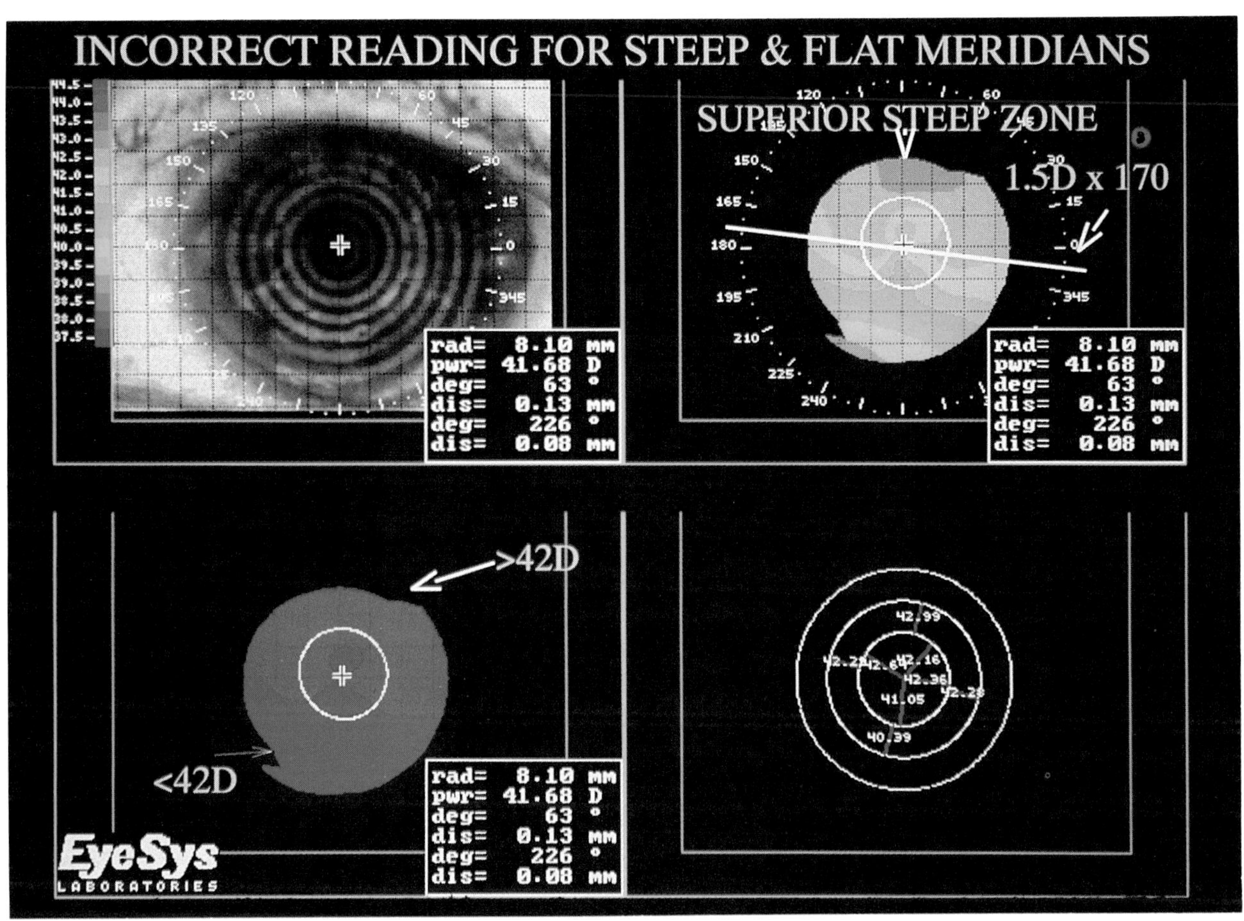

Figure 1.7: Preoperative cataract case with unusual asymmetric cornea. The keratometer localized the astigmatism to the 170° meridian. Topography shows the steepest portion of the cornea to be superiorly at 90°.

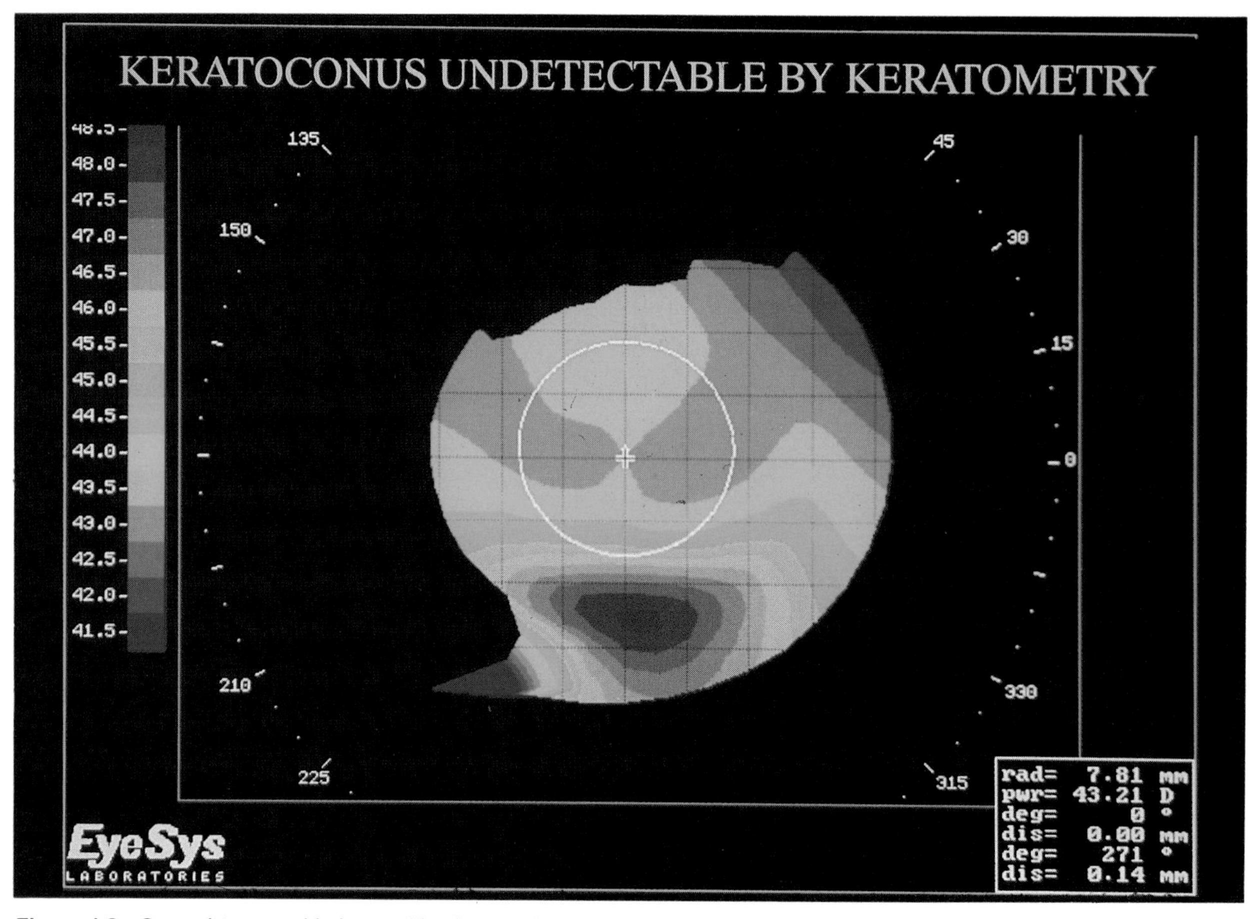

Figure 1.8: Corneal topographic image 30 minutes after removal of rigid gas permeable contact lens in a case with suspected keratoconus. Note that the inferior steepening is outside of the pupillary area (white circle) and outside of the 3 mm optical zone and thus undetectable by routine keratometry.

classic article[2] (Figure 1.10). These devices offer the advantages of low cost and rapid use, and they facilitate analysis of large regional differences in corneal curvature, such as high astigmatism following penetrating keratoplasty. However, detection of small but clinically important topographic features and quantitative measurements are not possible.

The CorneaScope (KERA Corporation) provides photographic images of Placido rings projected onto the cornea[2] (Figure 1.11). The introduction of this unit in the early 1980's was an important catalyst in the explosive progress in this field. Corneascope photographs permit qualitative analysis of corneal topography (Figures 1.12, 1.13), but quantitative analysis is cumbersome and accuracy is limited to ± 1 to 2 D.

Computerized Videokeratography: The Breakthrough in Corneal Topographic Analysis

The introduction of the Corneal Modeling System ushered in the new era of corneal topographic analysis.[3] This instrument and

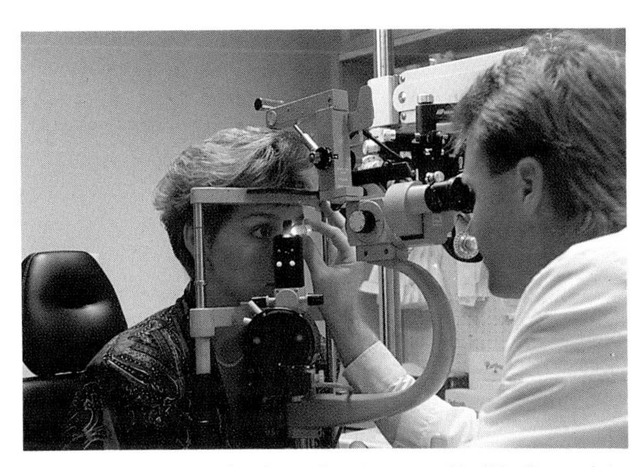

Figure 1.9: The von Loehnan keratoscope (JedMed) consists of a translucent white cylinder with Placido rings lining its inner surface. The device is held close to the patient's cornea and is illuminated by a bright oblique slit beam, thereby projecting the Placido rings onto the cornea.

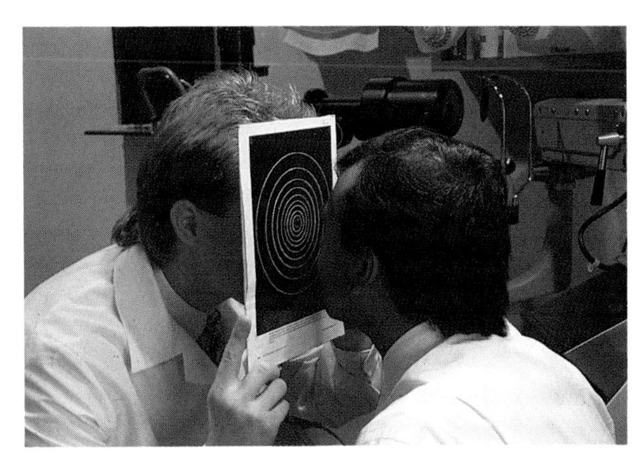

Figure 1.10: Use of the Placido image published in Rowsey and colleagues' article.[2] The spacing of the rings on the curved face plate of the CorneaScope has been preserved by transposition onto a flat plane. A 15 to 20 D lens is taped behind a small hole made in the center of the rings, and the reflected image is used for qualitative keratoscopy.

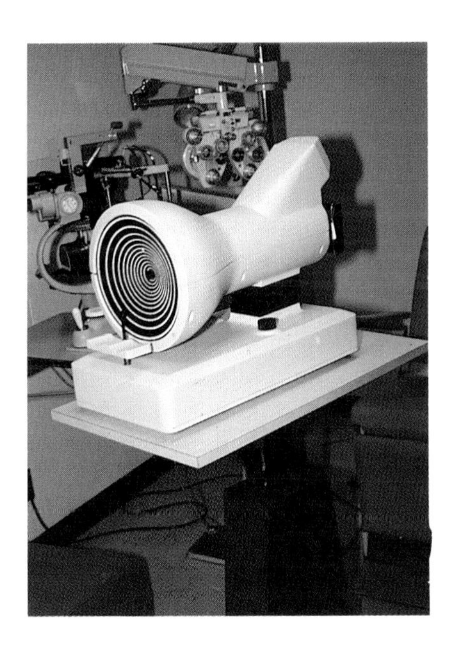

Figure 1.11: The CorneaScope (KERA Corporation) provides Polaroid photographic images of Placido rings projected onto the cornea.

its successors have completely changed our ability to measure and modify corneal curvature. The remainder of this book is devoted to the burgeoning contributions of these instruments to our understanding of the cornea and vision.

Computerized videokeratographs (CVK's) share certain common features:

1) some form of light is projected onto the cornea,
2) the modification of this light by the cornea is captured by a video camera,
3) this information is analyzed by computer software, and
4) the data are displayed in a variety of formats.

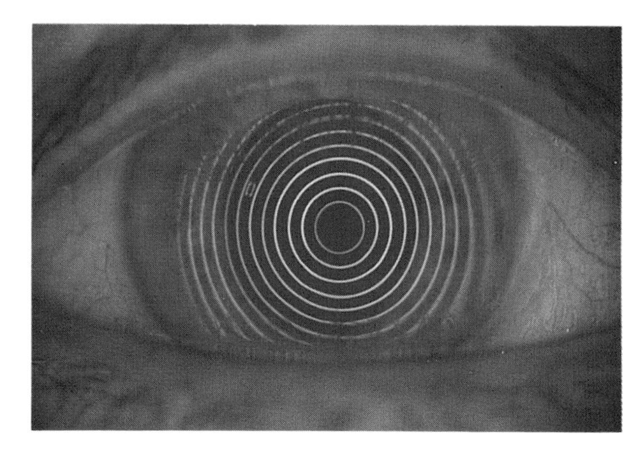

Figure 1.12: CorneaScope photograph of a cornea with against-the-rule astigmatism following cataract surgery. Note the vertically oval shape of the rings.

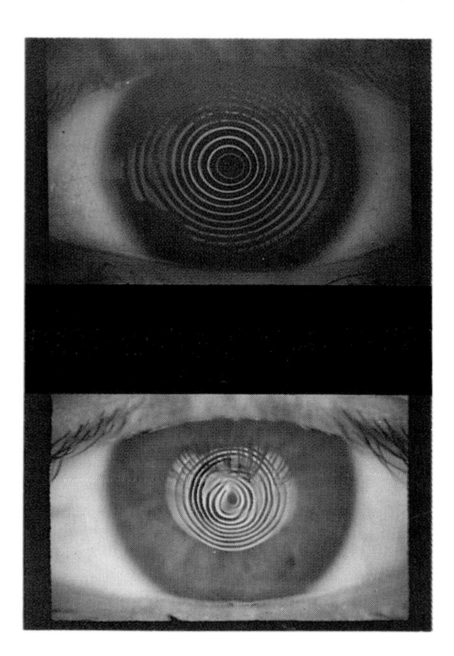

Figure 1.13: Top, CorneaScope photograph showing moderate keratoconus, with inferotemporal steepening. Bottom, CorneaScope photograph of advanced keratoconus, showing marked central steepening (compare ring sizes to those in Figure 1.12) and distortion of the ring pattern.

There are a variety of ways to measure corneal curvature, and several have been utilized in currently available and prototype devices.

Computerized videokeratographs: Placido-based devices

The prevalent approach in these new devices is the use of Placido disk imaging, which is an extension of the single mire used in the keratometer. A series of rings is projected onto the cornea, and the reflected images are detected by a video camera. (The virtual image of these reflected rings is located just anterior to the iris.) Curvature data are derived from the measured distances between rings. The algorithms for this analysis assume that the cornea is spherical, and small errors are introduced as a result. However, this type of imaging has the potential for excellent accuracy and reproducibility.[4] Three devices are currently available.

EyeSys system. The EyeSys Corneal Analysis System (CAS) (EyeSys Laboratories)

(Figure 1.14A, B) is the system that we use in clinical practice and with which we are most familiar. It will therefore be described in greatest detail with the differences between it and the other available systems pointed out as appropriate.

On the right side of the tabletop is mounted a corneoscope projecting a 16-ring (8 light and 8 dark rings) conical Placido disc that is positioned 92 mm in front of the cornea[5] (Figure 1.14A), and a chin rest for patient examination (Figure 1.14B). The patient examination portion of the procedure typically takes two minutes for both eyes. Within the housing of the corneoscope is a CCD camera for image capture. The computer mounted vertically below the tabletop on the left-hand side digitizes or converts the data obtained from the video output into a form that can be analyzed. A typical corneoscope image obtained by the instrument is shown in Figure 1.15A.

For a 42.5 D cornea, the diameter of the measured region is 0.9 to 9.2 mm. An edge detection program identifies the white to black (yellow dotted lines) and black to white (red dotted lines) interfaces of the corneoscope pattern (Figure 1.15B). Each of the 16 interfaces is measured at 1° intervals for 360° for a total of 5,760 points. Simple observation of the alternating yellow and red line pattern will verify if the edges were appropriately detected. Since the human brain is markedly superior as a pattern recognition system to any computer, the EyeSys unit allows the operator to edit the computer's pattern recognition findings. A new program option uses special image subtraction and enhancement techniques to find the patient's pupil (Figure 1.15C). This feature has been found to be critical for detecting proper centration of refractive surgical techniques.

Once the ring edges and the pupil have been properly identified, a number of highly sophisticated programs convert the data into a series of user selectable color graphics displays. Hard copy output can be obtained from a color PaintJet printer, Polaroid camera, or even as a 35 mm slide.

Besides the standard color topographic maps, a number of other types of visual and

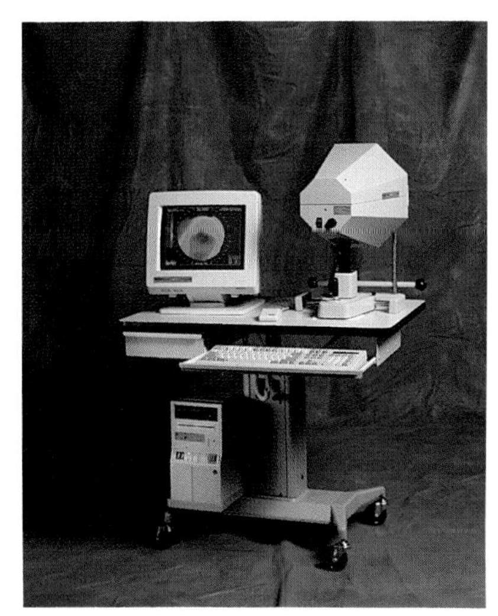

Figure 1.14A.

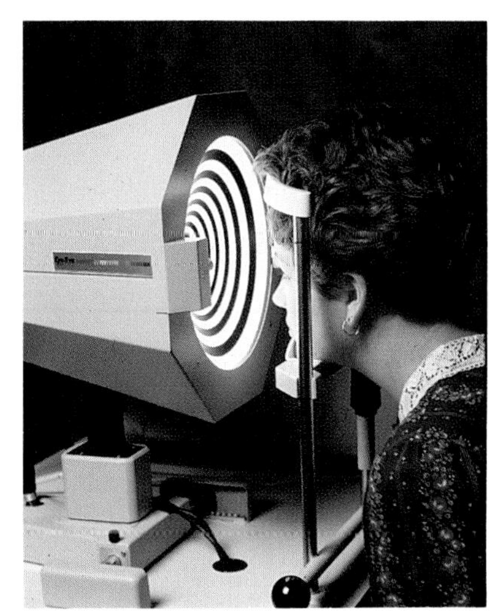

Figure 1.14B.

Figure 1.14: EyeSys Corneal Analysis System. (A) View from examiner's side. (B) View from patient's side during examination.

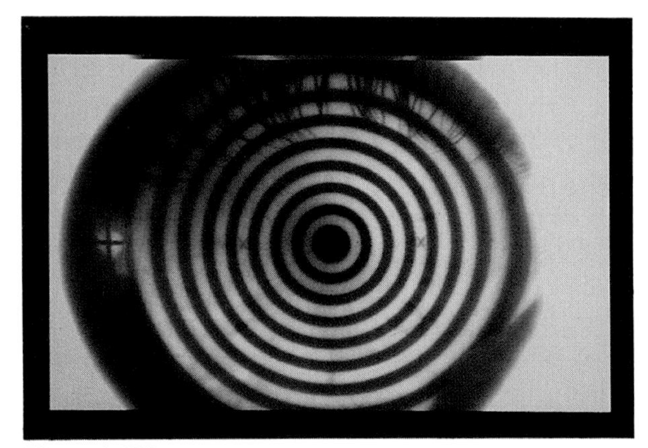

Figure 1.15A.

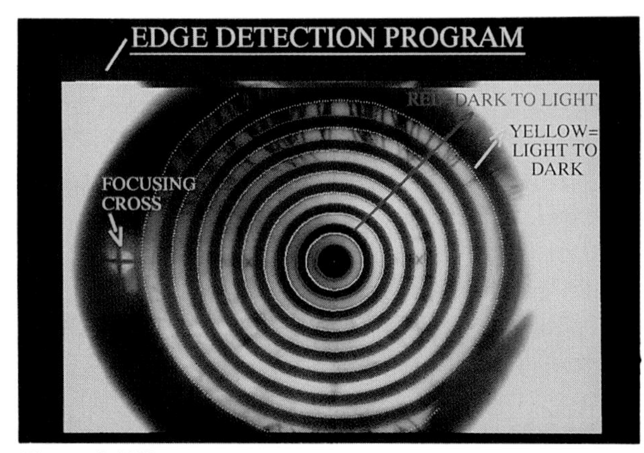

Figure 1.15B.

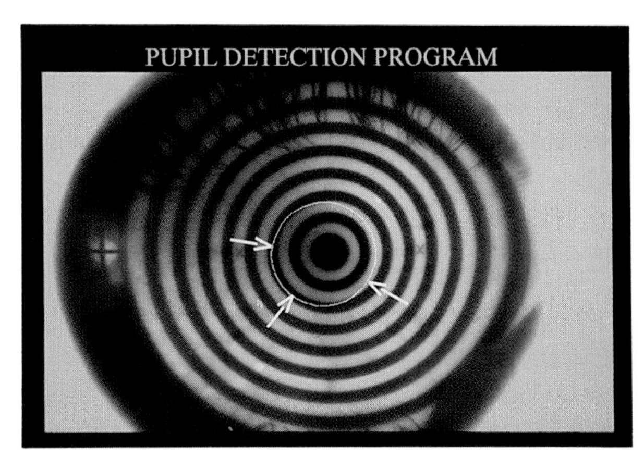

Figure 1.15C.

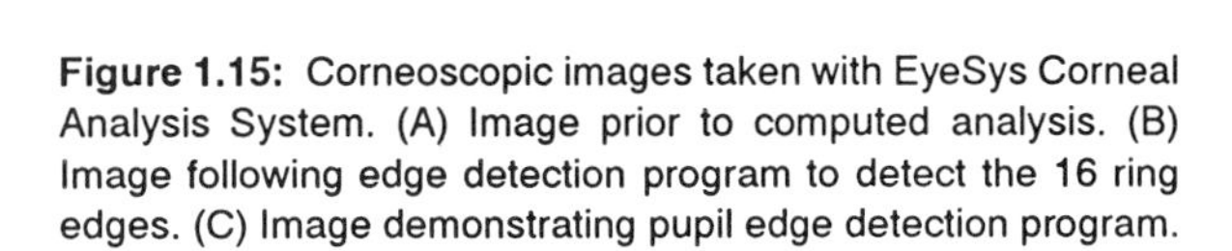

Figure 1.15: Corneoscopic images taken with EyeSys Corneal Analysis System. (A) Image prior to computed analysis. (B) Image following edge detection program to detect the 16 ring edges. (C) Image demonstrating pupil edge detection program.

data arrays are available. To follow patients serially, up to four different color maps can be displayed together on the same scale. A preoperative, postoperative, and difference or delta map display can be generated to determine procedure-induced changes.

An astigmatic profile graph, a data overview display, and a keratometric display provide detailed information regarding astigmatism. Data fusion combines various available views, and a contact lens data display helps the contact lens fitter further understand the relationship between the contact lens and corneal surface.

A new topographical display weights corneal power as a function of the Stiles-Crawford effect. This display provides an estimate of the actual refractive effect of the measured corneal curvatures. The usefulness of these various displays will be demonstrated throughout the book with clinical examples.

Computed Anatomy system. The Topographic Modeling System (TMS) (Computed Anatomy, Inc.) (Figure 1.16) projects 25 or 31 rings onto the cornea from a cylindrical Placido (Figure 1.17) at a distance of 32 mm from the 12th ring.[6] The TMS measures 256 meridians for a total of 7,000 points. For a

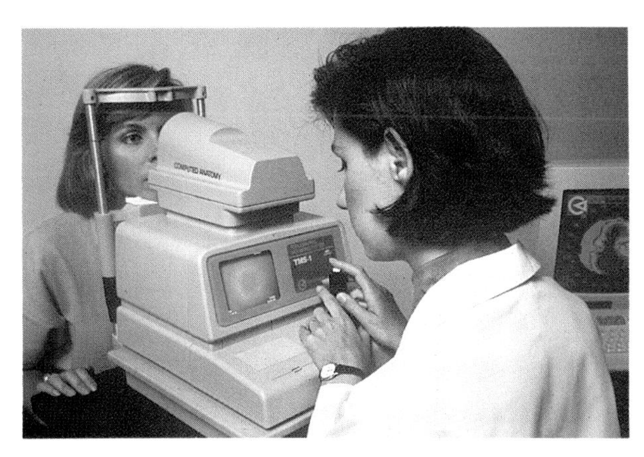

Figure 1.16: Patient and technician using the TMS-1 (Photograph courtesy of Computed Anatomy, Inc.).

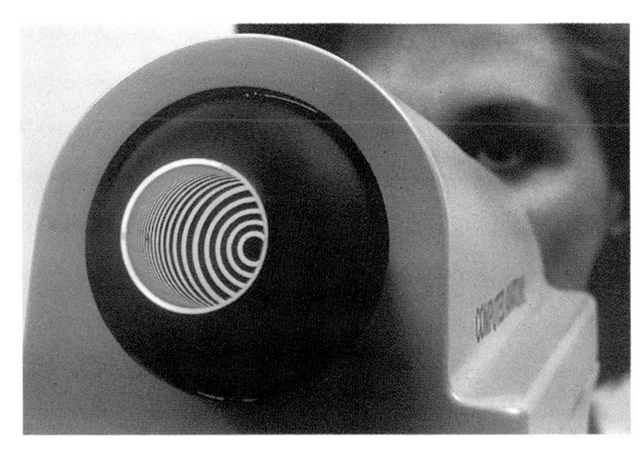

Figure 1.17: The TMS-1 Light Cone (TM) (Photograph courtesy of Computed Anatomy, Inc.).

42 D cornea, the diameter of the measured zone is 0.4 to 8.9 mm. A wide variety of displays are available (Figures 1.18A, B), including a contact lens program that mimics fluorescein pooling under any given hypothetical lens.

Visioptic system. The Visio EH-270 (Figure 1.19) projects 23 rings onto the cornea from a conical Placido at a distance of 20 mm from the outermost ring.[7] This unit measures 828 points over 360 meridians. Eleven different color-coded displays are available (Figure 1.20).

Computerized videokeratographs: Other technologies

A variety of other technologies are being utilized in devices that are currently under development. These present new possibilities and limitations in the design of clinically useful devices.

Par Technology system. The Par Corneal Topography System (CTS) (Par Technology Corporation) (Figure 1.21) uses raster photogrammetry, in which a two-dimensional grid pattern is projected onto the cornea (Figure 1.22) and then imaged from a different orientation.[8] Approximately 1,700 points are imaged. To counteract corneal transparency, fluorescein dye must be instilled to visualize the grid. Corneal curvature alters the grid spacing, and these changes are detected by a video camera and converted into true elevation measurements of the corneal surface (Figure 1.23). Corneal curvature values are then calculated from the elevation data (Figure 1.24). Early studies have shown excellent accuracy and reproducibility for measurements of entire rings of calibrated spheres. Advantages of this approach are coverage of the entire corneal surface and the greater ability to quantify abrupt surface changes and irregularities that are difficult to interpret with Placido system algorithms.

Kerametrics system. The KM-1000 CLAS Corneal Topography Unit (Kerametrics, Inc.) uses laser holography to image the anterior corneal surface (Figure 1.25). This technology has exquisite sensitivity to detect subtle local differences in curvature (Figure 1.26), but the software needs are complex. This initial clinical device uses fringe detection to acquire information about topographic changes. A newer device uses phase modulation techniques to more accurately and repeatedly assess the

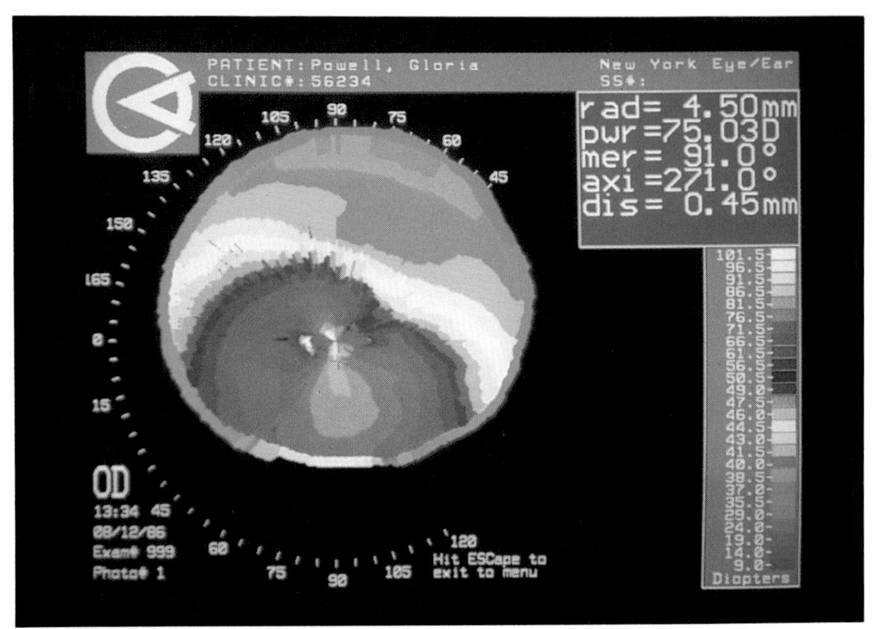

Figure 1.18A.

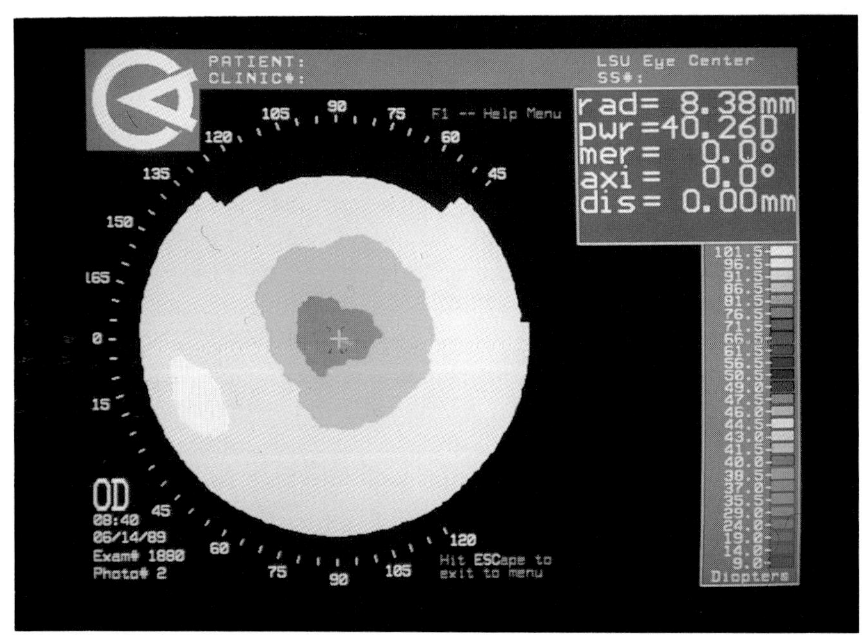

Figure 1.18B.

Figure 1.18: TMS-1 topographic maps. (A) Advanced keratoconus. (B) Persistent contact lens induced corneal warpage with central corneal flattening after six-month abstinence from contact lenses (Photograph courtesy of Computed Anatomy, Inc.).

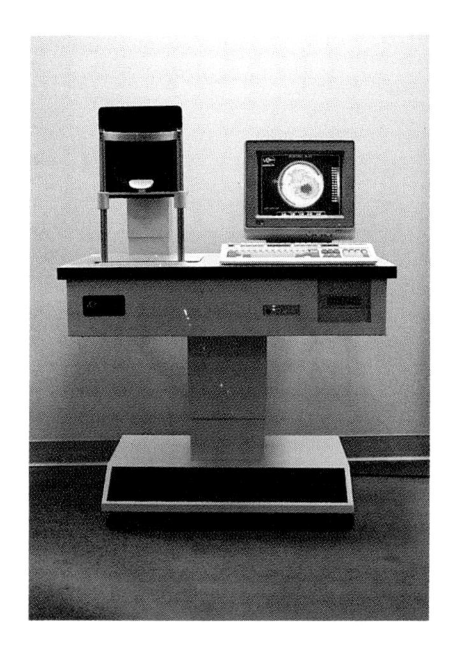

Figure 1.19: The EH-270 Computerized Corneal Topographer (Photograph courtesy of Visioptic, Inc.).

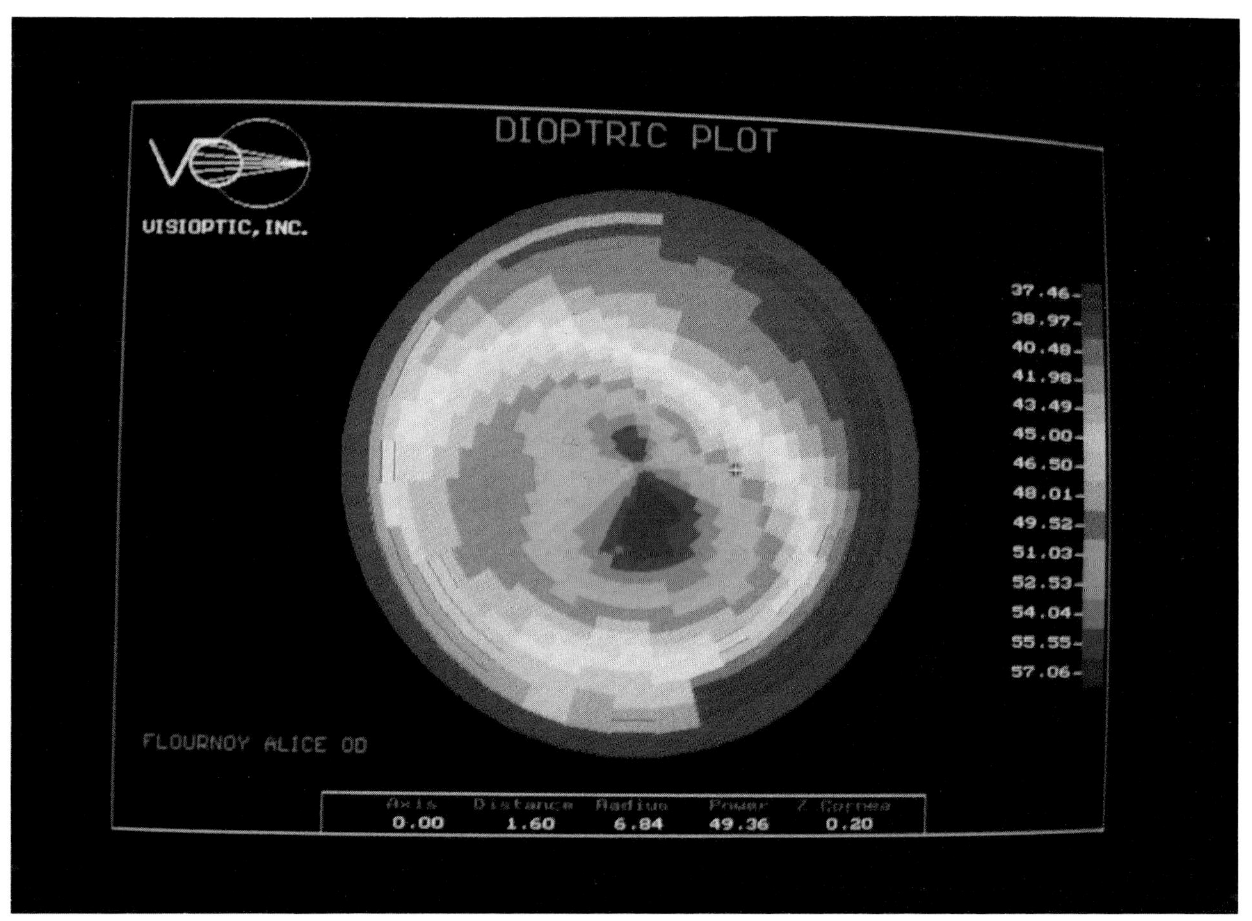

Figure 1.20: Photograph of the screen of the EH-270 with a topographic map of keratoconus. This device uses a color scheme directly opposite that of the CAS and TMS-1; thus the cooler colors (e.g., blue) represent steeper regions and the warmer colors (e.g., red) indicate flatter regions (Photograph courtesy of Visioptic, Inc.).

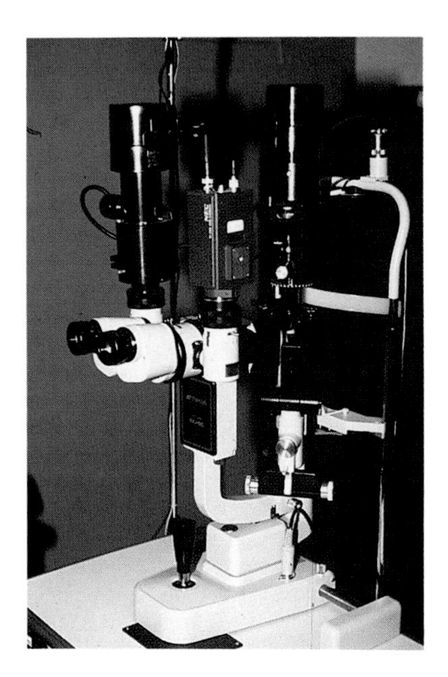

Figure 1.21: The Par Corneal Topography System showing the projection unit (black cylinder) mounted on the left side of the binoculars, with the camera (gray rectangular box) mounted on the right side. The unit works through the optics of the slit-lamp (Photograph courtesy of PAR Technology Corporation).

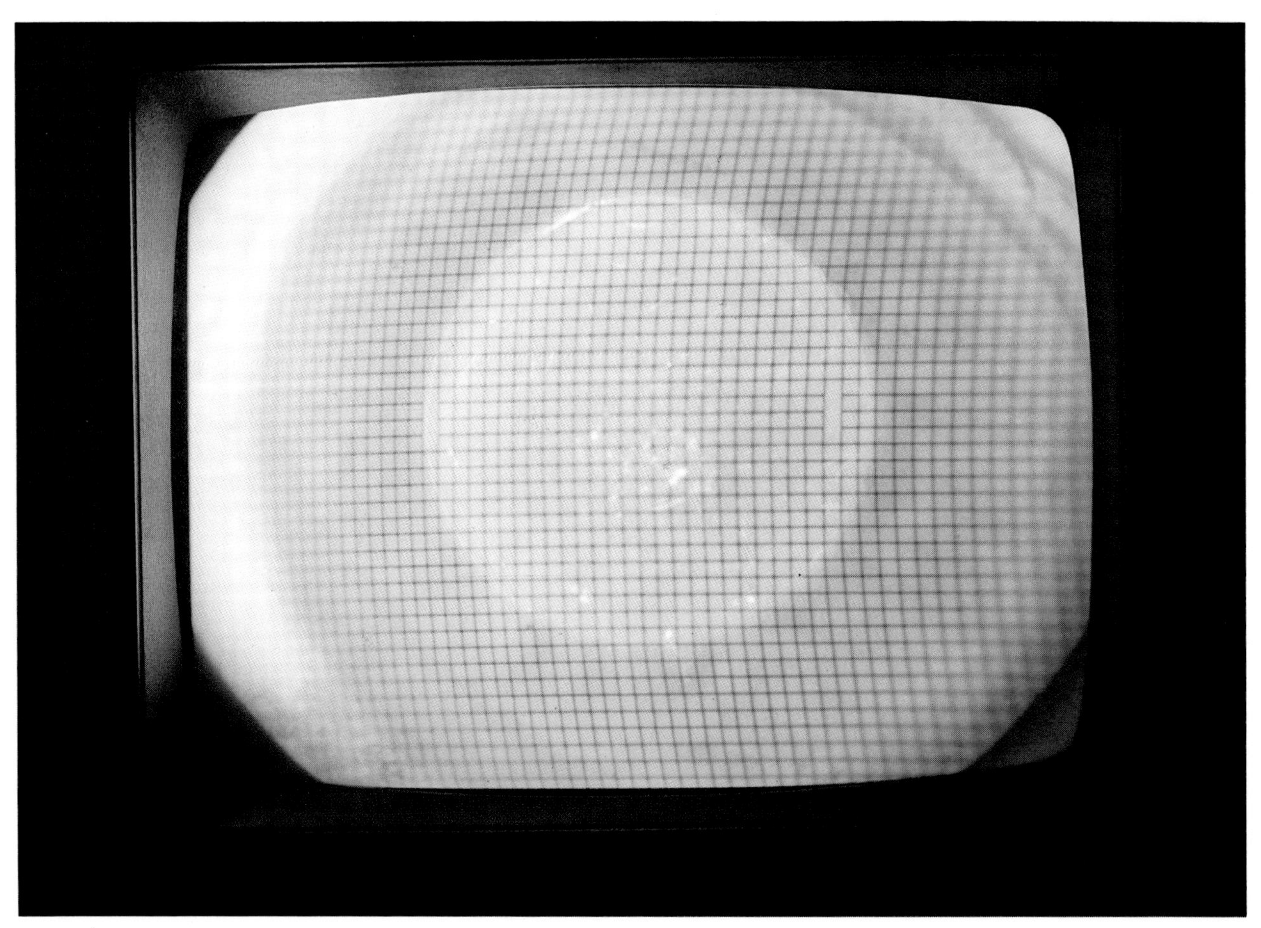

Figure 1.22: The Par Corneal Topography System projects a grid onto the fluorescein-coated cornea. This cornea has just undergone lamellar keratectomy; note the ability to image both on intact epithelium and bare stroma. (Photograph courtesy of Michael W. Belin, MD, Department of Ophthalmology, The Albany Medical College.)

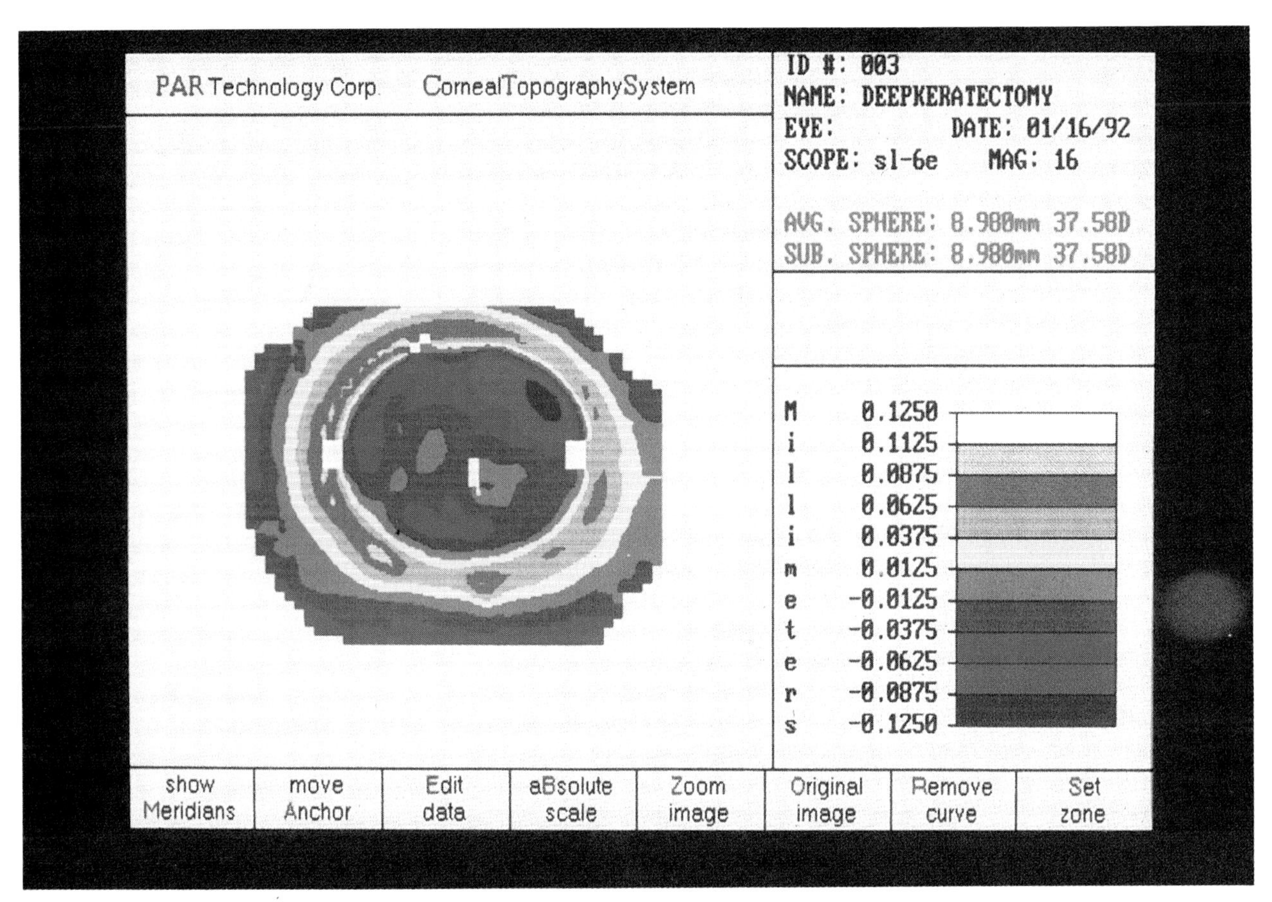

Figure 1.23: Par system spherical subtraction map of the lamellar keratectomy cornea shown in Figure 1.20. The dark area corresponds to keratectomized region. Note the color scale at right using elevation data relative to a reference point. This corneal map shows corneal height, not curvature. (Photograph courtesy of Michael W. Belin, MD, Department of Ophthalmology, The Albany Medical College.)

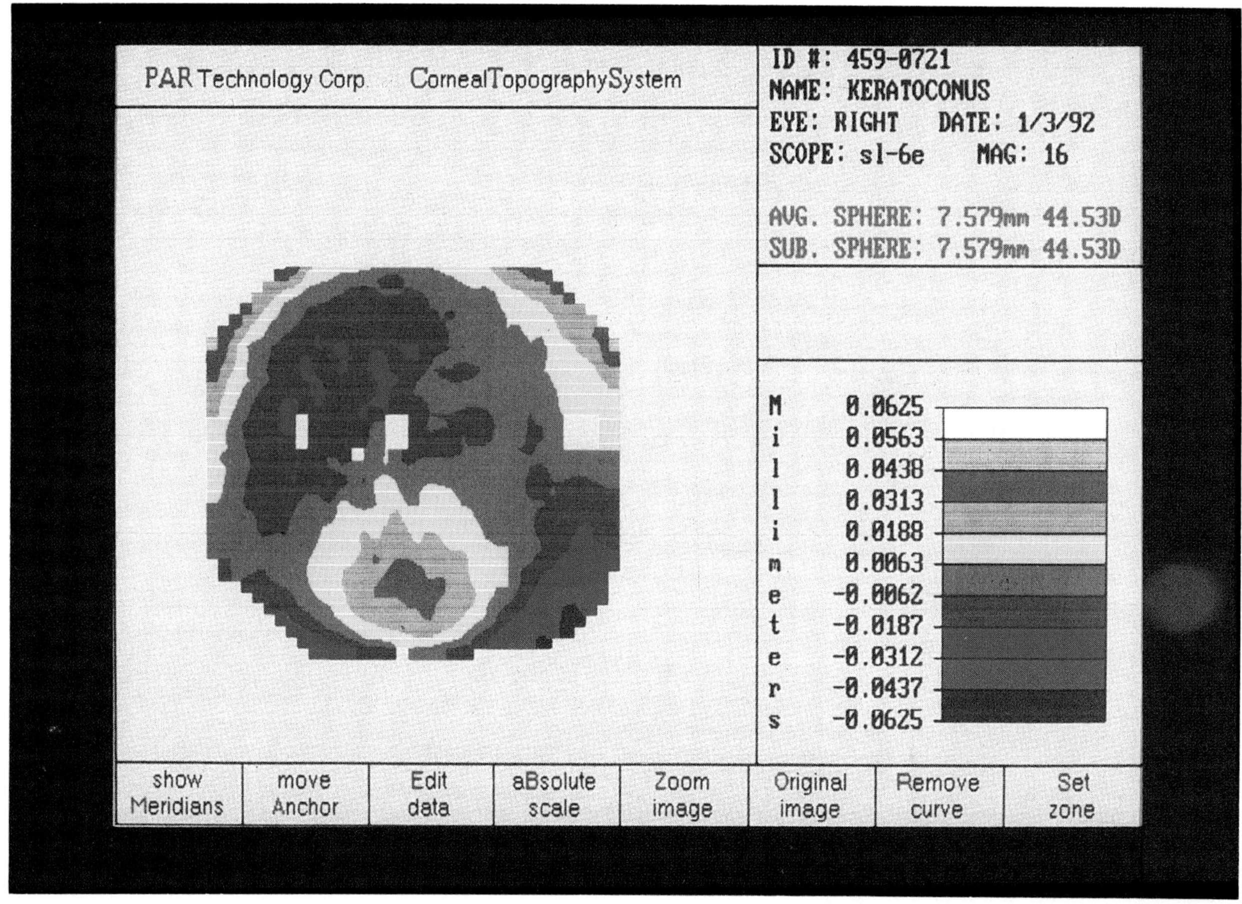

Figure 1.24: Par spherical subtraction map of a cornea with keratoconus; the cone is inferior, with the red and yellow colors showing the elevation in the area of the cone. (Photograph courtesy of Michael W. Belin, MD, Department of Ophthalmology, The Albany Medical College.)

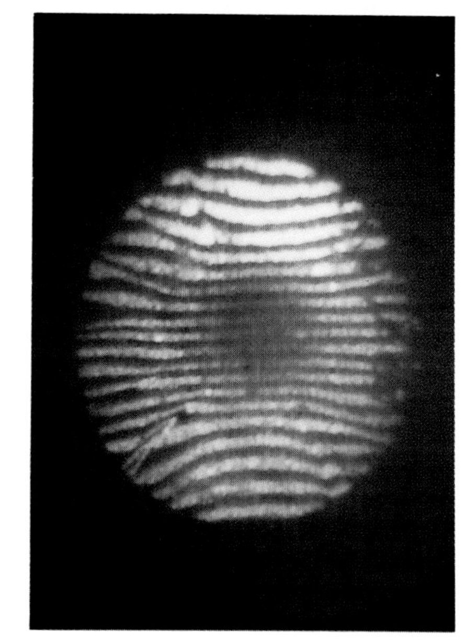

Figure 1.25: Fringe destructive and constructive interference pattern made by the KM-1000 CLAS Corneal topography unit (Kerametrics) from a cornea that has undergone 4-incision RK. Note the convergence of the pattern centrally, indicating central flattening, as well as the local changes over the incisions. (Photograph courtesy of Phillip Baker, MS, President, Kerametrics, Inc.)

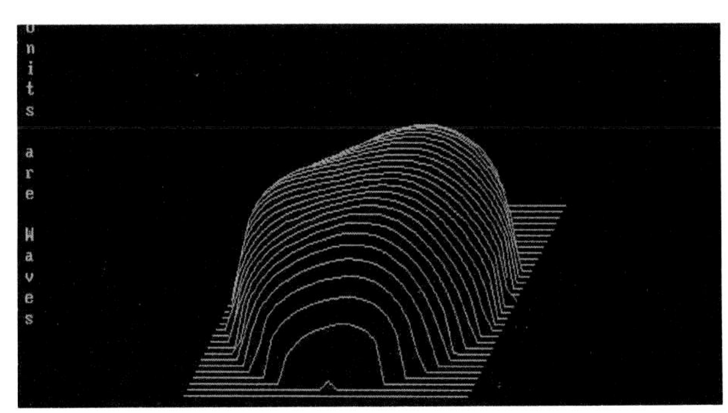

Figure 1.26: KM-1000 CLAS three-dimensional isometric analysis of pig cornea following implantation of intrastromal corneal ring. Note the slightly tilted central plateau representing asymmetric central flattening. (Photograph courtesy of Phillip Baker, MS, President, Kerametrics, Inc.)

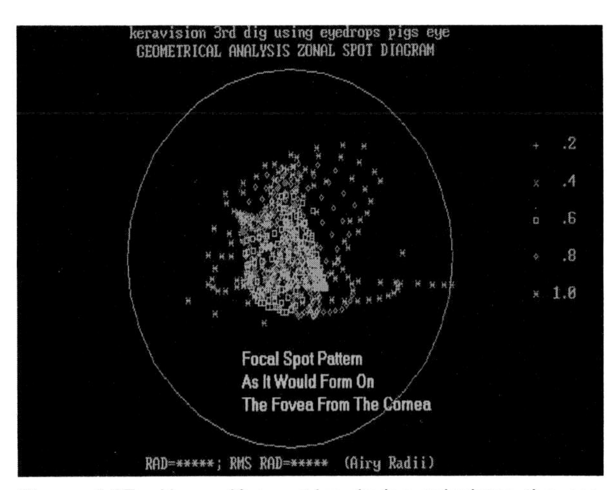

Figure 1.27: Newer Kerametrics device calculates the cornea's refraction of light from the measured corneal topographic changes. This figure shows the light pattern from the cornea analyzed in Figure 1.24. Note that the refracted light is uniformly distributed over the region inside the circle. A normal eye has a strongly compacted distribution of light roughly 1/20th the size of this pattern. Different patterns are seen with different corneal refractive procedures. (Photograph courtesy of Phillip Baker, MS, President, Kerametrics, Inc.)

topographic contour (Figure 1.27). It is anticipated that this device will be available by late 1992.

Other technologies under investigation include laser tomography and Moiré fringe detection, and undoubtedly new technologies will emerge.

Applications of Computerized Videokeratography

In subsequent chapters, this book will describe at length various applications of computerized videokeratography in different clinical settings. As our understanding of these devices and the interpretation of their data have advanced, the range of uses has multiplied, particularly in surgical patients. Two fundamental applications have been the elucidation of normal corneal topography, described below, and the detection of corneal topographic abnormalities, discussed in further chapters in this book.

Normal corneal topography

Using the Corneal Modeling System, Bogan and colleagues provided the first classification of CVK patterns of normal corneal topography.[9] These patterns are:

1) round: 22.6% (Figure 1.28);
2) oval: 20.8% (Figure 1.29);
3) symmetric bow-tie: 17.5% (Figure 1.30);
4) asymmetric bow-tie: 32.1% (Figure 1.31); and
5) irregular: 7.1% (Figure 1.32).

As the authors point out, this classification represents positions along a spectrum of topographic patterns. Corneas classified as "irregular" undoubtedly include anomalies that have previously not been detected and can only now be evaluated using CVK (Figure 1.33A, B). Our own experience with the CAS suggests that fewer corneas have round or oval patterns than Bogan reported, which is likely attributable to hardware and software advances in the newer Placido-based devices. The remainder of this book will be dedicated to documenting in a very visual fashion the uses of corneal topography in present clinical practice.

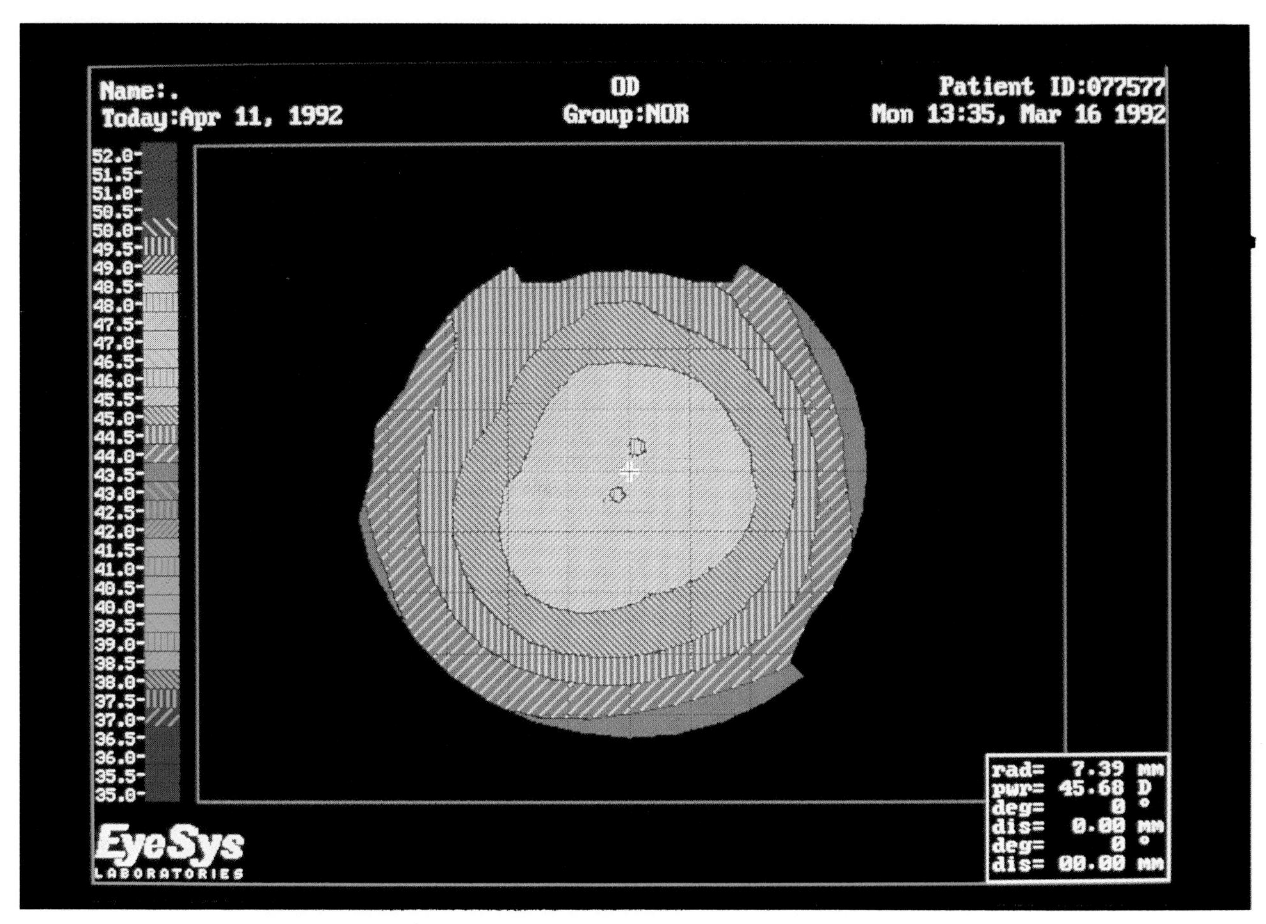

Figure 1.28: Round corneal topographic pattern using the absolute scale.

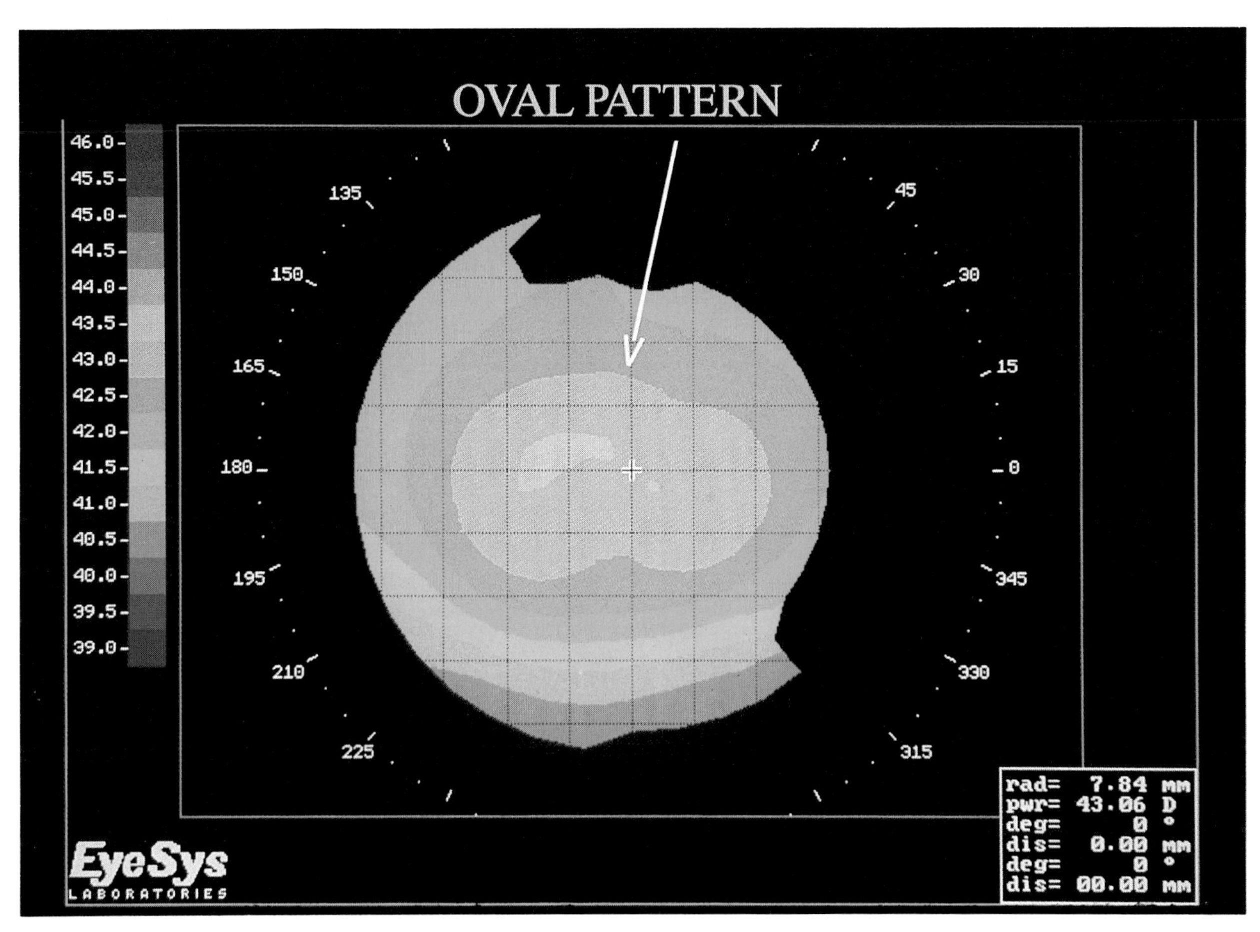

Figure 1.29: Oval corneal topographic pattern of the central topographic zone. Using dioptric scales as small as 0.5 D, it is relatively uncommon to find pure oval or round patterns; bow-tie patterns are much more common.

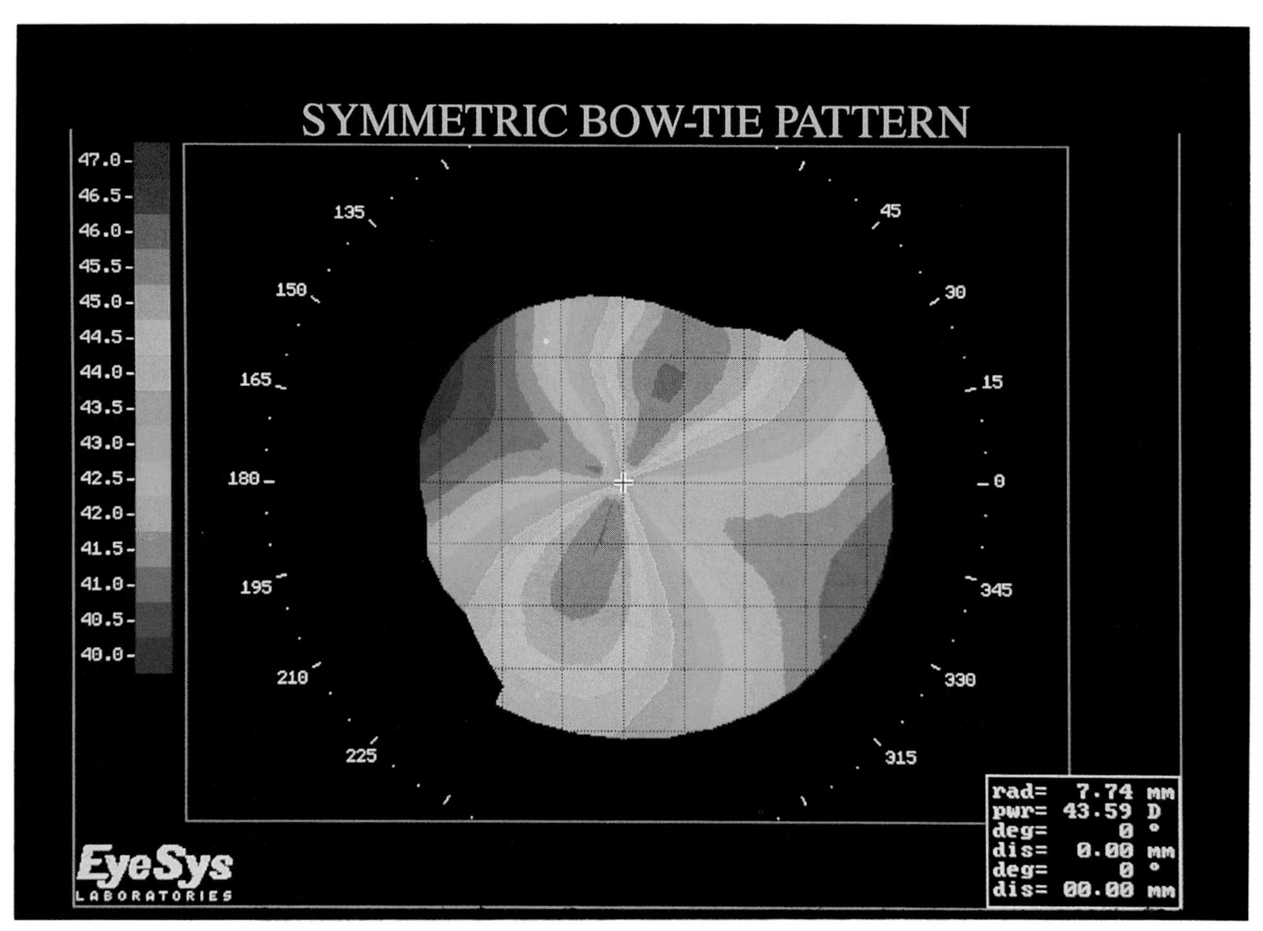

Figure 1.30: Symmetrical bow-tie pattern of astigmatism.

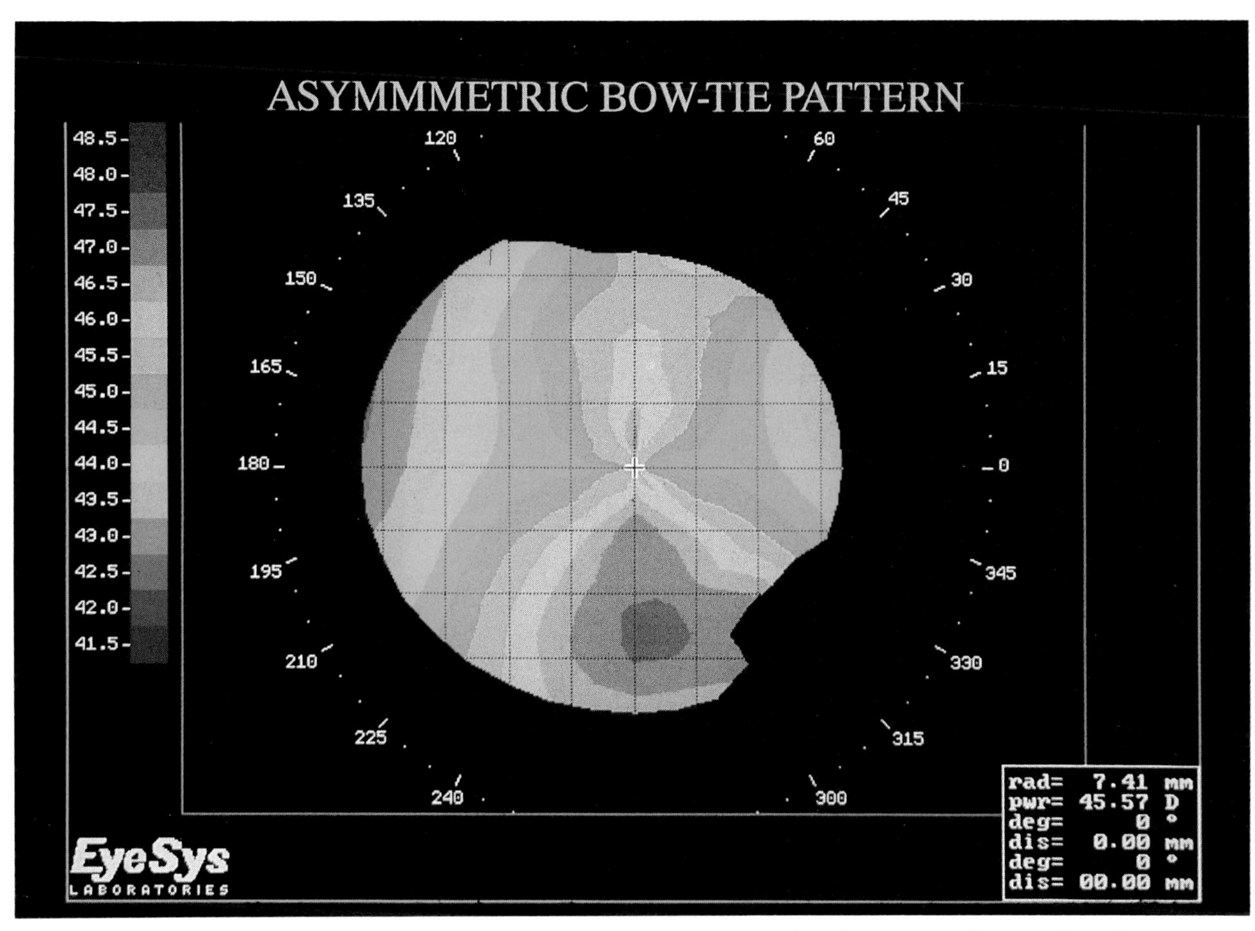

Figure 1.31: Asymmetric bow-tie pattern. The inferior cornea is generally steeper than the corresponding superior regions.

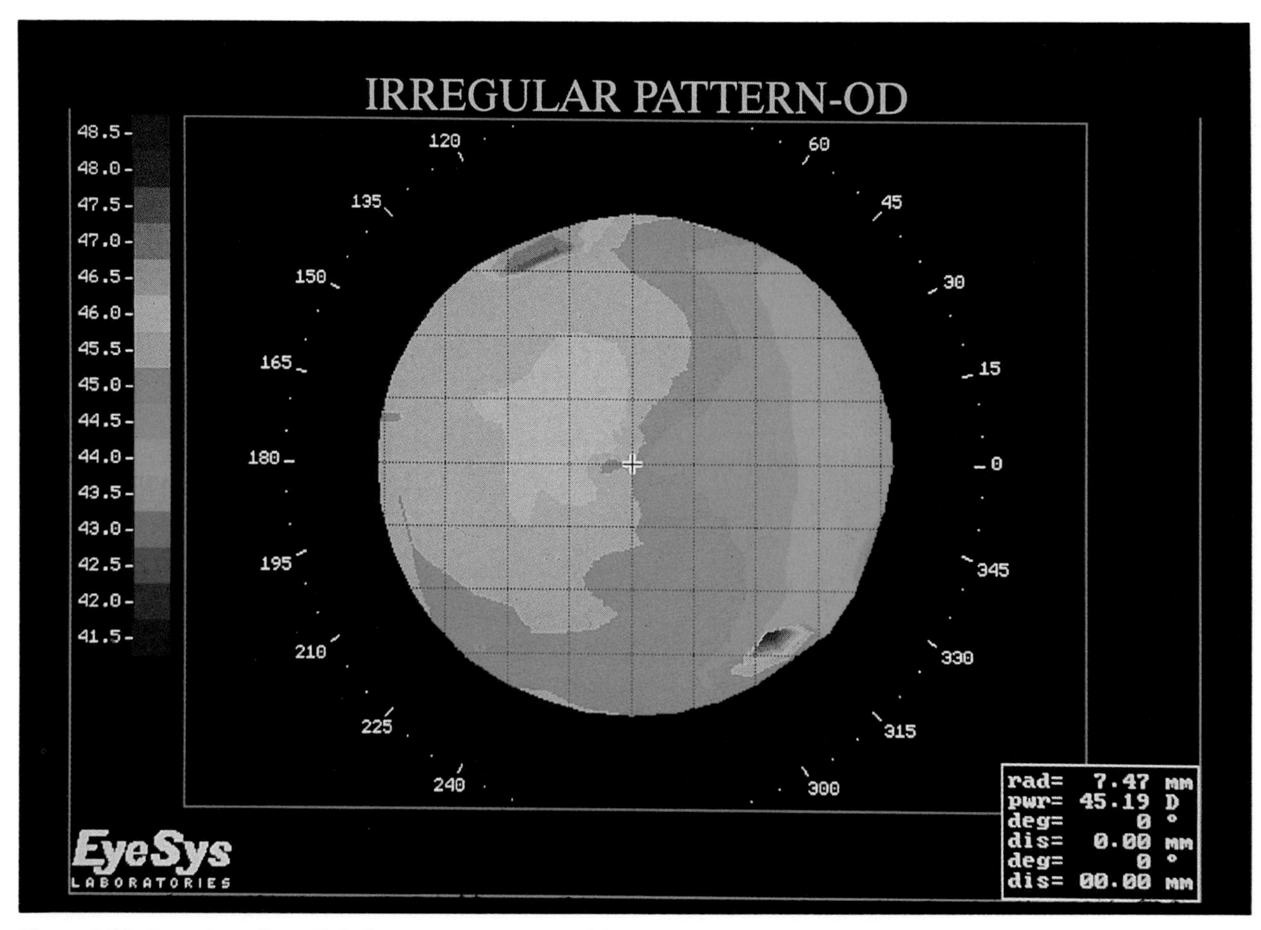

Figure 1.32: Irregular pattern. Note the greater steepness of the temporal cornea. For example, at corresponding points along the horizontal meridian 1.5 mm from the corneal center, corneal curvature is 45.98 D temporally and 44.58 D nasally.

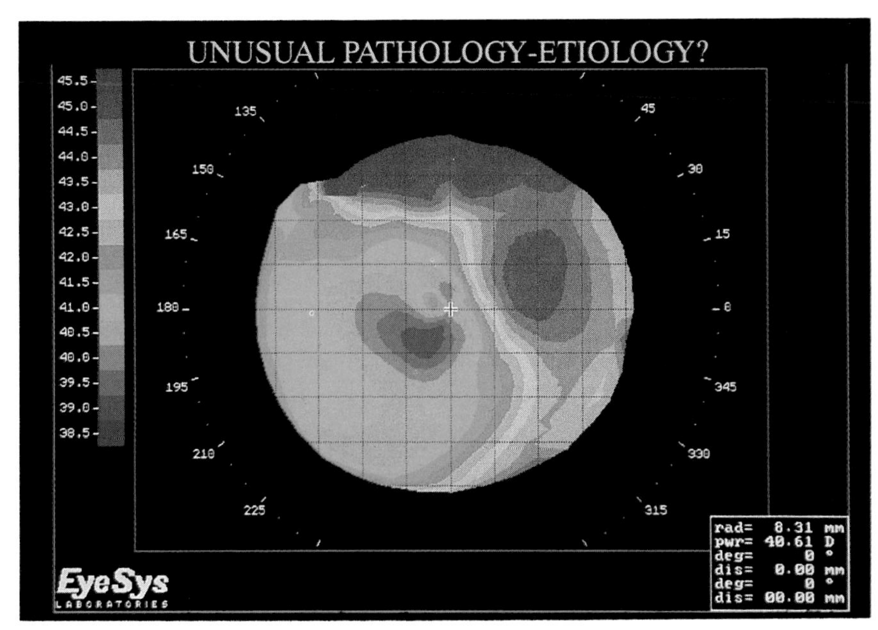

Figure 1.33A.

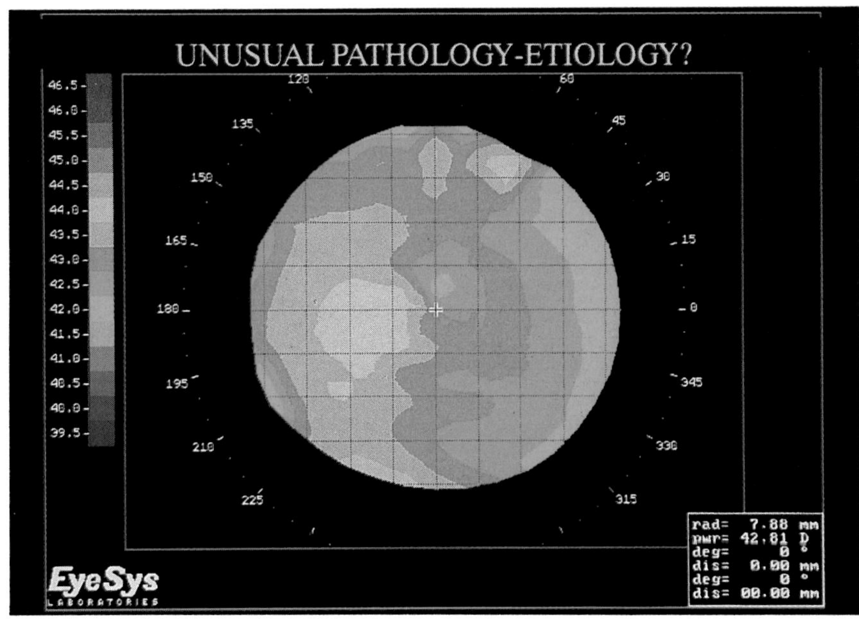

Figure 1.33B.

Figure 1.33: Unusual irregular topographic patterns in fellow eyes of 53-year-old male who presented complaining of blurred vision OD. Refraction one year earlier had been +1.00 D OU; new refraction was +4.00 D OD and +1.00 D OS, giving 20/20 OU. (A) Right eye, note the large flat zone inferotemporally, extending into the central cornea. (B) Left eye, the inferotemporal cornea is slightly flatter than other regions. The etiology of these topographic findings is unknown.

References

1. Moon P, Spencer DE: On the Stiles-Crawford effect. *J Optical Society America* 34:319-329, 1944.
2. Rowsey JJ, Reynolds AE, Brown R: Corneal topography. *Arch Ophthalmol* 99:1093-1100, 1981.
3. Gormely DJ, Gersten M, Koplin RS, Lubkin V: Corneal modeling. *Cornea* 7:30-35, 1988.
4. Heit LE, Franco CM, Graham KT, Koch DD: Corneal topographical measurements of spheric, aspheric and bicurved surfaces. *Invest Ophthalmol Vis Sci* 33/4(suppl):996, 1992.
5. Koch DD, Wakil JS, Samuelson SW, Haft EA: A comparison of the EyeSys Corneal Modeling System with standard keratometry. *J Cat Refract Surg*, in press.
6. Wilson SE, Verity SM, Conger DL: Accuracy and precision of the corneal analysis system and the topographic modeling system. *Cornea* 11:28-35, 1992.
7. El Hage SG: Computerized corneal topographer. *Contact Lens Spectrum* 45-50, 1989.
8. Belin MW, Litoff D, Strods SJ, Winn SS, Smith RS: The PAR technology corneal topography system. *Ref & Corn Surg* 8:88-96, 1992.
9. Bogan SJ, Waring GO, Ibrahim O: Classification of normal corneal topography based on computer-assisted videokeratography. *Arch Ophthalmol* 108:945-949, 1990.

2

DOUGLAS D. KOCH, MD

Detection and Characterization of Corneal Pathology

Keratoconus

Computerized videokeratography (CVK) has become essential in various aspects of the diagnosis and management of keratoconus and related corneal topographic disorders. First and foremost, CVK is sometimes required to diagnose keratoconus. Maguire and Bourne first described nine eyes of seven patients in which keratoconus was diagnosed only by CVK, having previously eluded clinical detection.[1] In eyes with early keratoconus, slit lamp corneal changes are too subtle for detection or have not yet occurred, keratometry may be normal, topographical keratometry may show only nonspecific peripheral steepening, and qualitative Placido systems may not reveal topographic abnormalities. The greater precision of CVK is required to make the diagnosis (Figures 2.1A, B).

Detection of subclinical keratoconus becomes a critical issue in patients who are potential candidates for refractive surgical procedures. Radial keratotomy, astigmatic keratotomy, and excimer laser photorefractive keratectomy are currently contraindicated in patients with keratoconus. Nesburn and colleagues recently reported that six of 91 consecutive patients screened for excimer laser PRK had subclinical keratoconus.[2] CVK may become an essential component of the preoperative evaluation of refractive surgical patients.

CVK has been essential in developing a classification scheme for keratoconus and in establishing diagnostic criteria. Using the Corneal Modeling System, Wilson and colleagues evaluated 85 eyes of 49 patients.[3] In the 61 eyes that could be accurately processed and had signs of keratoconus, two types of patterns were noted. Forty-four of the cones (72%) were peripheral, typically either inferiorly or inferotemporally (Figures 2.2A, B). The remainder of the cones were central with or without a superimposed asymmetric pattern of bow-tie astig-

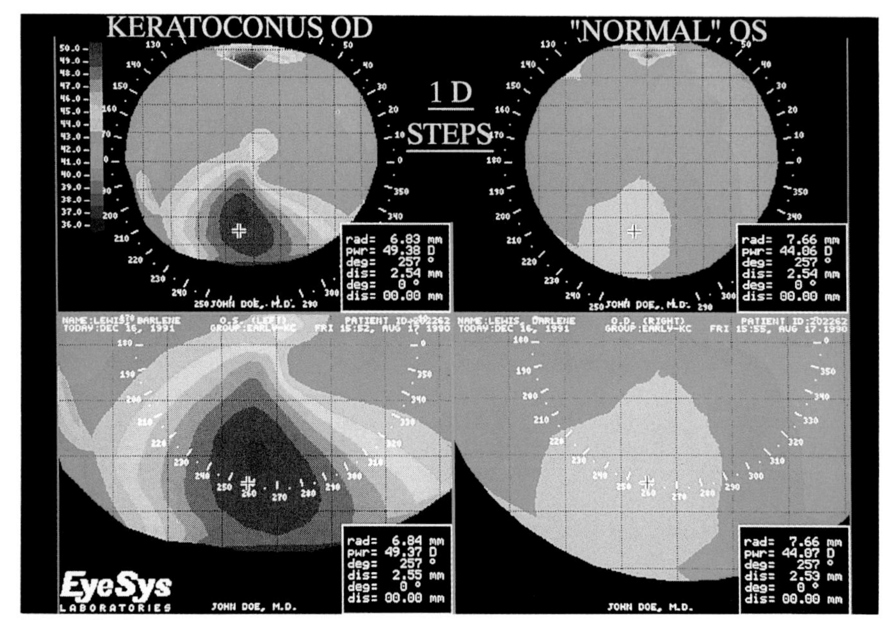

Figure 2.1A.

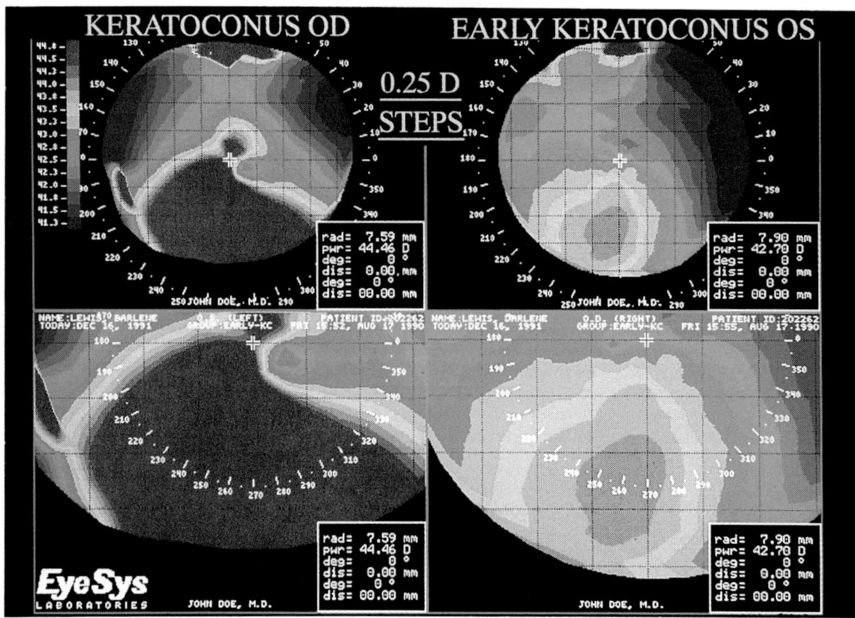

Figure 2.1B.

Figure 2.1: Right and left eyes of a patient with clinical keratoconus in the right eye and a clinically normal left eye. There was no distortion of keratometer mires with keratometry of 42.5 × 43 at 90° in the left eye. The bottom images are magnified views of the inferior cornea. (A) Topography scaled in 1 D steps to emphasize the obvious keratoconus in the right eye. There is a suspect area in the inferior cornea of the left eye but the power in that area is only 44 D. (B) Topography scaled in 0.25 D steps clearly demonstrates the early keratoconus in the left eye.

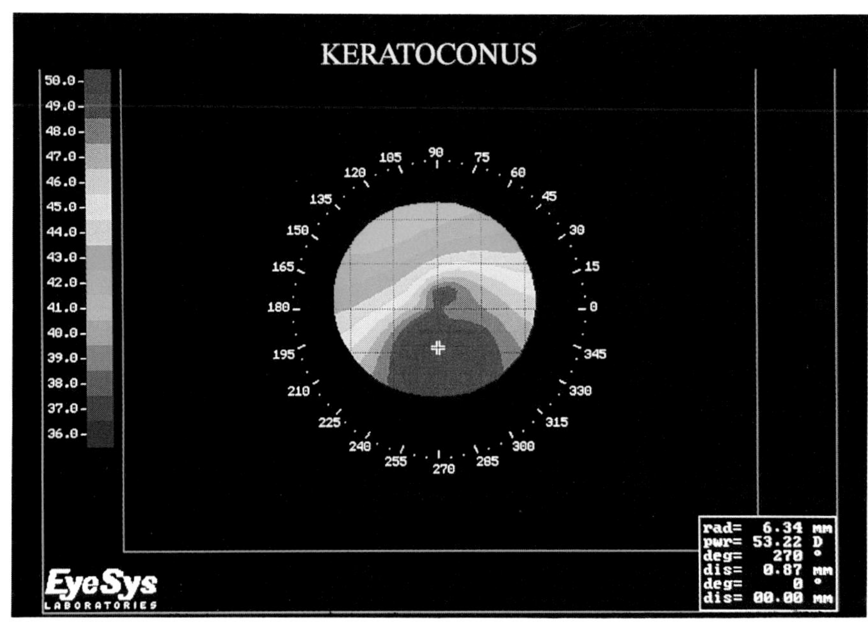

Figure 2.2A.

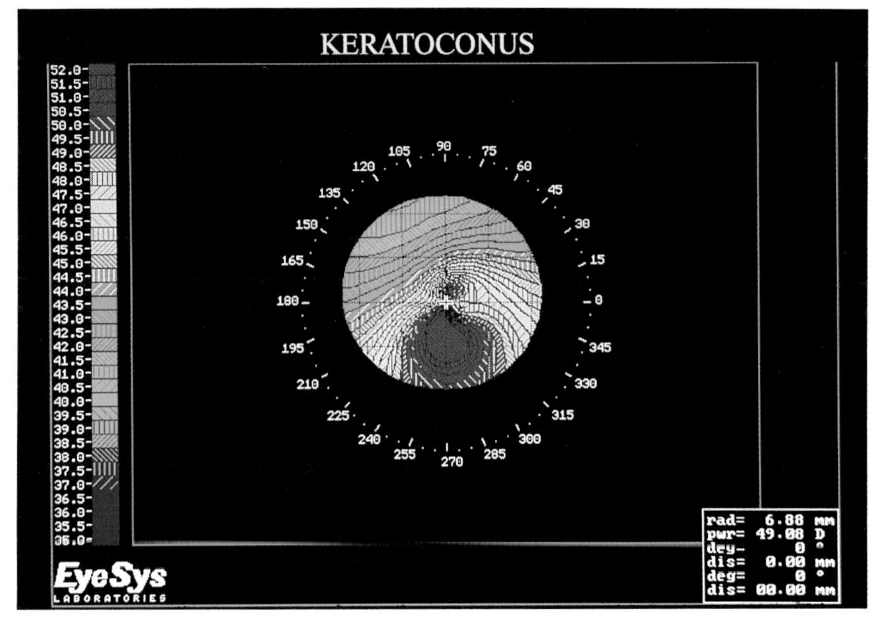

Figure 2.2B.

Figure 2.2: Peripheral keratoconus left eye. There is inferior steepening extending toward the limbus. Note also the superonasal flattening. (A) Normalized scale in 1 D steps. (B) Absolute scale in 0.5 D steps.

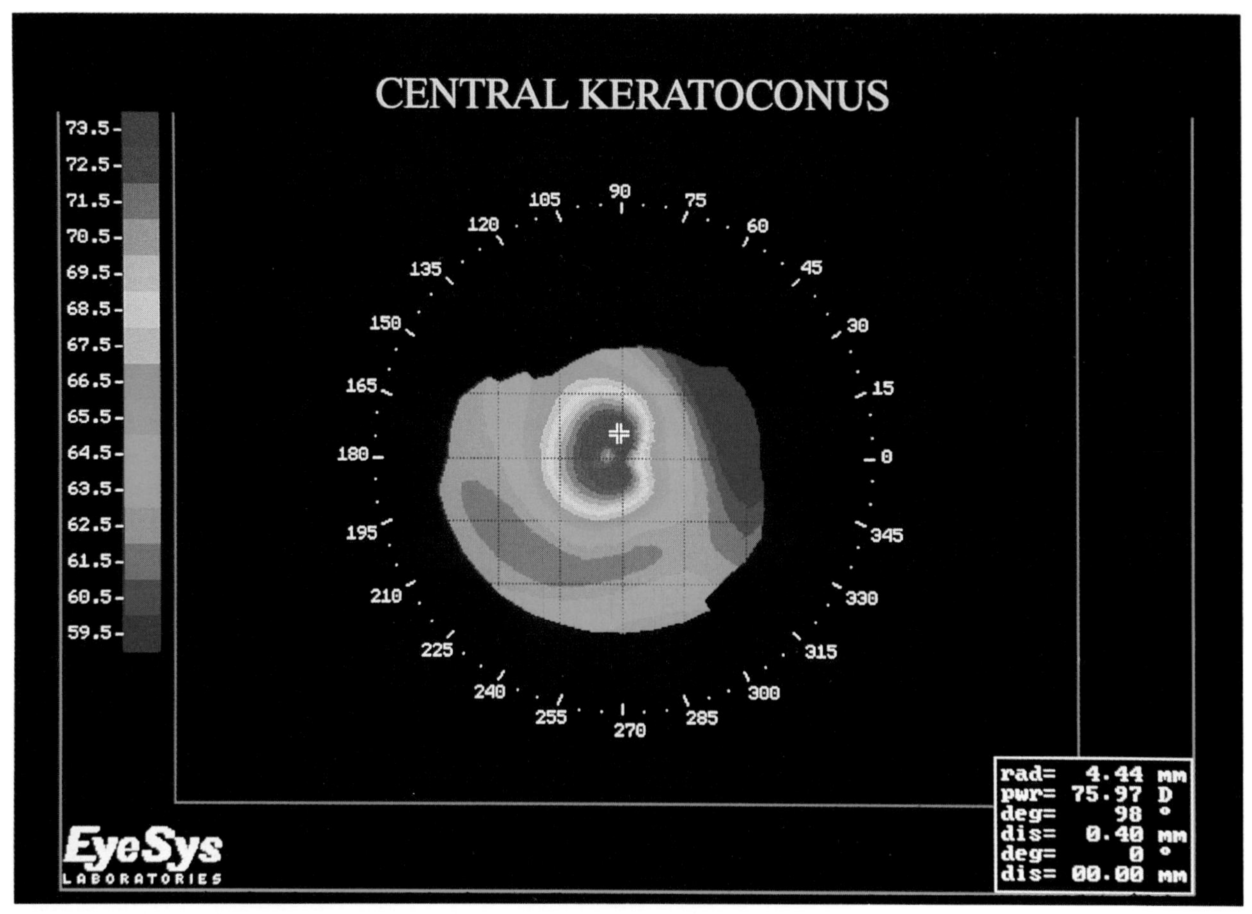

Figure 2.3: Central keratoconus. In this cornea there is remarkably little asymmetry around the apex of this nipple cone.

matism (Figure 2.3). In an earlier study, Rabinowitz and McDonnell similarly noted these two types of keratoconus, and they described three diagnostic CVK features of keratoconus:

1) central corneal power greater than 47 D,
2) a difference of 3 D or more in corneal power comparing points 3 mm inferior to the center to points 3 mm superior to the center (I - S), and
3) asymmetry between central corneal power of fellow eyes in excess of 1 D[4] (Figures 2.4A-C).

Further work is being done to develop definitive criteria for the diagnosis of keratoconus.

CVK is also helpful in evaluating progression of keratoconus,[5] in detecting unusual forms of keratoconus (Figure 2.5), in fitting contact lenses and monitoring their effects in keratoconus (Figure 2.6), and in diagnosing and evaluating related disorders such as keratoglobus (Figures 2.7 and 2.8A, B) and pellucid marginal degeneration.

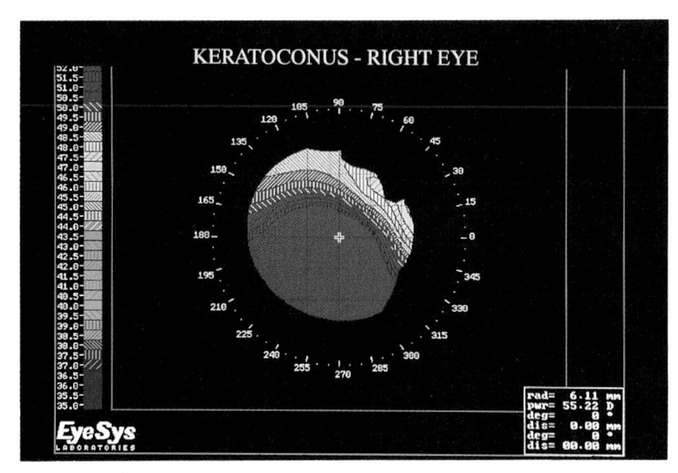

Figure 2.4A.

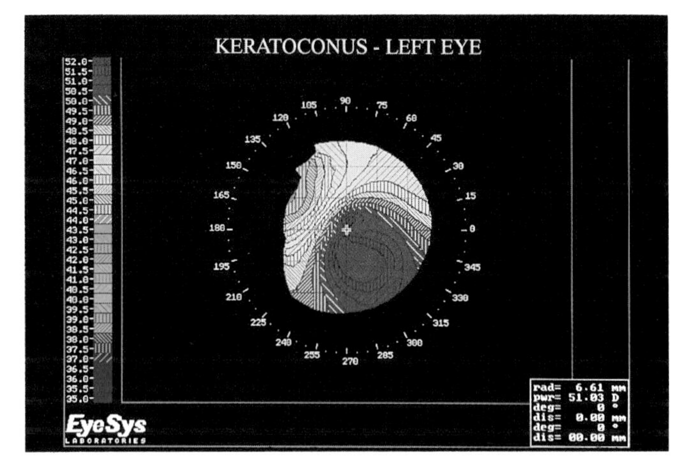

Figure 2.4B.

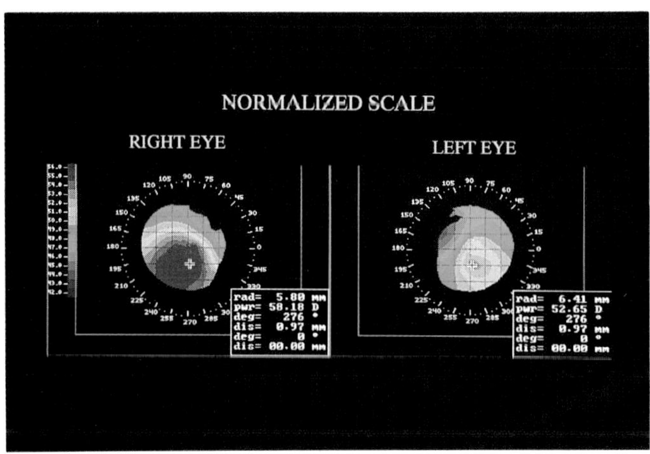

Figure 2.4C.

Figure 2.4: Topographic maps of right and left corneas of a 31-year-old male with bilateral keratoconus. All of the diagnostic features of keratoconus described by Rabinowitz and McDonnell[4] are present. Note the marked central steepness OU (55.00 D OD and 51.00 D OS), the (I – S) disparity due to the greater inferior steepness, and the marked difference in central power between the two corneas. (A) Right eye: absolute scale. (B) Left eye: absolute scale. (C) Both eyes: normalized scale.

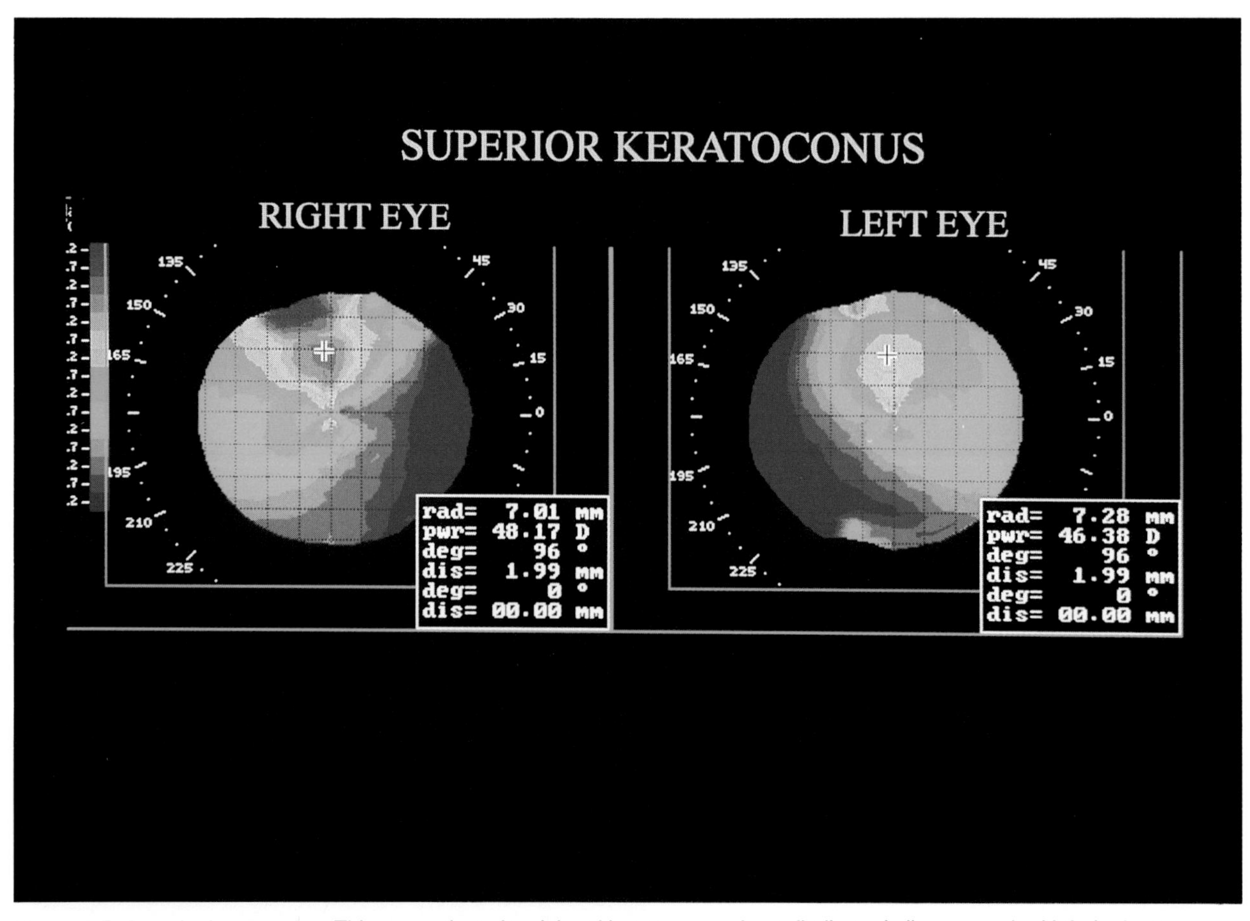

Figure 2.5: Superior keratoconus. This rare variant of peripheral keratoconus shows findings similar to standard inferior keratoconus, except the steepening is present superiorly and slightly temporally. Note the nasal flattening, which is classic for keratoconus, although in these corneas the flattening is centered below the horizontal meridian.

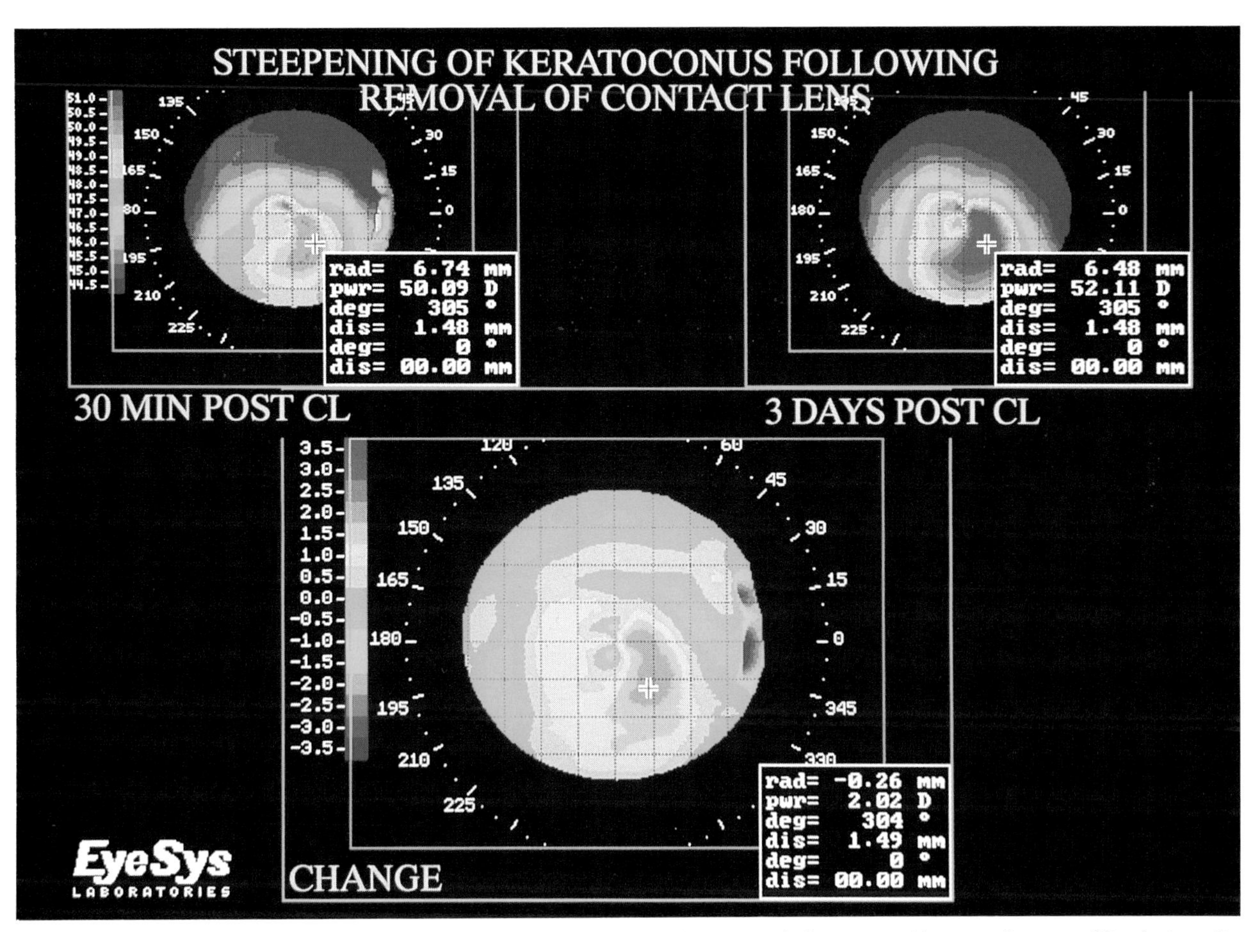

Figure 2.6: Flattening of keratoconus by rigid gas permeable contact lens wear. Left, topographic map of cornea 30 minutes after removing contact lens. Right, after three days of contact lens abstinence, the cone has steepened 2.02 D. Bottom, difference map showing the steepening of the cone.

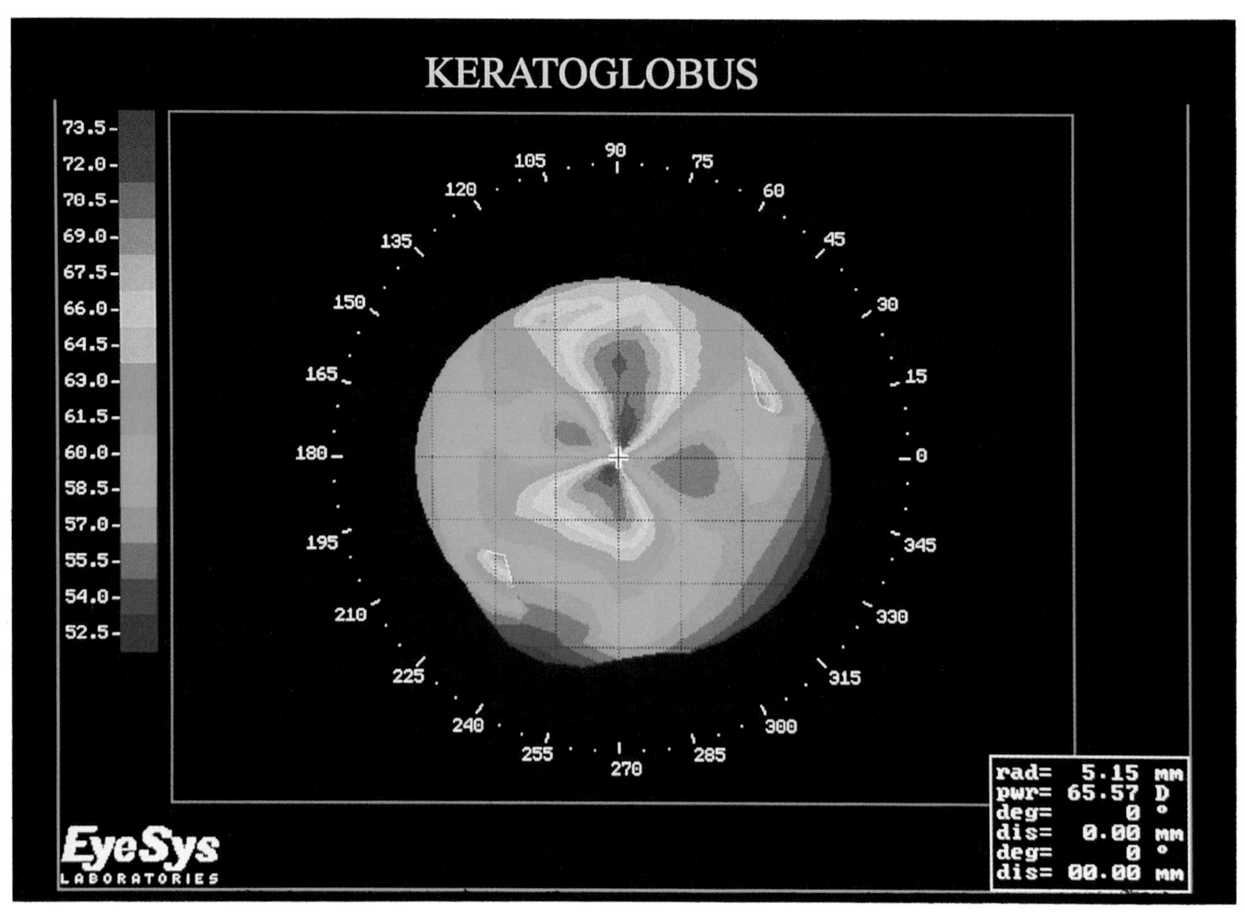

Figure 2.7: Keratoglobus using a normalized scale in 1.5 D steps. The entire cornea is above the range of the absolute scale (>52 D).

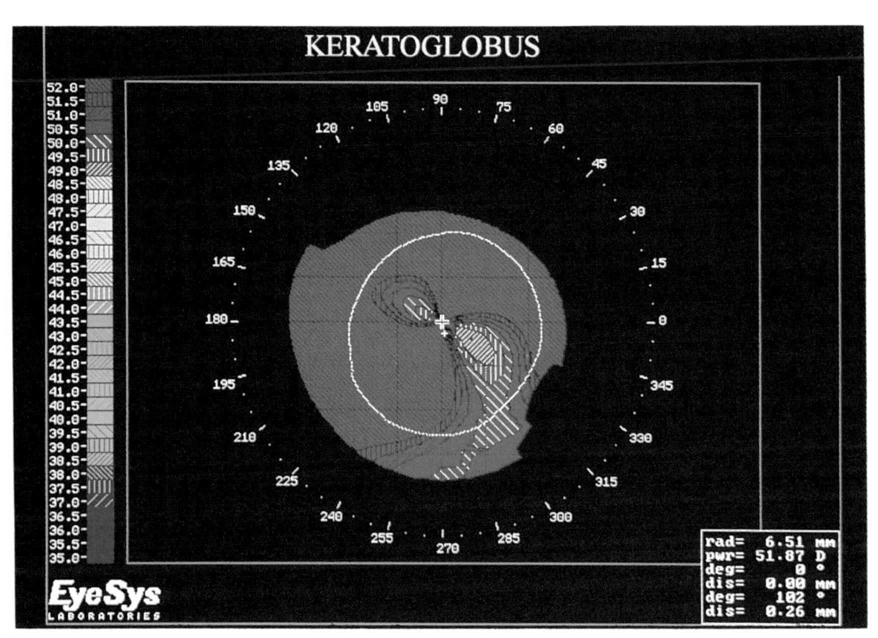

Figure 2.8A.

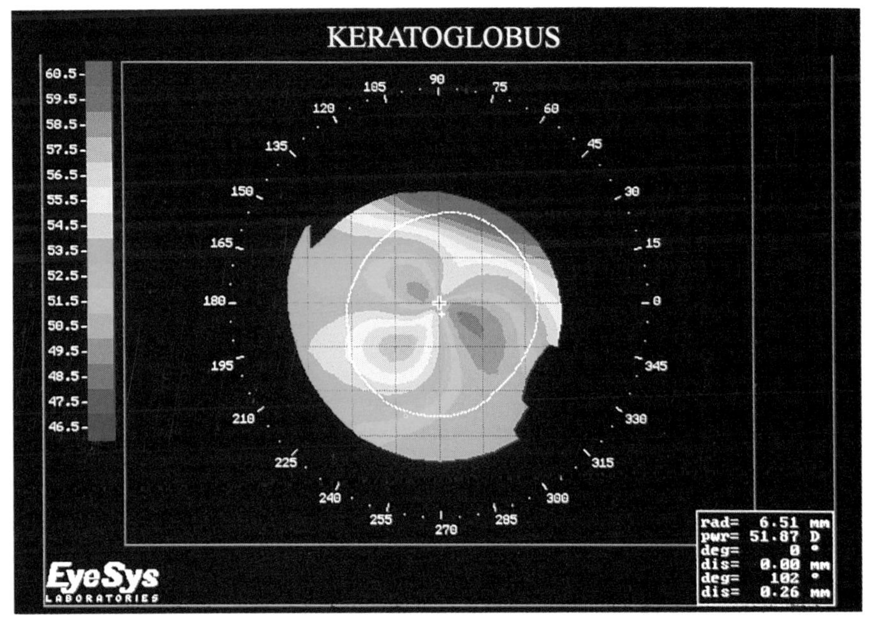

Figure 2.8B.

Figure 2.8: Corneal topographic map of the right eye of a 56-year-old white male with keratoglobus. Note the steep overall curvature with negligible flattening towards the periphery; superimposed is an irregular bow-tie pattern of astigmatism. Corneal ultrasonic pachymetry measured 0.47 mm centrally, and, adjacent to the limbus, 0.45 mm superiorly and 0.51 mm inferiorly. The fellow eye had corneal hydrops. (A) Absolute scale. The whole cornea is at the most extreme end of this scale. Green and yellow ranges are normal. (B) Normalized scale in 1 D steps emphasizing the central irregular bow-tie pattern.

References

1. Maguire LJ, Bourne WM: Corneal topography of early keratoconus. *Amer J Ophthalmol* 108:107-112, 1989.
2. Nesburn AB, Bahri S, Berlin M, et al: Computer assisted corneal topography (CACT) to detect mild keratoconus (kc) in candidates for photorefractive keratectomy. *Invest Ophthalmol Vis Sci* 33/4(suppl):995, 1992.
3. Wilson SE, Lin DTC, Klyce SD: Corneal topography of keratoconus. *Cornea* 10:2-8, 1991.
4. Rabinowitz YS, McDonnell PJ: Computer-assisted corneal topography in keratoconus. *Refract Corneal Surg* 5:400-408, 1989.
5. Maguire LJ, Lowry JC: Identifying progression of subclinical keratoconus by serial topography analysis. *Am J Ophthalmol* 112:41-45, 1991.

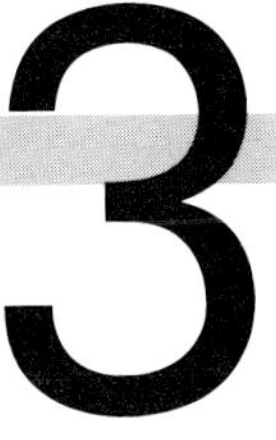

DONALD R. SANDERS, MD, PhD
JAMES P. GILLS, MD
ROBERT G. MARTIN, MD

Characterizing Astigmatism

Introduction

Until now, corneal astigmatism has routinely been measured by keratometry. Keratometry uses only four data points, each approximately 1.5 mm from the center of the cornea, two on the apparently steepest axis and two on the axis 90° away. Astigmatism is defined as the difference in the two axes in diopters. In many cases, this measurement is adequate.

However, this definition of astigmatism depends on the implicit assumption that the cornea is symmetrical, although not spherical. Unfortunately, many corneas are asymmetrical, and the greater the asymmetry, the greater the potential for keratometric error.

Corneal topography maps the entire surface of the cornea with slightly less than 6,000 data points and thus provides an extremely detailed picture of the shape of the cornea. This visual image of the cornea can provide more data than keratometry, and often reveals that keratometry can be misleading.

Symmetrical Astigmatism

Of course, conventional keratometry often describes the shape of the cornea quite accurately. For example, the corneal topography image in Figure 3.1 shows symmetrical, with-the-rule astigmatism in the typical bow-tie pattern. Keratometry indicates 2.5 D of astigmatism at 90°, which is consistent with this image.

In another case, keratometry was 1.5 D at 180°, indicating against-the-rule astigmatism. The topographical image, Figure 3.2, indeed shows against-the-rule astigmatism of the classic bow-tie pattern. Another, less typical pattern of against-the-rule astigmatism is shown in Figure 3.3. Notice that the steepest areas are wedge-shaped.

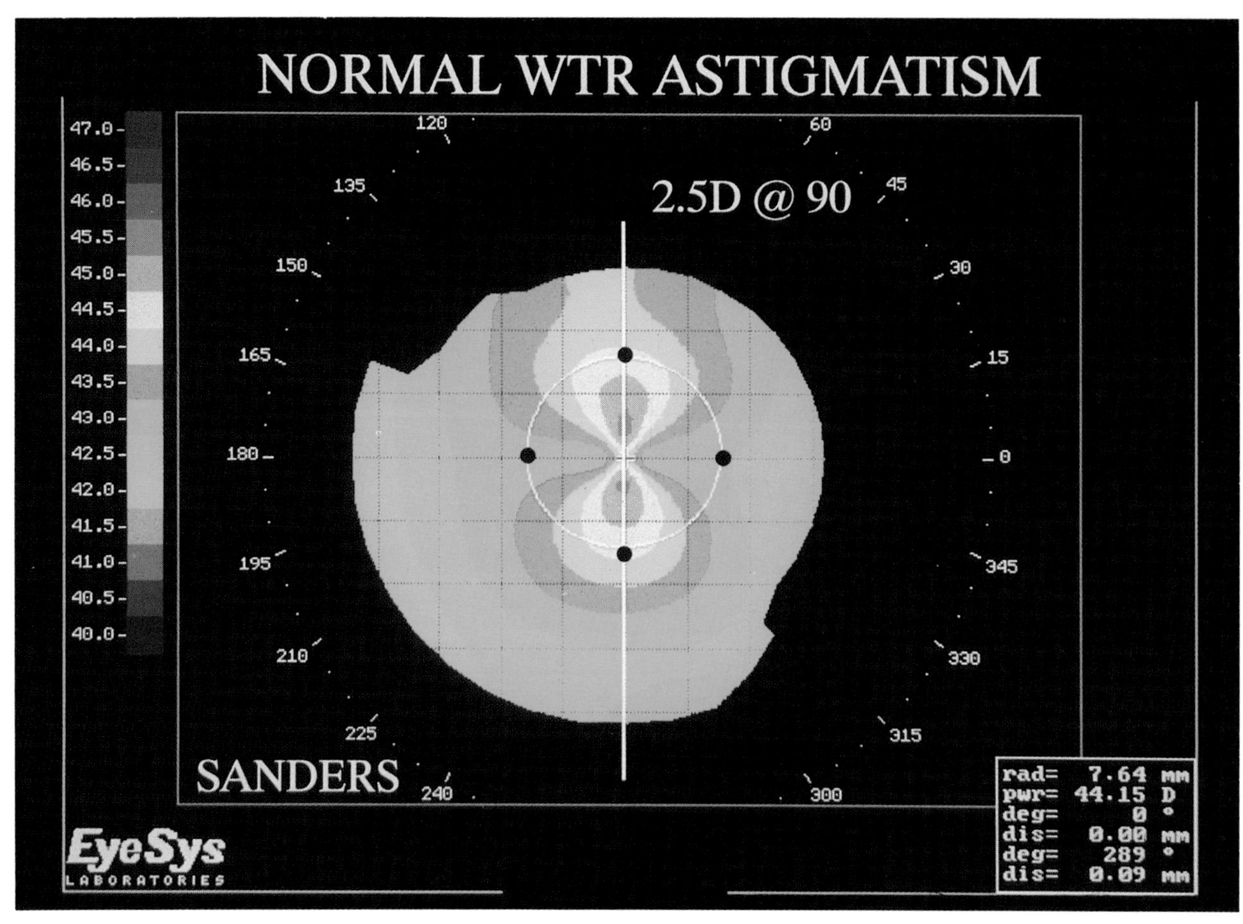

Figure 3.1: Symmetrical with-the-rule astigmatism at 90° (vertical line). Black circles indicate keratometric data points.

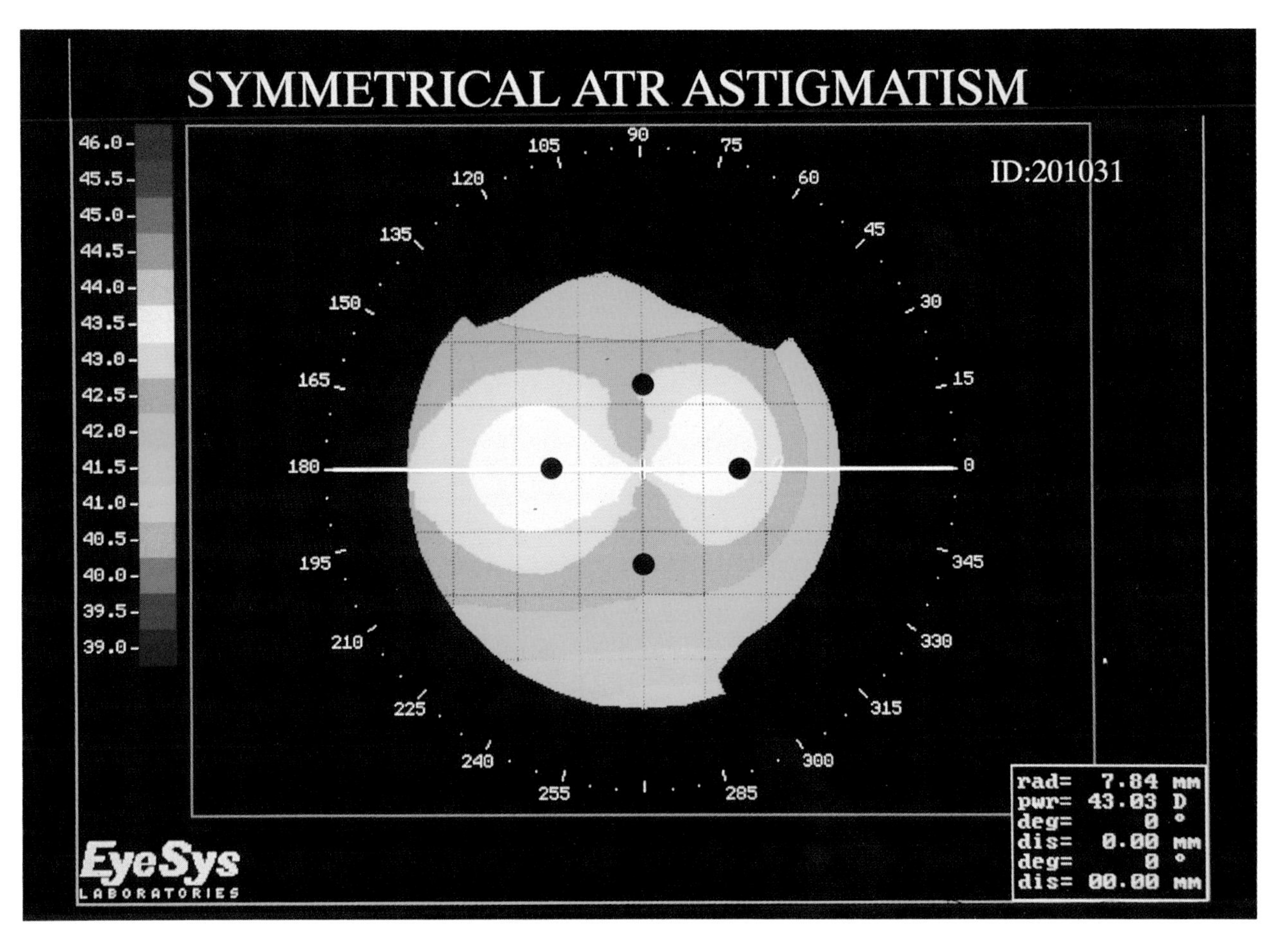

Figure 3.2: Symmetrical against-the-rule astigmatism at 180° (horizontal line). Black circles indicate keratometric data points.

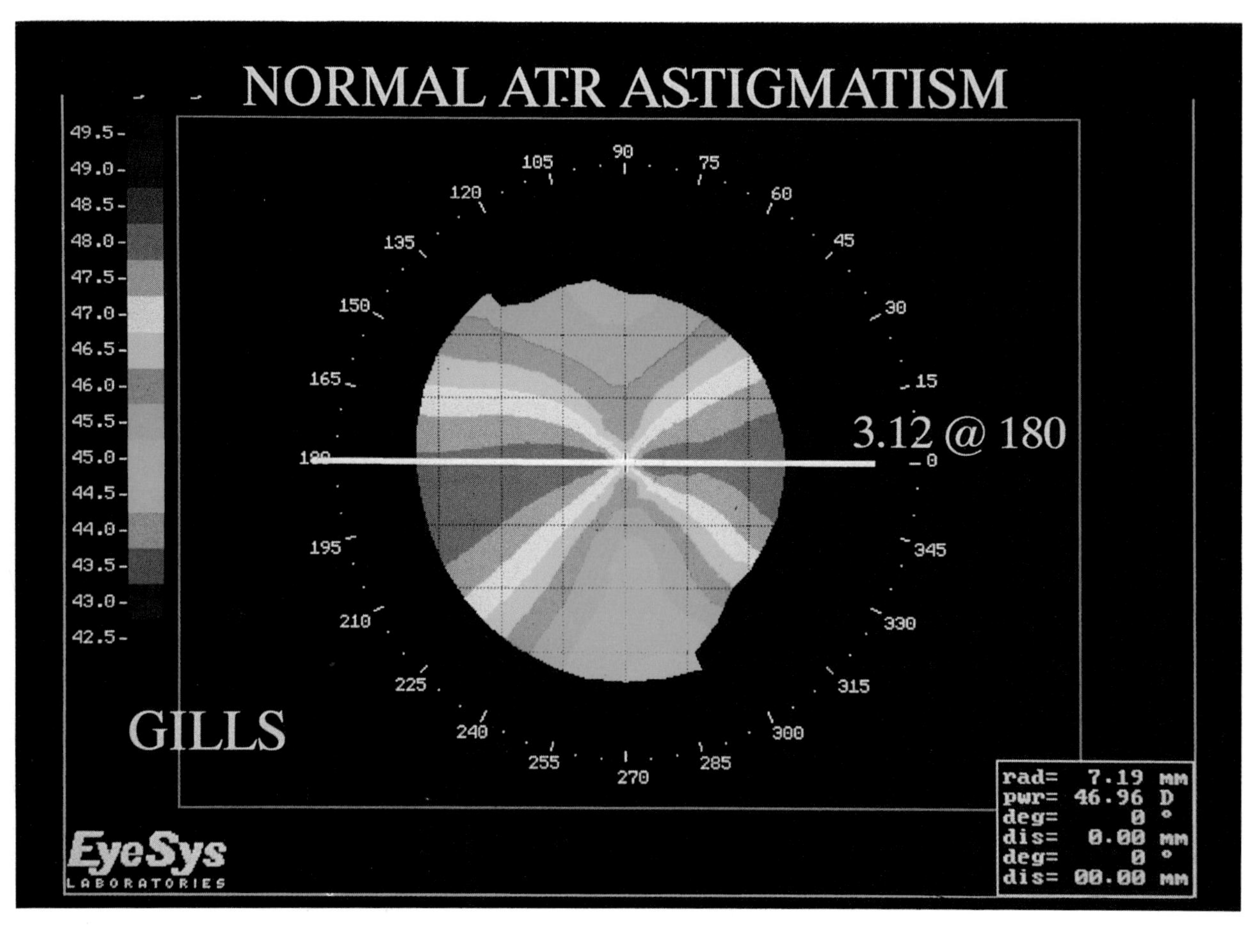

Figure 3.3: Unusual against-the-rule astigmatism with wedge-shaped steep areas. Horizontal line indicates steep keratometric meridian measured at 180°.

Figure 3.4 shows the topographical images of the right and left eyes of another patient. Note the common finding of nonsuperimposable mirror symmetry (enantiomorphism). In all of the preceding examples of symmetrical astigmatism, keratometry provided an adequate, if not always complete, description of the astigmatism present.

Asymmetrical Astigmatism

However, in cases of asymmetrical astigmatism, corneal topography often yields data that is not apparent from keratometry, even when the keratometry provides a reasonable estimate of the degree of astigmatism. For example, Figure 3.5 shows another case of with-the-rule astigmatism. Keratometry indicates 3.5 D of astigmatism at 108°, but the topographic image reveals more information than just the magnitude and direction of the astigmatism, namely that this cornea is steeper superiorly than inferiorly.

Figure 3.6 demonstrates the same case with some other display options. In the upper left is the color-coded contour map showing some asymmetrical astigmatism, with greater astigmatism superiorly. In the

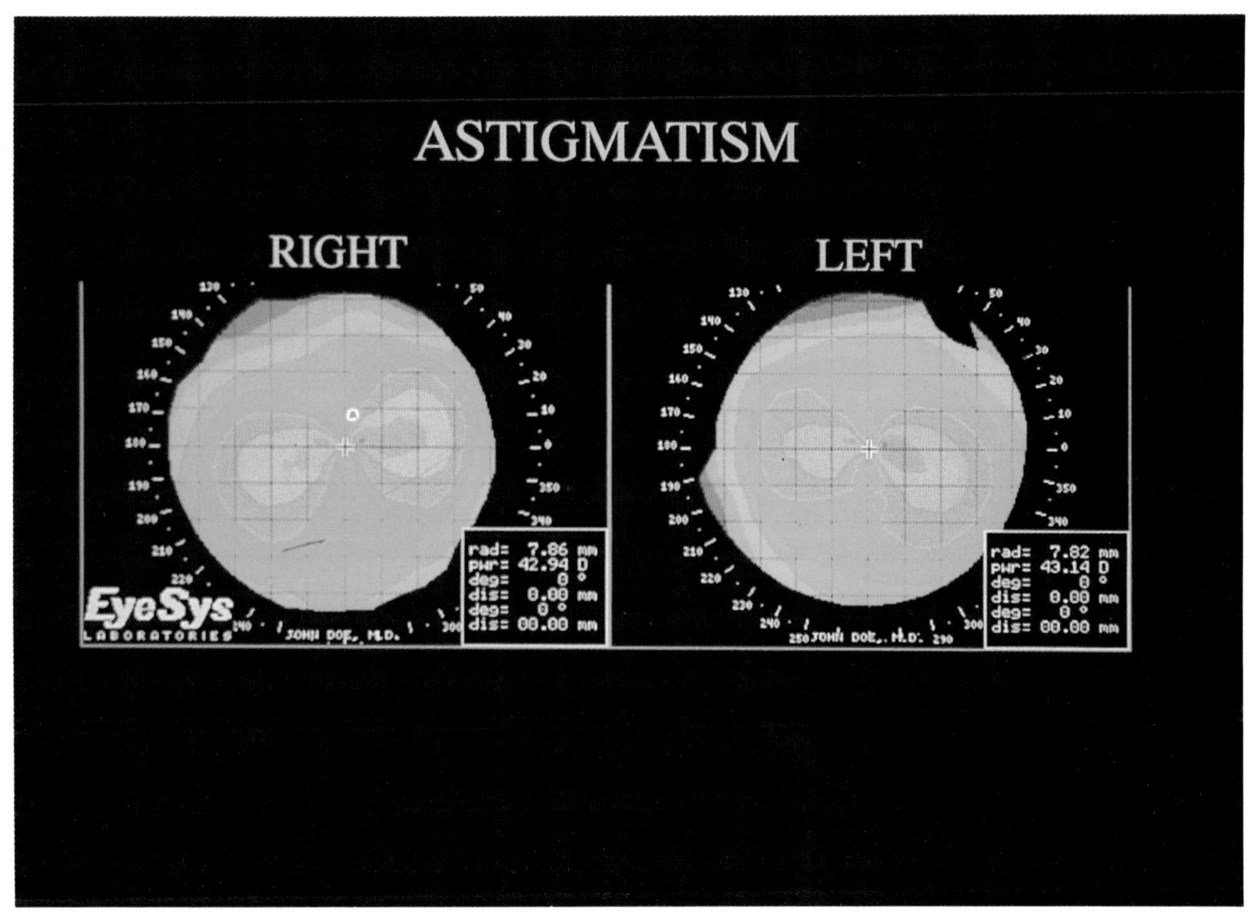

Figure 3.4: Mirror-image astigmatism in right and left eyes of same patient.

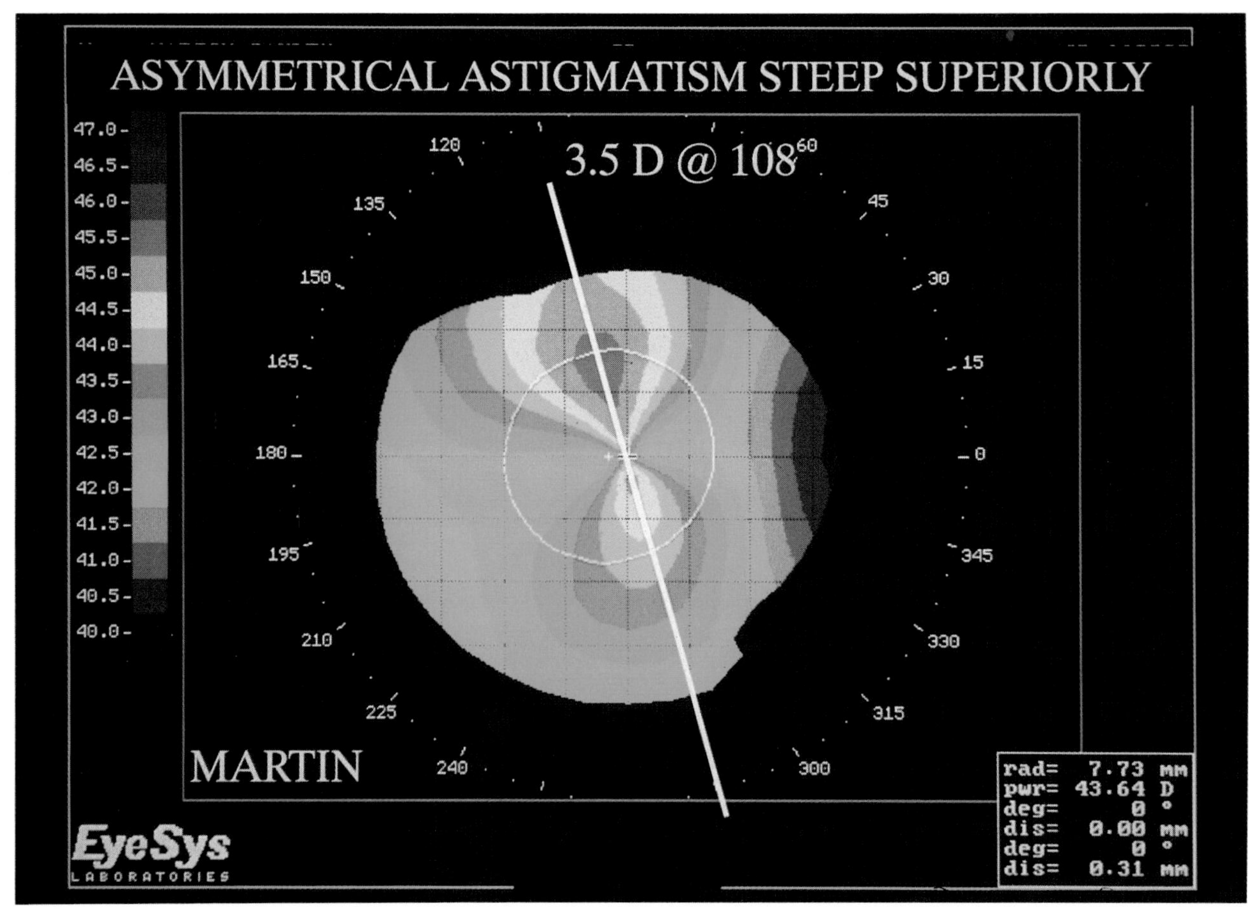

Figure 3.5: Asymmetrical with-the-rule astigmatism, steeper superiorly. Line indicates steep keratometric meridian measured at 108°.

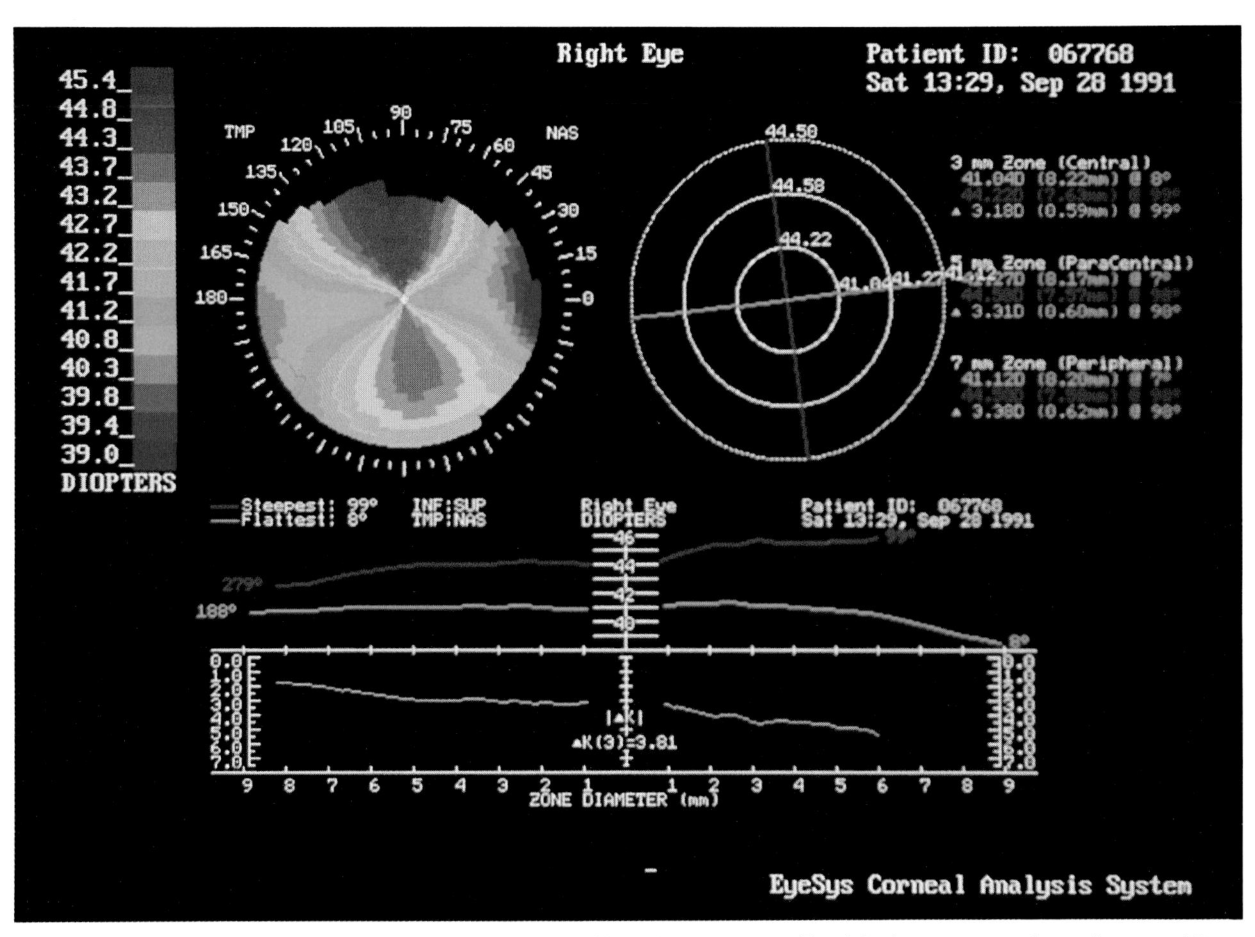

Figure 3.6: Other display options for case shown in Figure 3.5. Top left: contour map. Top right: keratometry at 3 mm, 5 mm, and 7 mm optical zones. Bottom: corneal profile map.

upper right are the average keratometry measurements at the 3, 5, and 7 mm optical zones. The bottom shows a corneal profile map with the corneal astigmatism asymmetry mapped out. Reading the 279° line from left to right, the power of the astigmatism is mapped from the 8 to 9 mm optical zone inferiorly through the center to the upper cornea, indicating an increase of astigmatism of almost 2 D. This information can only be obtained by corneal topography and could be crucial in determining a surgical plan, as one might want to consider more surgery superiorly in this case.

Figure 3.7 demonstrates another asymmetrical cornea. The steep areas are very discrepant in size. For the patient in Figure 3.8, the keratometry reading is 1.62 D at 180°, but the corneal topography image clearly shows asymmetrical astigmatism with the steepest area at the 340° meridian.

The left eye in Figure 3.9 has a flat central cornea, shown in blue, with asymmetrical regions of steepness on either side. It is clearly much steeper nasally than temporally, indicated by orange areas. Figure 3.10 is another example of a relatively flat central cornea, the blue and green areas, surrounded by steeper, orange regions. In all of these examples so far, the keratometric

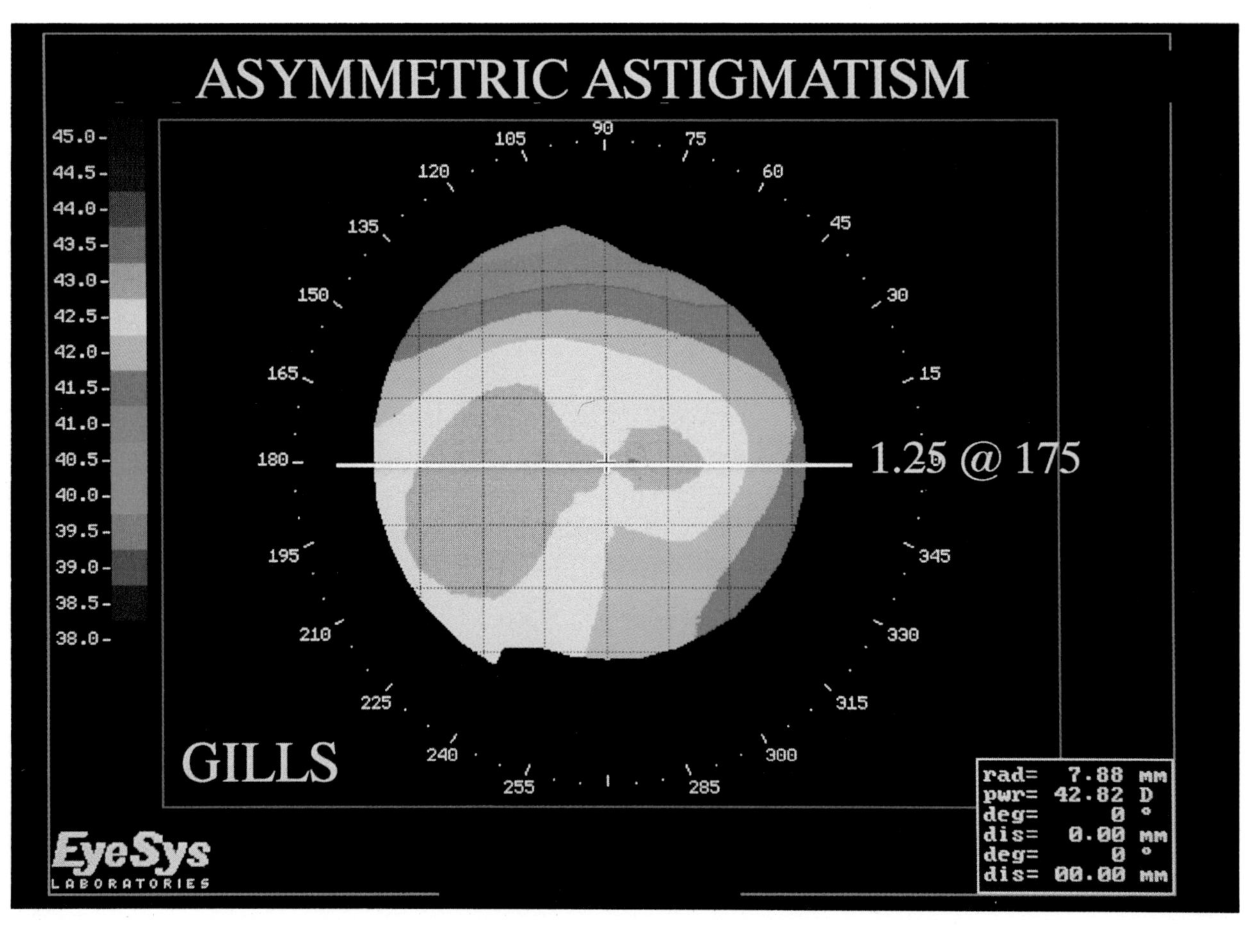

Figure 3.7: Asymmetrical astigmatism with steep areas of discrepant size. Line indicates steep keratometry meridian measured at 175°.

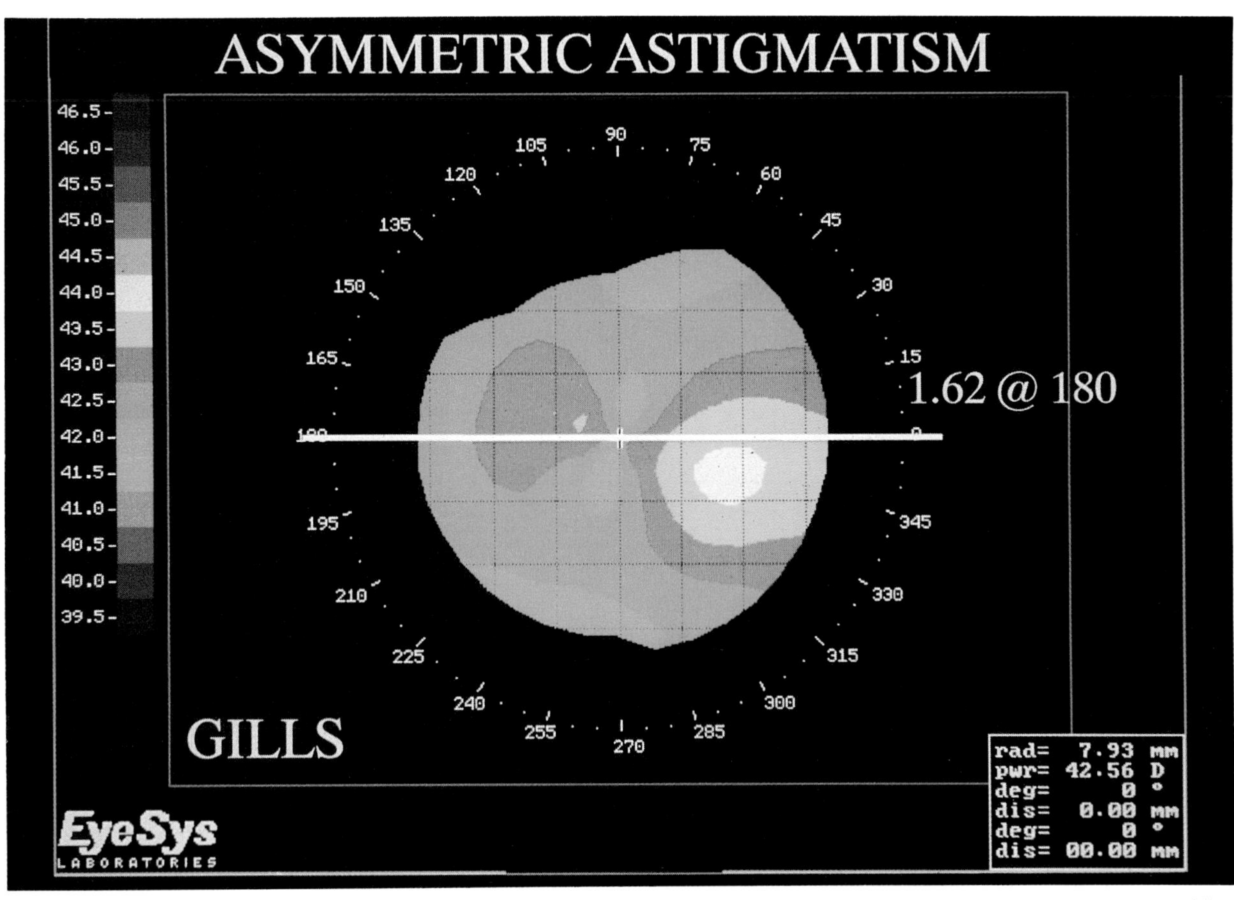

Figure 3.8: Asymmetrical astigmatism OD, steeper nasally with flat central cornea. Line indicates steep keratometric meridian measured at 180°.

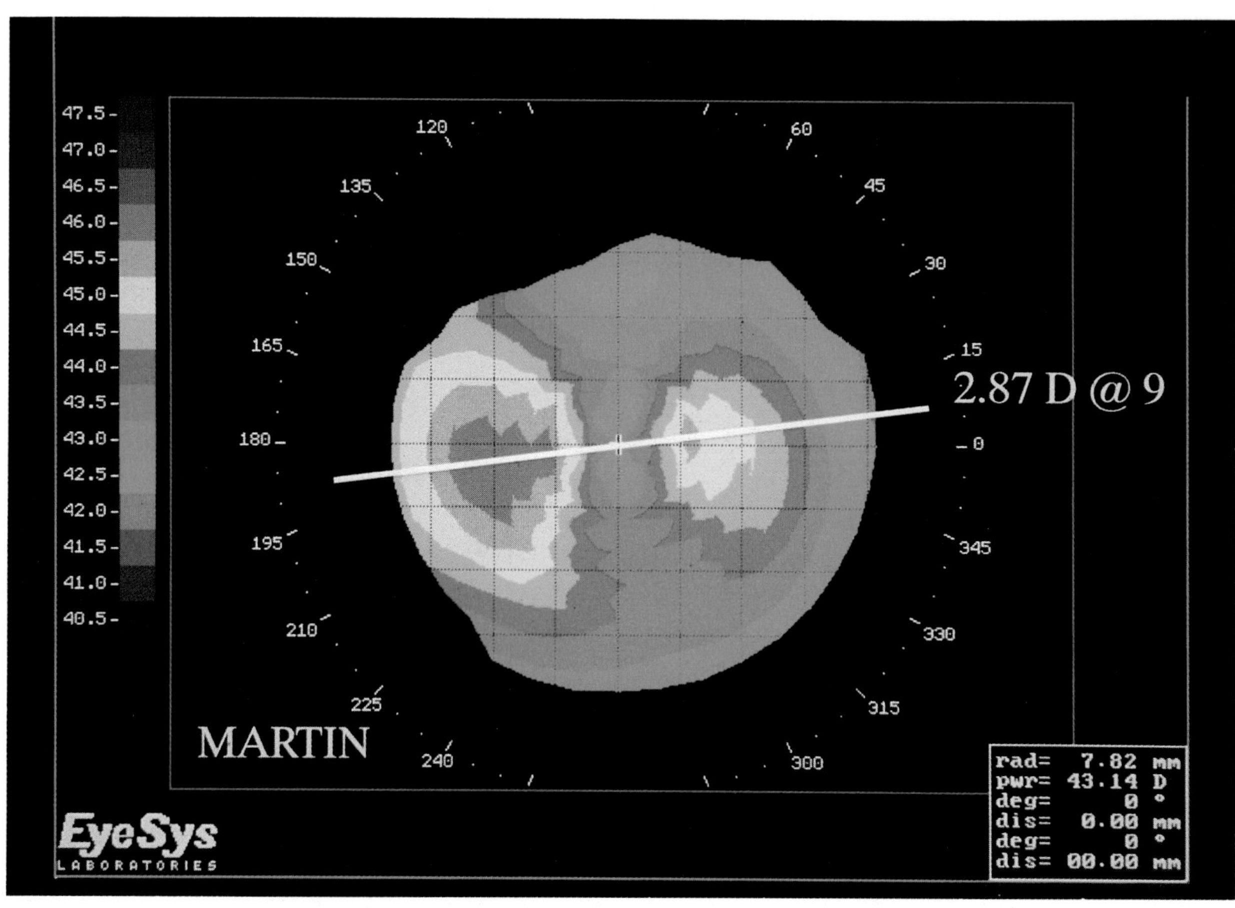

Figure 3.9: Asymmetrical astigmatism, steeper nasally, with flat central cornea. Line indicates steep keratometric meridian measured at 9°.

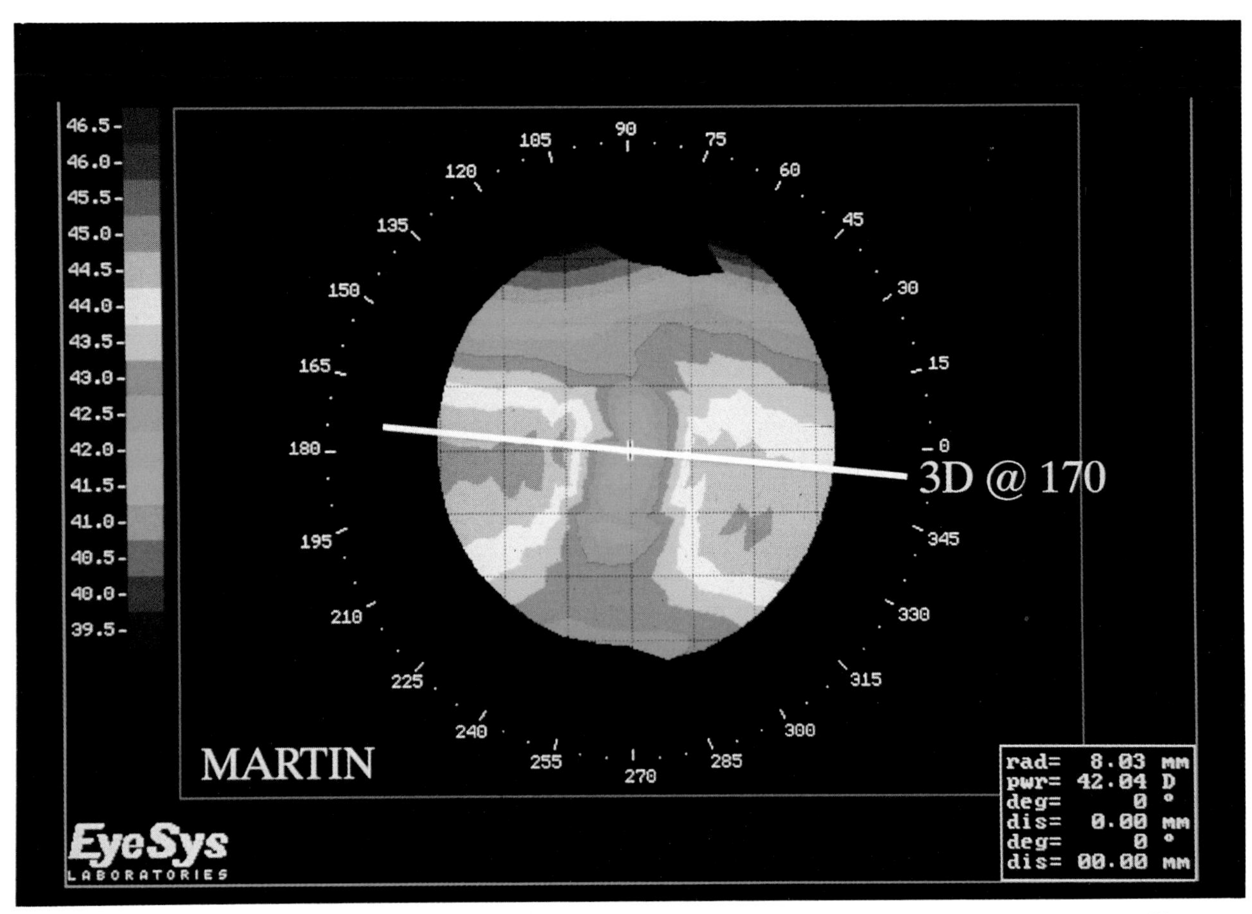

Figure 3.10: Flat central cornea surrounded by steeper regions. Line indicates steep keratometric meridian measured at 170°.

cylinder meridian has roughly corresponded to the corneal topographic appearance.

Misleading Keratometry

Figures 3.11, and 3.12 show corneas in which no true astigmatic pattern can be identified on the topographic images, yet both have non-trivial keratometric astigmatism. Figure 3.11 has keratometric astigmatism of 0.87 D at 18°. However, the topographic image clearly shows that the cornea is steep superiorly, with a gradient of 2 D from the top to the bottom of the cornea. Figure 3.12 has keratometric astigmatism of 1.37 D at 179°. The cornea is in fact steep inferotemporally and flat superonasally, with a gradient of 2.5 D. Clearly, the keratometry measurements do not reflect the corneal surface characteristics.

Figure 3.13 illustrates the value of corneal topography in avoiding possible inappropriate surgery. The keratometric measurements demonstrated 1.5 D of astigmatism at 170°. Corneal topography reveals a very unusual pattern of superior steepness and inferior flatness. The gradient of 4 D lies approximately 90° away from the steep keratometric meridian. If a surgeon attempted

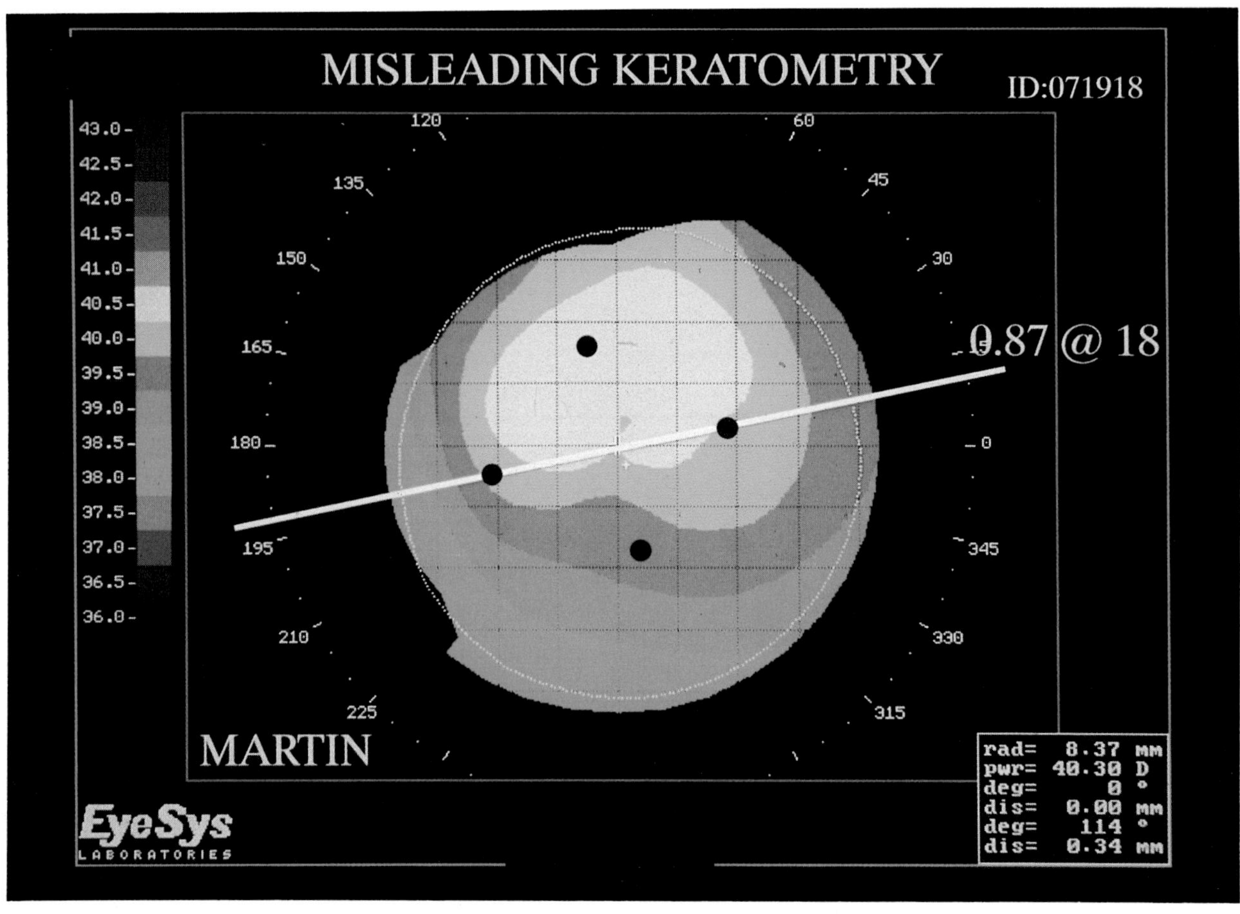

Figure 3.11: Misleading keratometry. The cornea is steep superiorly, with a 2 D gradient from top to bottom. Keratometry indicated astigmatism of 0.87 D at 18° (line). Black circles indicate keratometric data points.

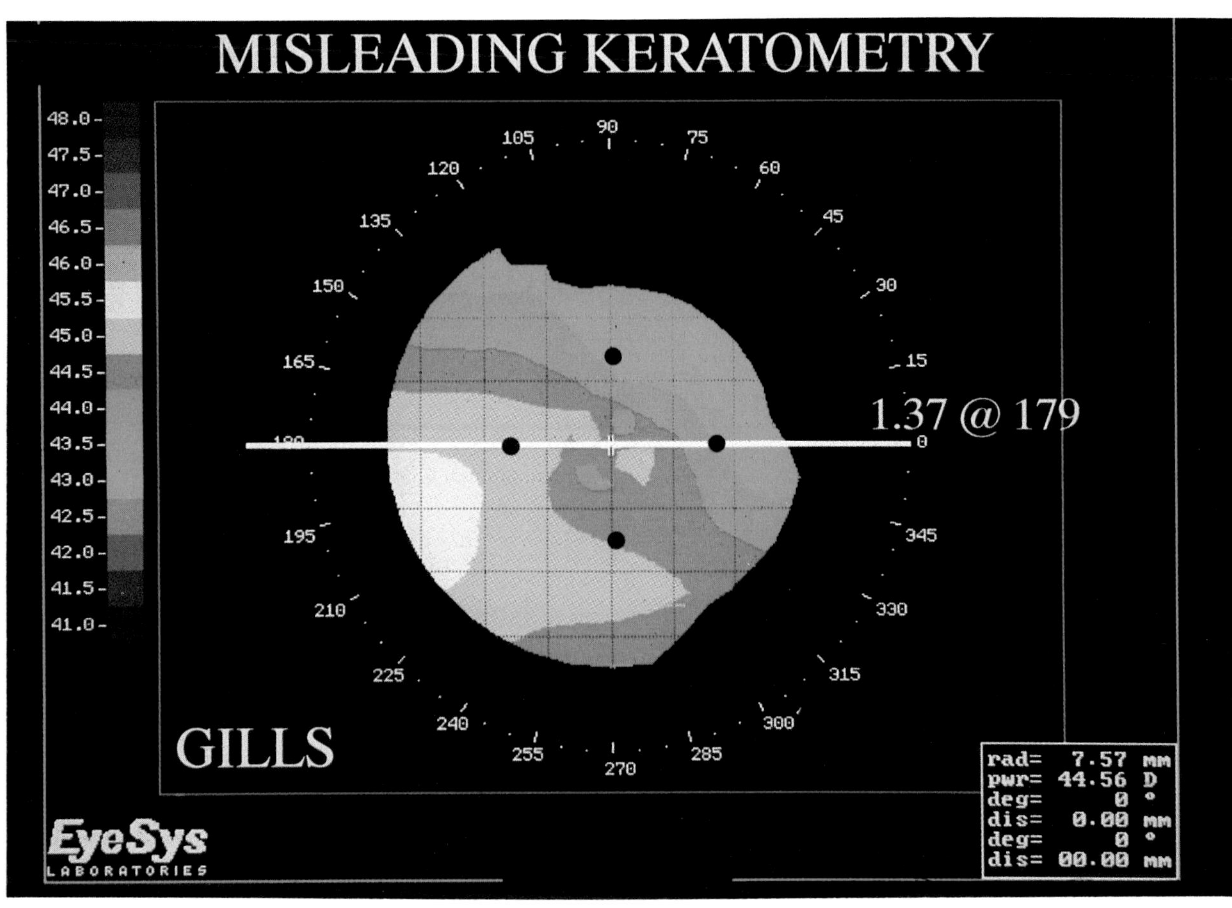

Figure 3.12: Misleading keratometry OD. The cornea is steep inferotemporally and flat superonasally. Keratometry indicates astigmatism of 1.37 D at 179° (line). Black circles indicate keratometric data points.

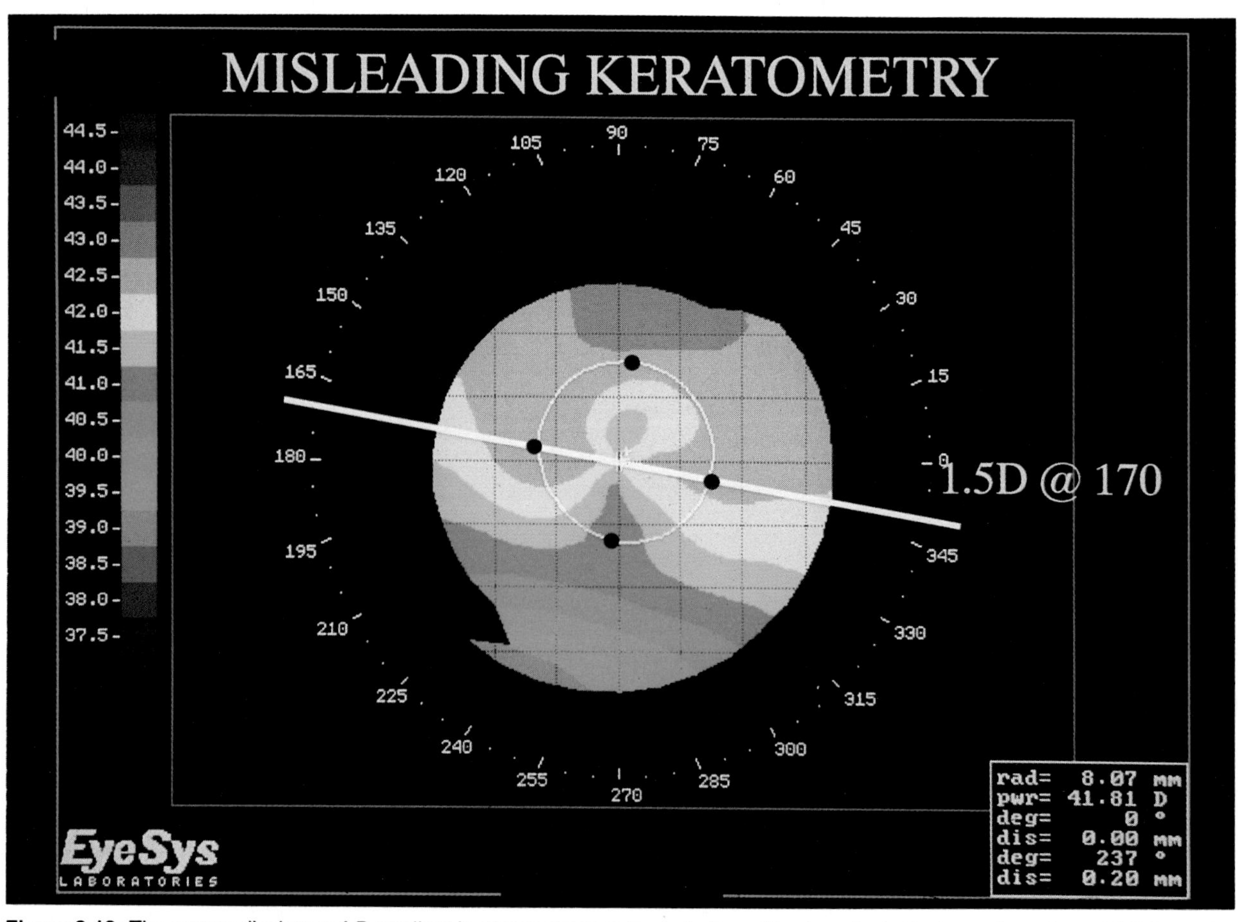

Figure 3.13: The cornea displays a 4 D gradient in steepness from top to bottom. Keratometry indicates astigmatism of 1.5 D at 170° (line), 90° away from the steepest area on the topographic image. Black circles indicate keratometric data points.

to correct the keratometric astigmatism by T-cuts at 170°, which is where the keratometer indicated the astigmatism to be, it would probably prove to be ineffective with this strange astigmatism pattern. In this case, making a single or two T-cuts superiorly with none inferiorly has the greatest probability of improving the astigmatism. Incisional refractive surgery should be approached with caution in such a case, however, as the response to incisional surgery in this type of cornea is unknown. Corneal topography is the only clinically available tool that could have detected this problem.

Figure 3.14 is a preoperative image that was unavailable to the surgeon, who placed corneal relaxing incisions at 70°, where keratometry indicated the steep astigmatic meridian to be. Unfortunately, this patient probably had an asymptomatic keratoconus without mire distortion, and corneal relaxing surgery resulted in further corneal distortion and an increase in the keratometric cylinder.

The next case, Figure 3.15, dramatizes how a case may have an abnormal response to astigmatic keratotomy and not be detected by keratometry. Preoperatively, the case had 1.75 D of against-the-rule astigmatism by keratometry. At 2 weeks postopera-

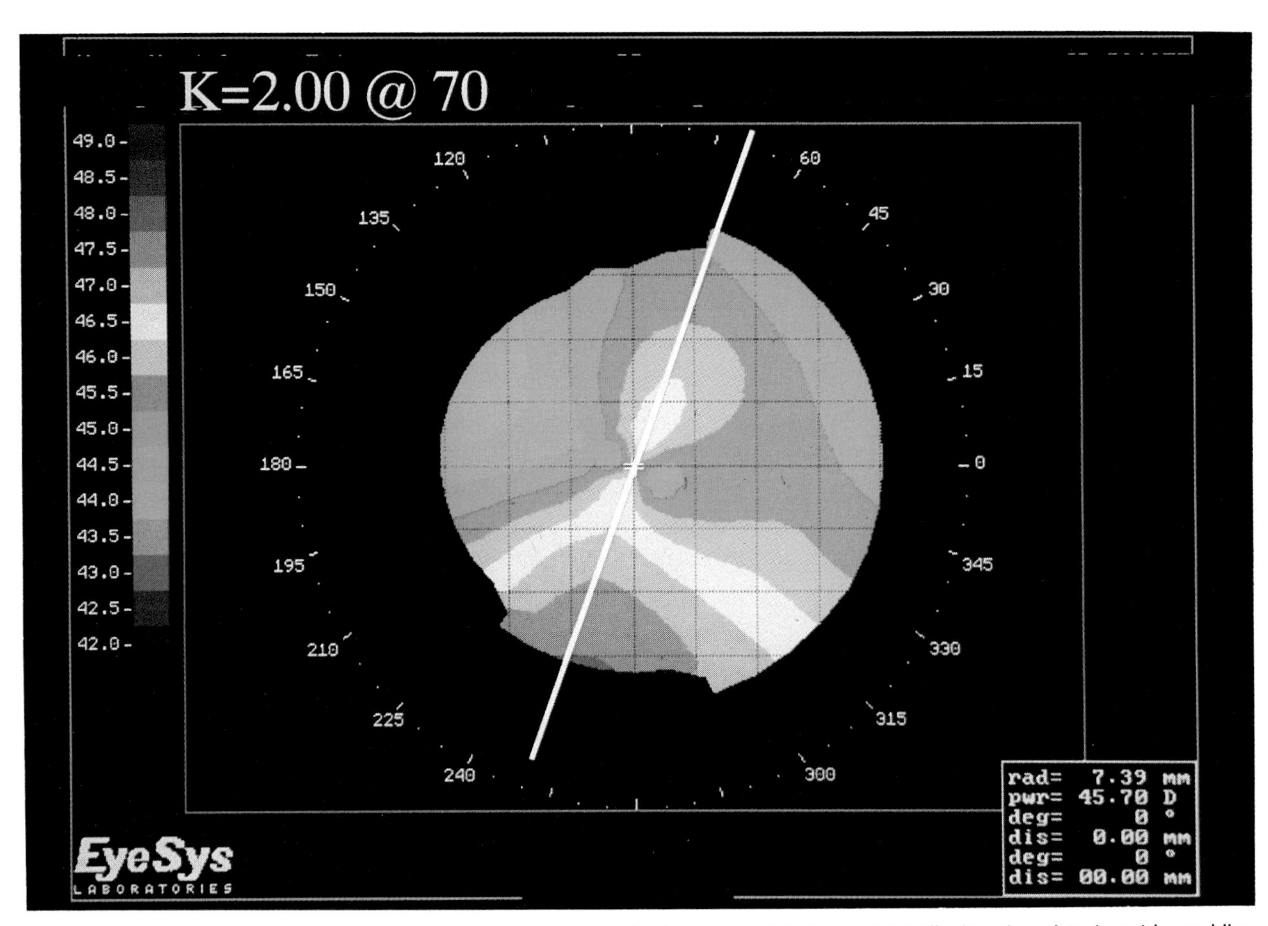

Figure 3.14: Possible asymptomatic keratoconus in patient who had no mires distortion. Line indicates steep keratometric meridian measured at 70°.

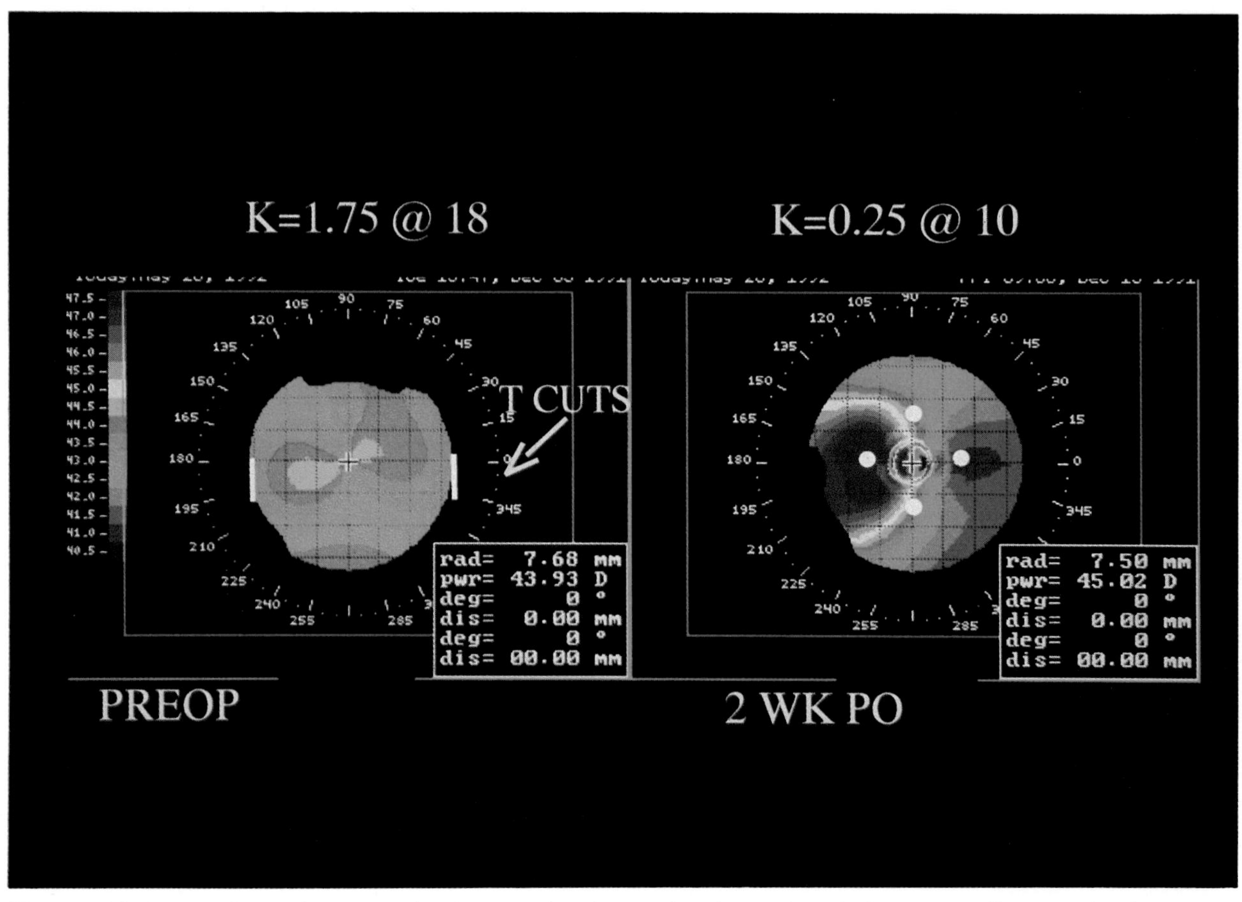

Figure 3.15: Preoperative and postoperative images of patient undergoing astigmatic keratotomy. Postoperative keratometry indicated little residual astigmatism. Lines indicate placement of T-cuts (corneal relaxing incisions) and white circles indicate keratometric data points.

tively, the keratometry readings indicate an excellent result with only 0.25 D of residual astigmatism. However, the 2-week postoperative corneal topography image is considerably abnormal, with marked steepening nasally and flattening temporally in this left eye. Since the keratometer averages two sets of points 180° away from each other, it averages the steep portion at 0° and the flat portion at 180° and detects little or no astigmatism. This reading may give the refractive surgeon a false sense of security. Corneal topography thus provides crucial information otherwise unobtainable to the refractive surgeon.

Conclusion

The examples presented in this chapter demonstrate the value of corneal topography to the clinician. Many corneas cannot be adequately described by keratometry because of their deviation from symmetry, underscoring the critical importance of topographic data in planning corneal relaxing surgery. These examples may explain much of the variability, and in some cases the ineffectuality or harmful results, of some incisional refractive procedures. The avoidance of ineffective or inappropriate surgery is a major contribution of corneal topography, but certainly not the only one. Research is now underway to explore the potential contribution of corneal topography to the predictability of refractive surgical procedures. In addition, corneal topography can be used to follow the postoperative course of surgery. In some cases, corneal topography may be used to explain apparent discrepancies between keratometric measurements of surgically modified astigmatism and postoperative visual acuity.

4

ROBERT G. MARTIN, MD
JAMES P. GILLS, MD

Evaluating Outcomes of Cataract Surgery

Using Corneal Topography with Cataract/IOL Surgery

Corneal topography is a useful tool for monitoring the postoperative course of cataract removal and intraocular lens implantation. For the clinician, corneal topography may reveal problems not apparent on routine examination. For the researcher, it is an essential adjunct to the investigation of the relative merits of sutureless and sutured surgery, and of small- vs. larger-incision surgery. Corneal topography makes important contributions to interpreting the visual rehabilitative results of these surgical options. The sequential image and change image display options are particularly useful for patient follow-up.

The sequential image option displays a preoperative and up to three postoperative images from the patient in the same scale. The resulting maps are directly comparable and postoperative changes in corneal shape can be monitored.

The change image, or delta map, option represents one of the most valuable features of computer-assisted video keratography, the ability to follow patients over time. The software will subtract point-for-point two maps from the same eye taken at different times. If the postoperative image is subtracted from the preoperative image, the change map visually demonstrates the surgically induced changes in corneal shape. Because each image is made up of slightly less than 6,000 data points across the entire surface of the cornea, the change map is extremely detailed, and is analogous to vector analysis of keratometric measurements. The change image is, however, much more precise and detailed.

Effect of Sutures

The classic pattern of early with-the-rule astigmatism that regresses within the first three months postoperatively is a pattern well known to the cataract surgeon.

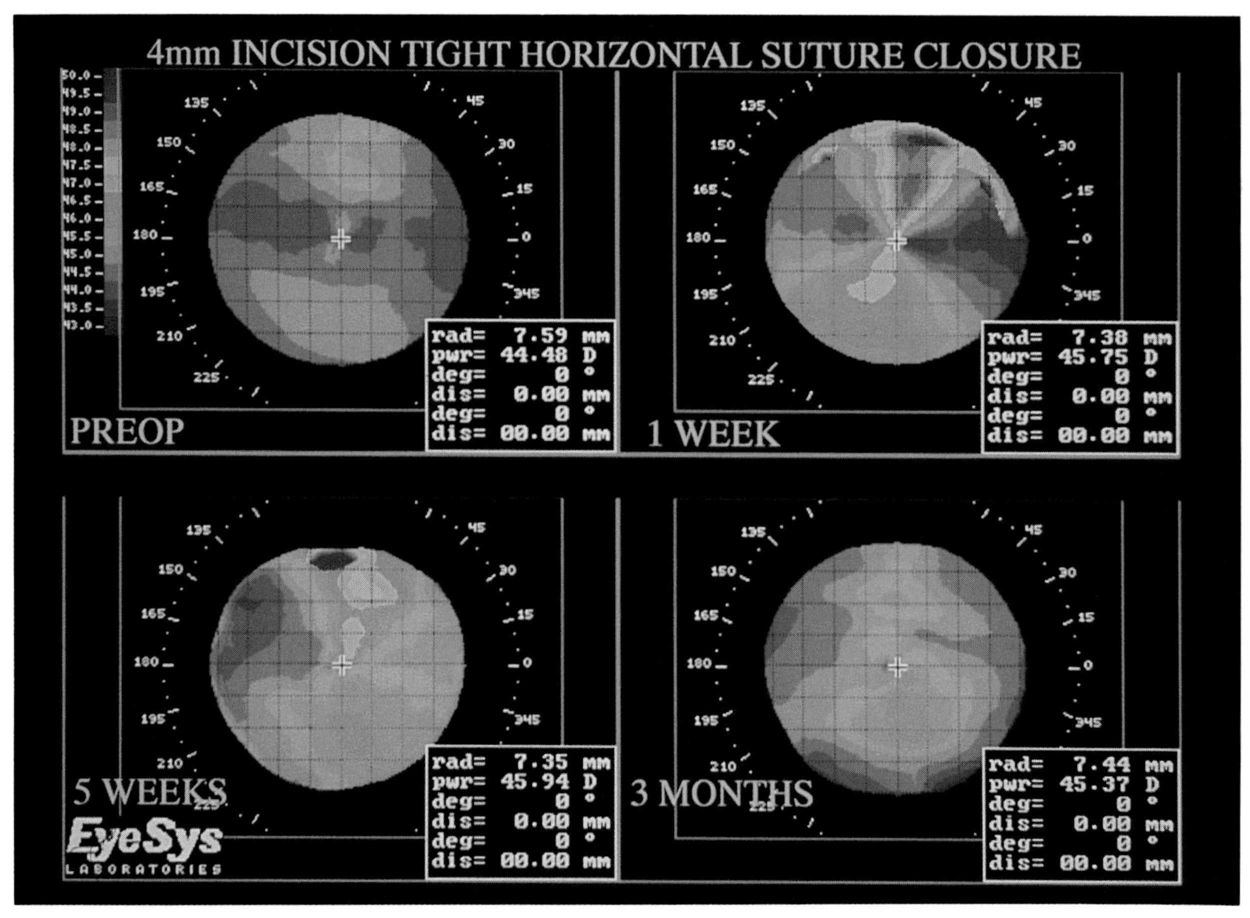

Figure 4.1: Preoperative and serial postoperative corneal topography of a case having a foldable IOL implantation, a 4 mm cataract incision and a too-tight horizontal suture in place.

Figure 4.1 shows preoperative, 1 week, 5 week and 3 month postoperative images from a patient who received a foldable lens inserted through a 4 mm incision closed with a too tight horizontal suture. The system automatically uses the same scaling for all four images. Note that the preoperative cornea is fairly flat relative to the postoperative images and it is fairly spherical.

At 1 week postoperatively, the patient had asymmetrical with-the-rule astigmatism, steeper superiorly near the suture. The two lower images in this figure show the same patient at 5 weeks and 3 months postoperatively. Having all images on the same dioptric scale facilitates tracking the patient's progress. Figure 4.2 shows the change image display option for the same

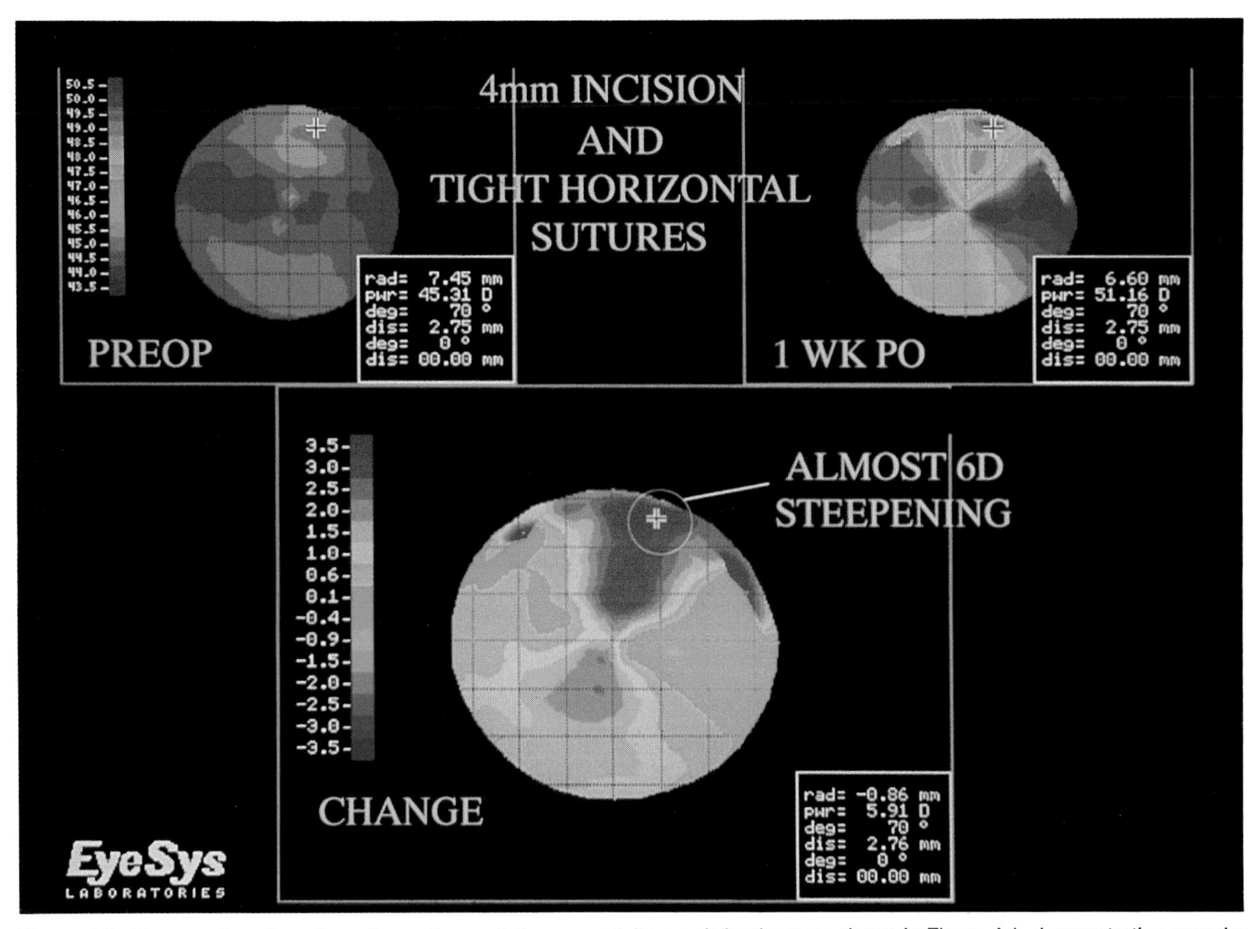

Figure 4.2: Preoperative, 1 week postoperative and change or delta graph for the case shown in Figure 4.1, demonstrating superior steepening and with-the-rule astigmatism due to tight suture placement.

patient comparing preoperative to one week postoperative. The change image (bottom) clearly shows the substantial superior steepening (red) associated with the tight suture. At this time period, the topographical image demonstrated that the superior cornea had been steepened by almost 6 D. Figure 4.3A shows the change image 3 months postoperatively, clearly depicting 2 D of residual steepness (orange) in the center of the cornea. Figure 4.3B is a magnified image of the central cornea at 3 months postoperatively. Two irregular areas of steepening can be seen within the central 2 mm of cornea, probably explaining the patient's persisting visual complaints.

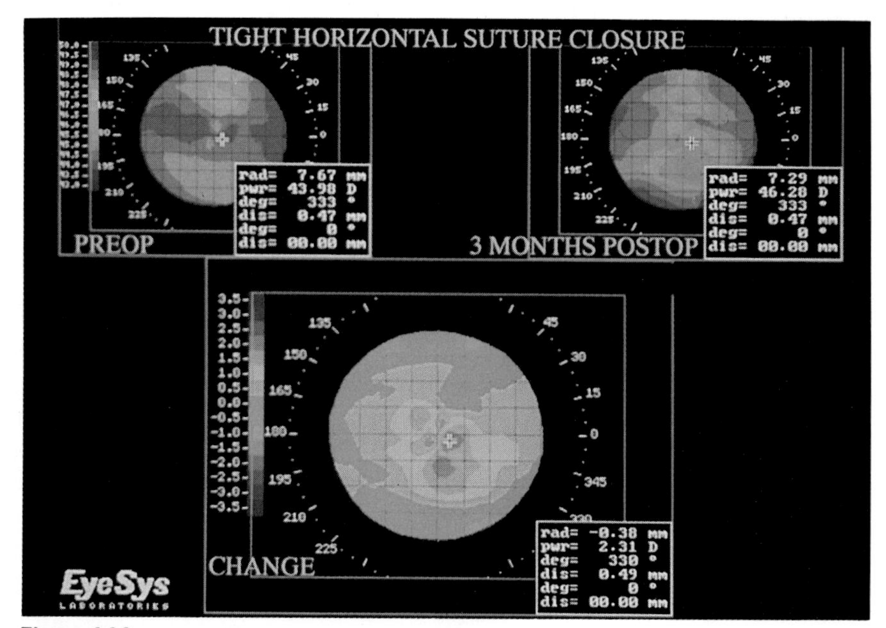

Figure 4.3A.

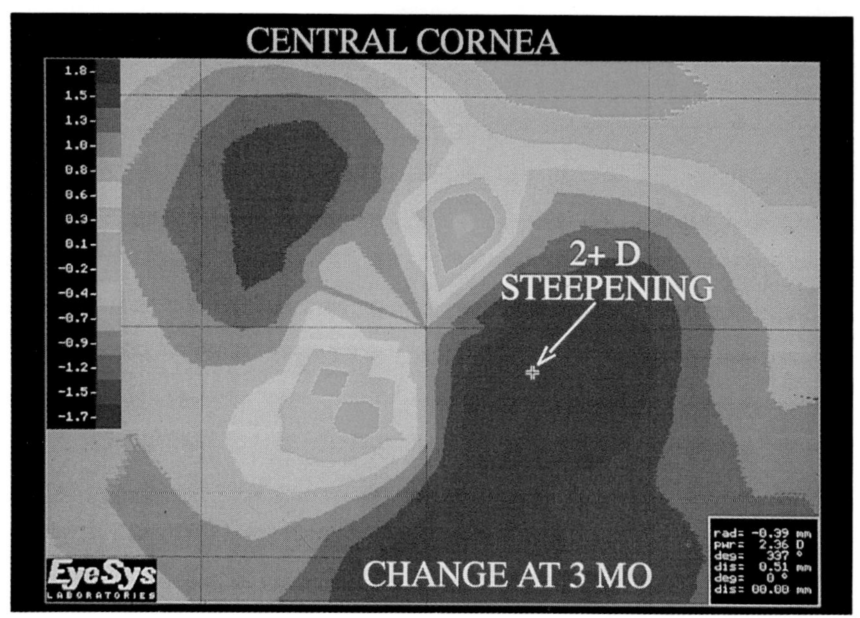

Figure 4.3B.

Figure 4.3: (A) Preoperative, 3 month postoperative and change or delta graph in same case as Figure 4.1 demonstrating residual central corneal steepening. (B) Magnified image of change map of (A) emphasizing central corneal changes. Each square is 1 mm by 1 mm. The scale of the change graph in (B) is in 0.25D steps to more clearly demonstrate the corneal changes.

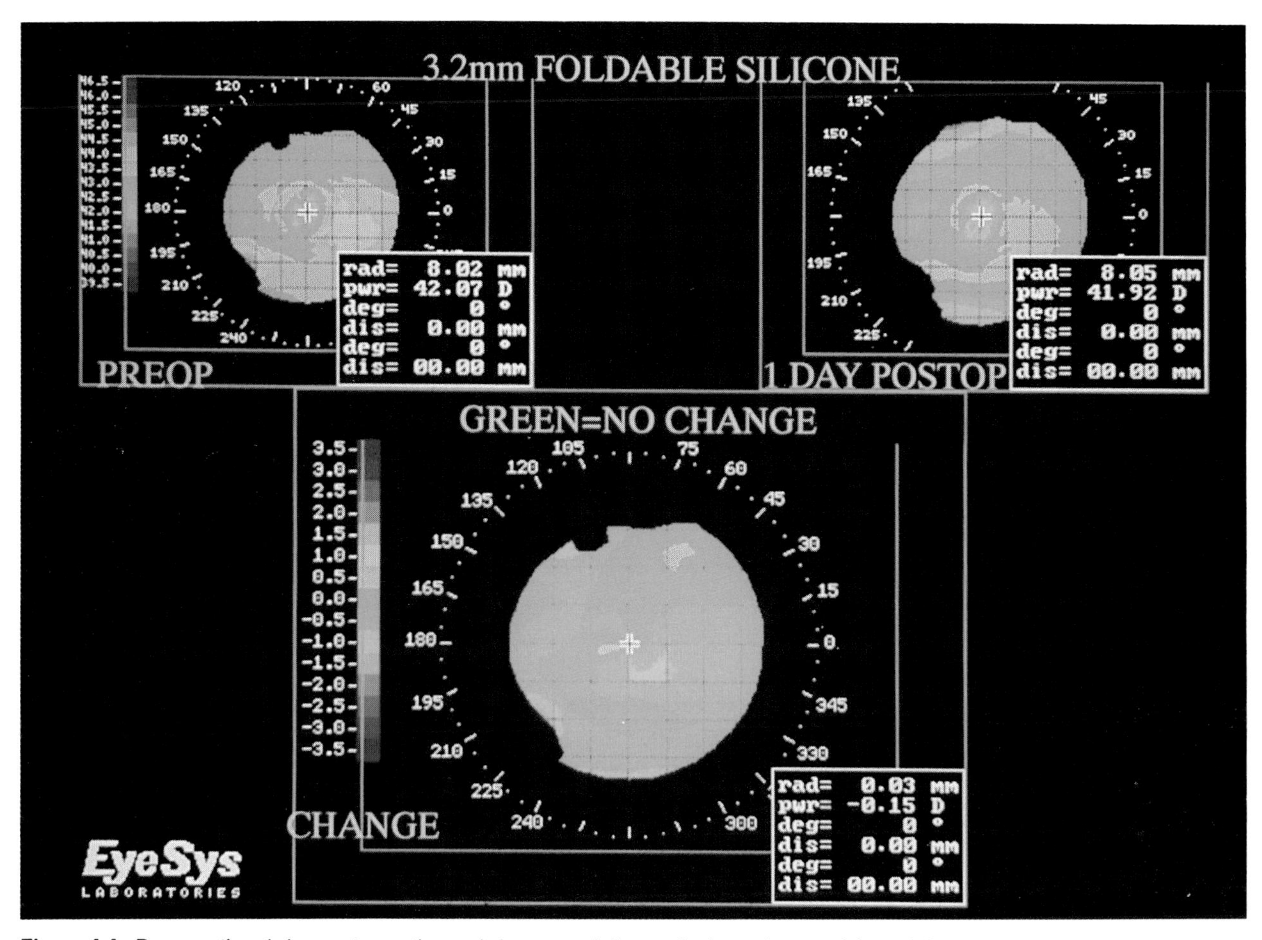

Figure 4.4: Preoperative, 1 day postoperative and change or delta graph of a patient receiving a 3.2 mm foldable silicone IOL with little change in corneal power due to surgery.

Effect of Incision Size: Sutureless Surgery

Figure 4.4 shows the preoperative, 1 day postoperative and change images for a patient receiving a Staar model AA-4203 foldable silicone lens through a 3.2 mm incision. The postoperative image closely resembles the preoperative image. Green areas on the change image indicate no difference between the preoperative and postoperative images. Figures 4.5A-C show the preoperative and 1 day, 2 week and 2 month postoperative and change images for a patient who received a round PMMA lens through a 6 mm incision. The 1 day postoperative image (Figure 4.5A) indicates little immediate change following surgery, except for some scattered central flattening of about 1.0 D. By 2 weeks postoperatively (Figure 4.5B), only two small areas of central flattening were apparent (blue), and these areas had regressed by 2 months postoperatively (Figure 4.5C).

Figures 4.4 and 4.5 demonstrate cataract wounds with incision sizes between 3 and 6 mm may result in little or no change in corneal topography. However central

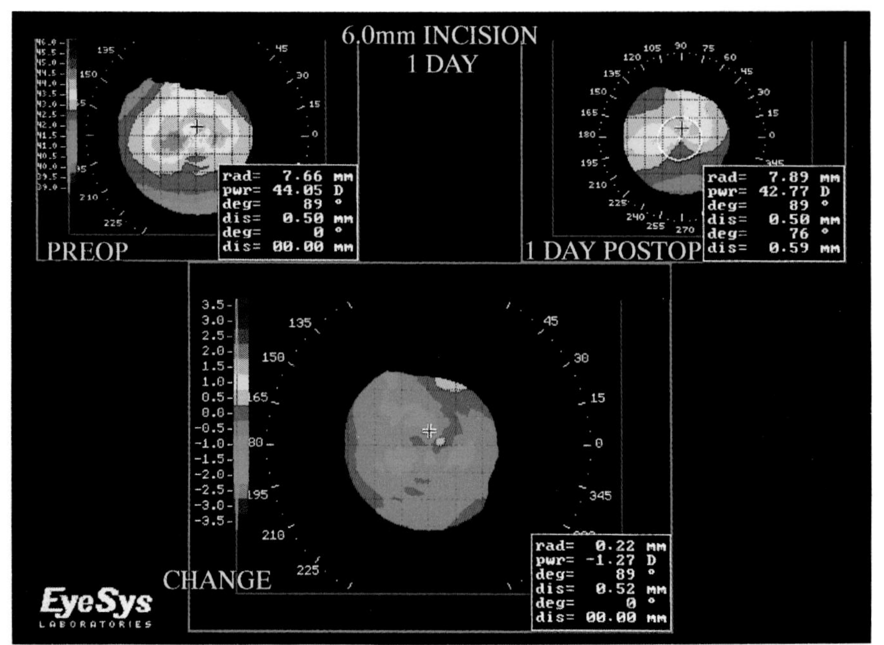

Figure 4.5A.

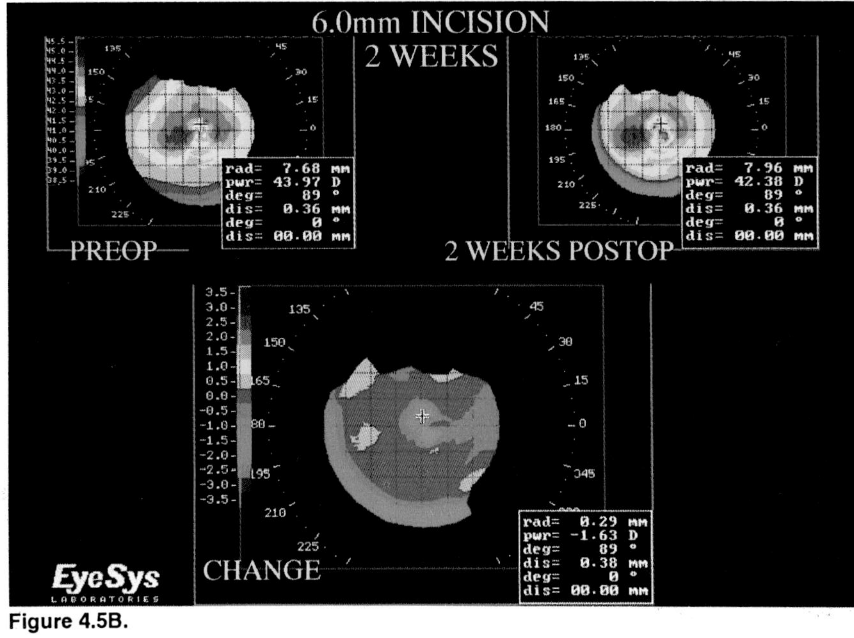

Figure 4.5B.

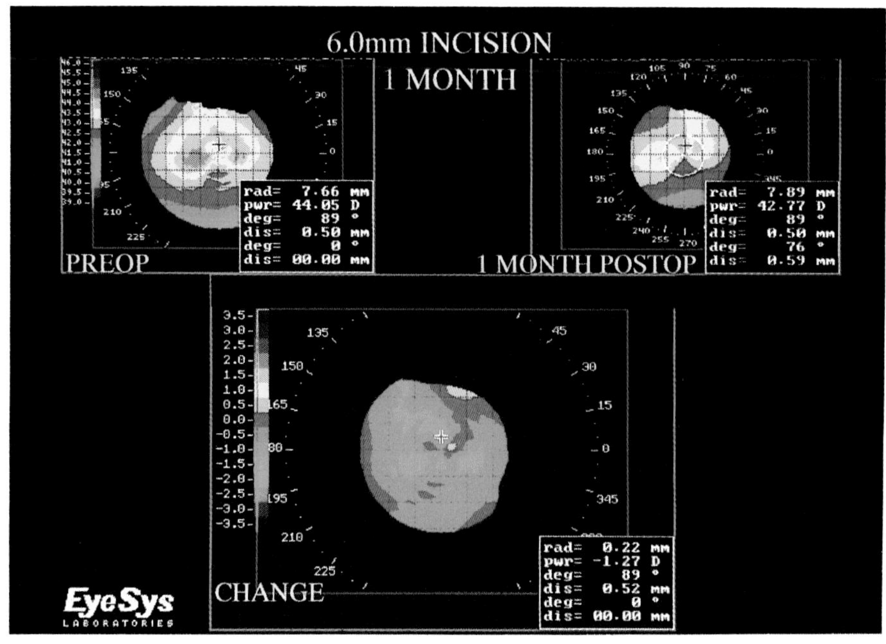

Figure 4.5C.

Figure 4.5: Corneal topography of a patient receiving a 6.0 mm sutureless cataract incision. (A) Preoperative and one day postoperative images. (B) Preoperative and 2 week postoperative images. Inferior blue crescent in the 2 week postoperative and change images is due to artifact. (C) Preoperative and 1 month images.

and peripheral corneal changes can sometimes occur.

We recently reported on a study comparing 3.2 mm, 5.0 mm and 6.0 mm sutureless cataract incisions using visual acuity, keratometry and corneal topography as efficacy variables.[1] The three groups did not differ significantly in mean keratometric cylinder preoperatively or at 1-2 days or 3-6 months postoperatively, nor did they differ significantly in surgically induced cylinder at either postoperative time period. At 1 to 2 days postoperatively, significantly more patients receiving 3.2 mm incisions had uncorrected visual acuity of 20/40 or better: 75% in the 3.2 mm group vs 50% and 47% in the 5.0 mm and 6.0 mm incision size groups, respectively.

In general, topographic images from patients receiving 3.2 mm incisions were rated as having fewer corneal changes than images from patients receiving 5.0 mm or 6.0 mm incisions (Figure 4.6). The 3.2 mm incision cases were characterized by less central steepening, less peripheral flattening, less peripheral steepening, less flattening originating from the wound site, and less induced astigmatism than the 5.0 mm or 6.0 mm incision cases. Only the differences in frequency of flattening at the wound site were statistically significant ($P < .05$), however, given the relatively small sample size studied in each group.

The most dramatic examples of flattening at the wound site are shown in Figures 4.7A, B, while milder cases are illustrated in Figures 4.8A, B. Central corneal changes were also noted. Figure 4.9A shows the 1

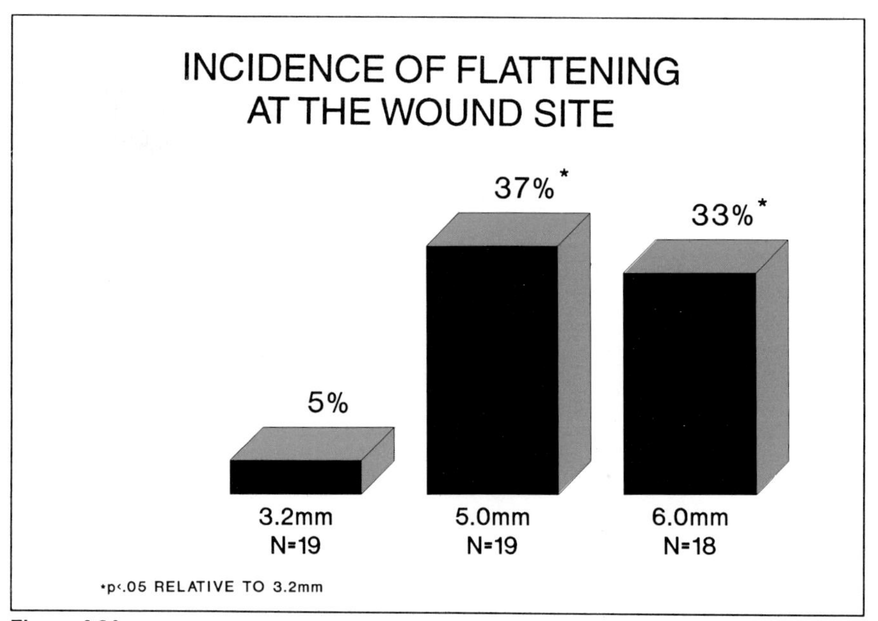

Figure 4.6A.

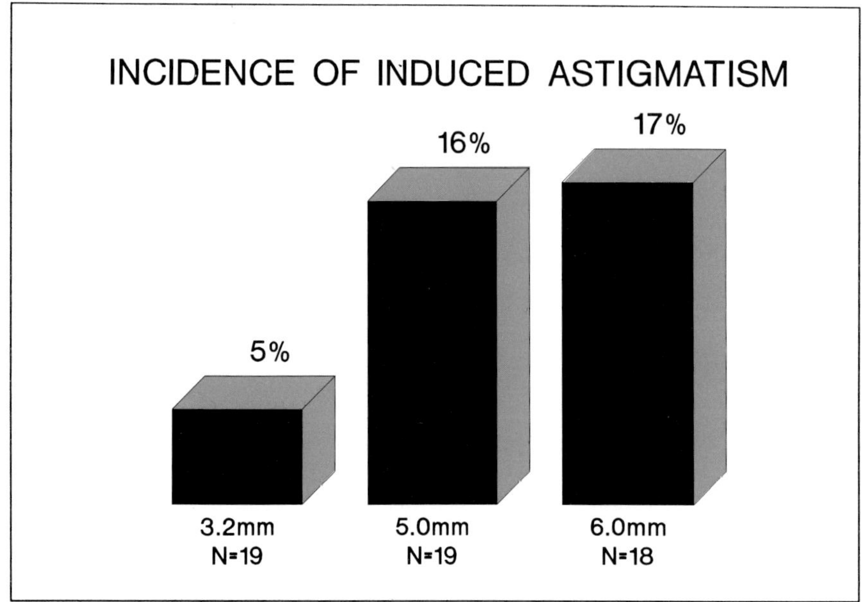

Figure 4.6B.

Figure 4.6: Histograms showing the major topographic differences between 3.2 mm, 5.0 mm and 6.0 mm sutureless incisions. (A) Incidence of flattening at the wound site. (B) Incidence of induced astigmatism.

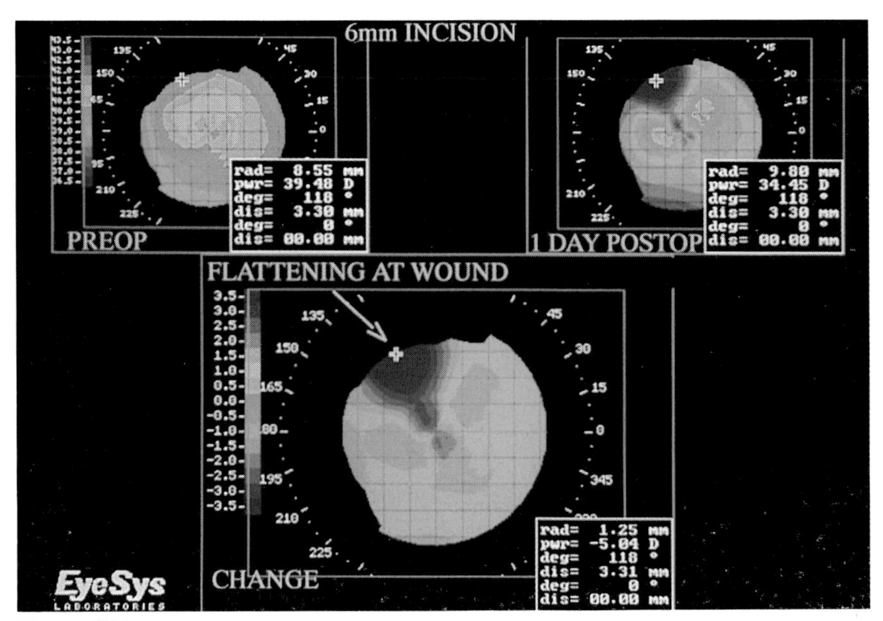

Figure 4.7A.

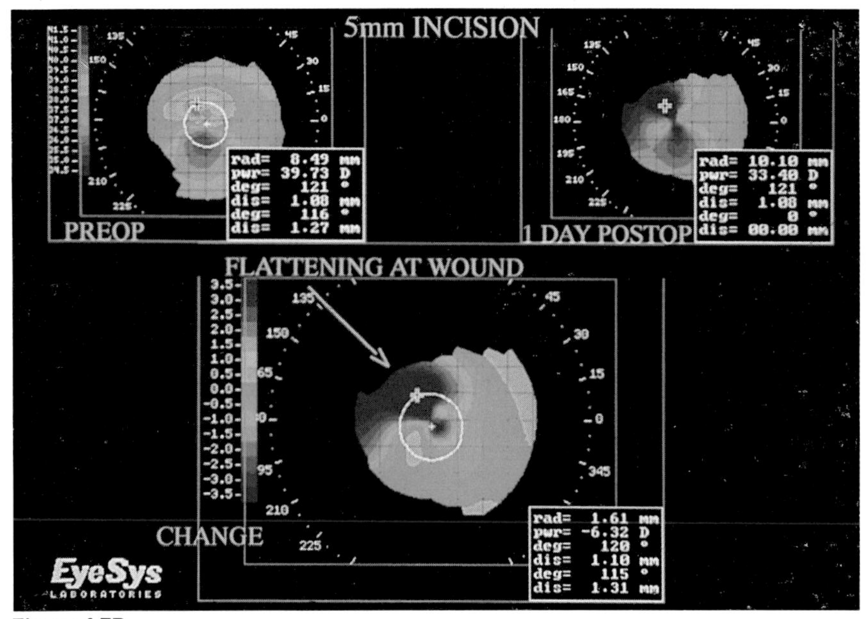

Figure 4.7B.

Figure 4.7: (A, B) Examples of large flattening at the wound site with 5.0 and 6.0 mm incisions. Over 5 D of flattening were seen in these cases.

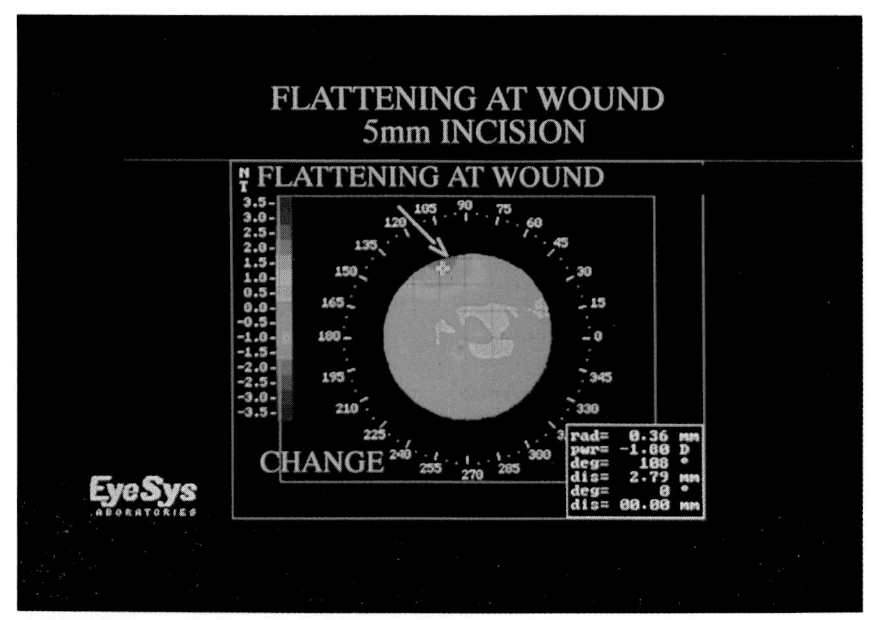

Figure 4.8A.

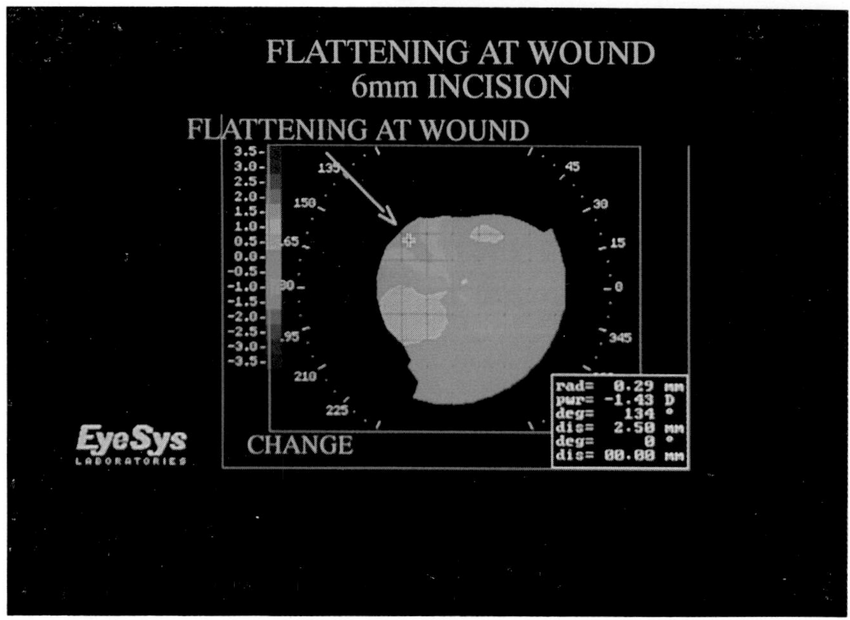

Figure 4.8B.

Figure 4.8: (A, B) Examples of mild flattening at the wound site, change or delta maps only.

day postoperative corneal topography picture of a patient who received a foldable silicone lens through a 3.2 mm incision. This patient exhibited slightly less than 3 D of central corneal flattening, shown in dark blue on the change (bottom) image. Because this flattening was largely confined to the central 2 mm of the cornea, keratometry failed to detect it. This flattening was unusual in a recipient of a foldable lens. The flattening was transient and by 2 weeks postoperatively (Figure 4.9B) regression had begun and by 6 weeks postoperatively the flattening had largely disappeared (Figure 4.9C).

Figures 4.10A, B show an example of extreme central corneal flattening, between 5 and 6 D, in a patient who received an unsutured 6 mm incision. Again, because the flattening is only in the very center of the cornea, keratometry failed to detect it. There was only a 0.2 D change in average keratometry. The applanation tension was 21 mm Hg, so this change could not be due to hypotony.

We also observed some mixed patterns: Figures 4.11A, B show peripheral flattening (blue) at the wound site and central steepening (yellow and orange). The concurrent flattening at the wound site in one upper quadrant with steepening in the opposite upper quadrant of the cornea was noted in four patients receiving 5.0 mm incisions and in three patients receiving 6.0 mm incisions, but not in any patient receiving a 3.2 mm incision. This pattern can be seen in Figures 4.12A, B.

In our study, keratometry indicated that 14 patients experienced surgically-induced astigmatism of one diopter or more. The EyeSys images from 12 of these patients did not indicate a true astigmatic pattern. Examples of the phenomenon are illustrated in Chapter 3.

One image clearly showed a greater increase in astigmatism that was missed by keratometry, with an incorrect steep meridian as well (Figure 4.13). Keratometry indicated only 0.56 D of surgically induced cylinder at 37°, but the image shows an increase in astigmatism of 1 D at 85°.

Other Uses for Corneal Topography with Cataract Surgery

One can monitor the effects of wound manipulation on resultant astigmatism. Figure 4.14 demonstrates a case with 3.75 D of preoperative with-the-rule astigmatism. Phacoemulsification and IOL implantation were performed with a deliberate 1.0 mm recession of the scleral flap. At 2 months postoperatively, the astigmatism was decreased by over 50% and vertical flattening and horizontal steepening are obvious on the topography change map.

Corneal topography may also be used to detect and monitor postoperative complications. Figure 4.15 demonstrates the left eye of a 71-year-old male with cataract and mild oblique astigmatism (Figure 4.15A upper left). Phacoemulsification with a 5 mm sutureless incision was performed. The incision was centered along the steep 50° meridian. At 5 weeks postoperatively, uncorrected vision was 20/200, and keratometry was 42.00/50.00 at 57°. Videokeratography shows a large amount of superior flattening with inferior steepening along the 57° semimeridian (Figure 4.15A upper left). The slit lamp examination revealed epithelial dysplasia superiorly extending nearly to the visual axis (Figures 4.15B, C). The patient was treated with scraping of the epithelium and cryotherapy of the superior limbus. Three weeks following treatment (Figure 4.15A lower left), there is minimal astigmatism and the corneal surface is quite regular.

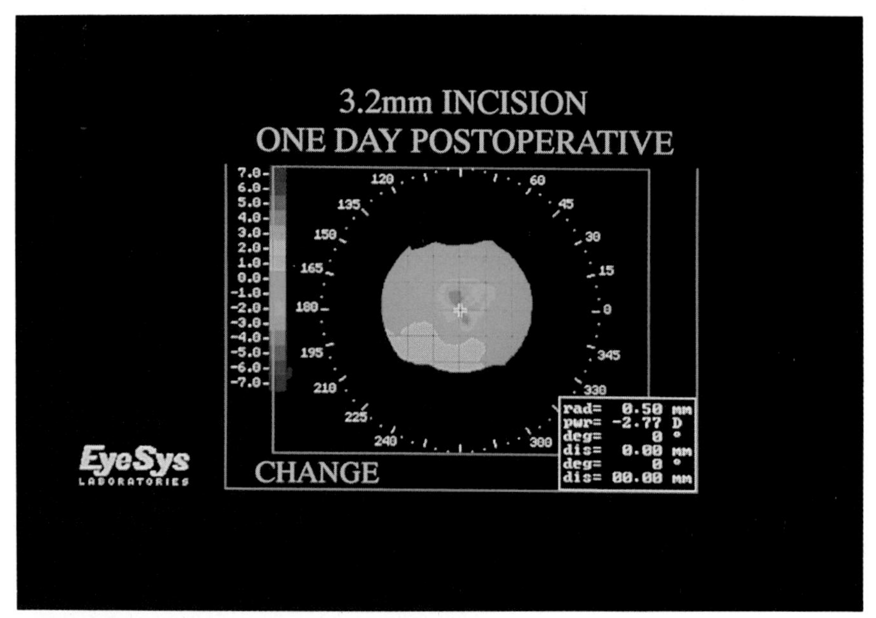

Figure 4.9A.

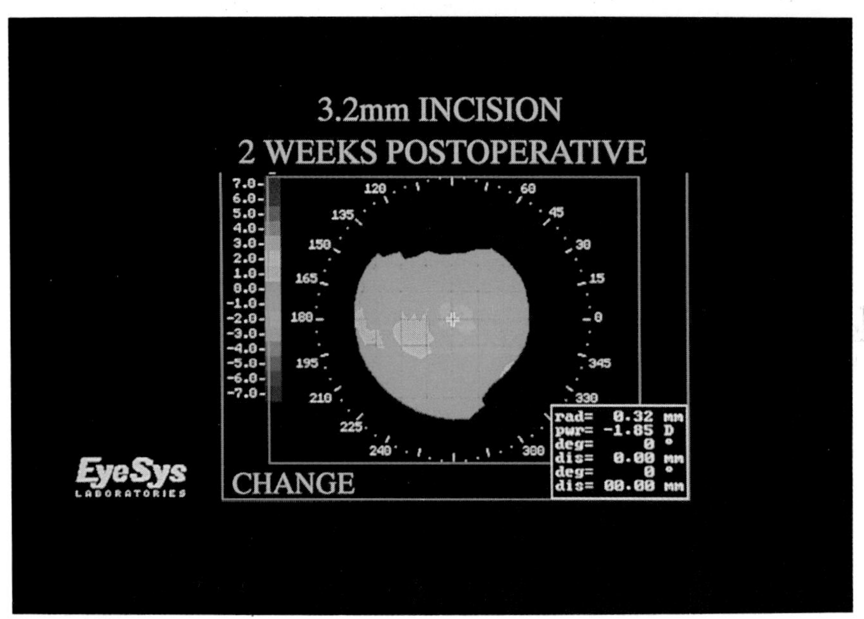

Figure 4.9B.

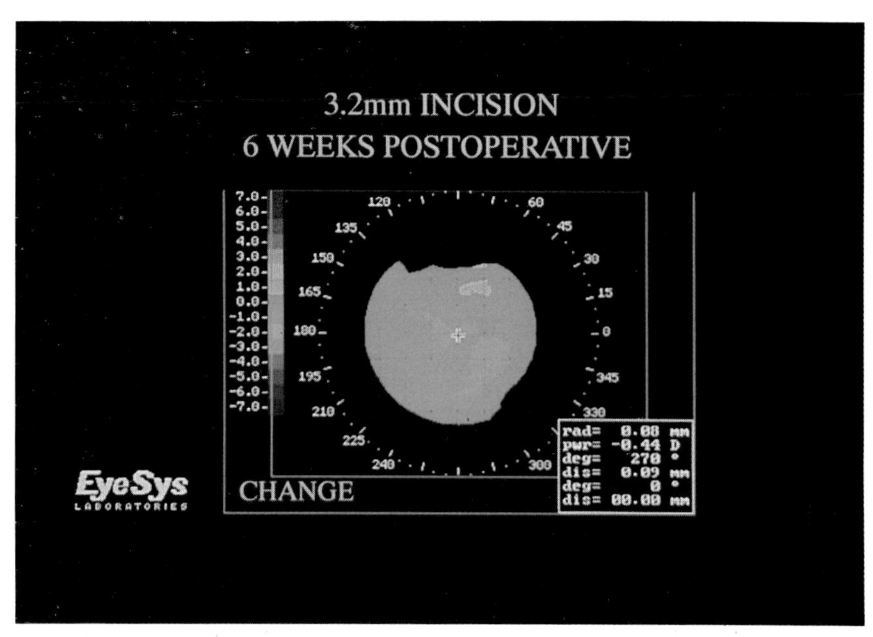

Figure 4.9C.

Figure 4.9: Corneal topography of a patient with a 3.2 mm incision. (A) One day postoperative change map shows area of central flattening of about 3 D. (B) Change map of same patient 2 weeks later demonstrates marked regression. (C) Change map of same patient at 6 weeks postoperatively demonstrates resolution of flattening.

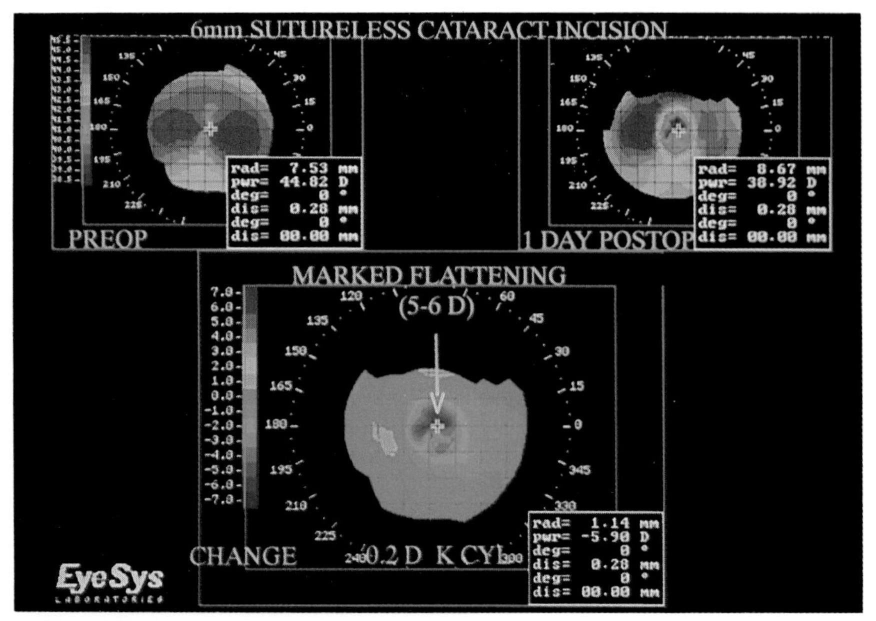

Figure 4.10A.

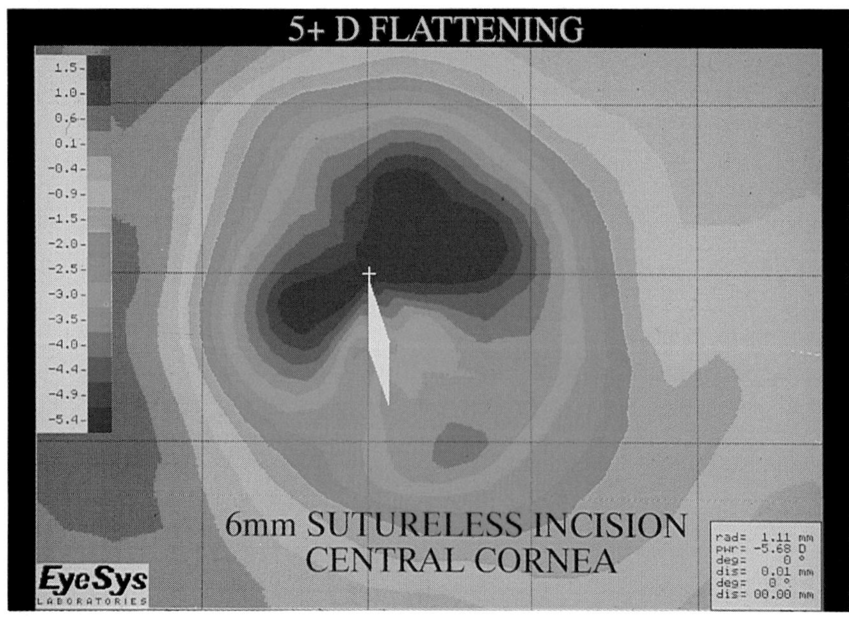

Figure 4.10B.

Figure 4.10: Corneal topography of a patient receiving a 6.0 mm sutureless incision. (A) One day postoperative change map indicates a large area of central flattening of 5 - 6 D. (B) Magnified image of change map of (A) demonstrating central corneal flattening.

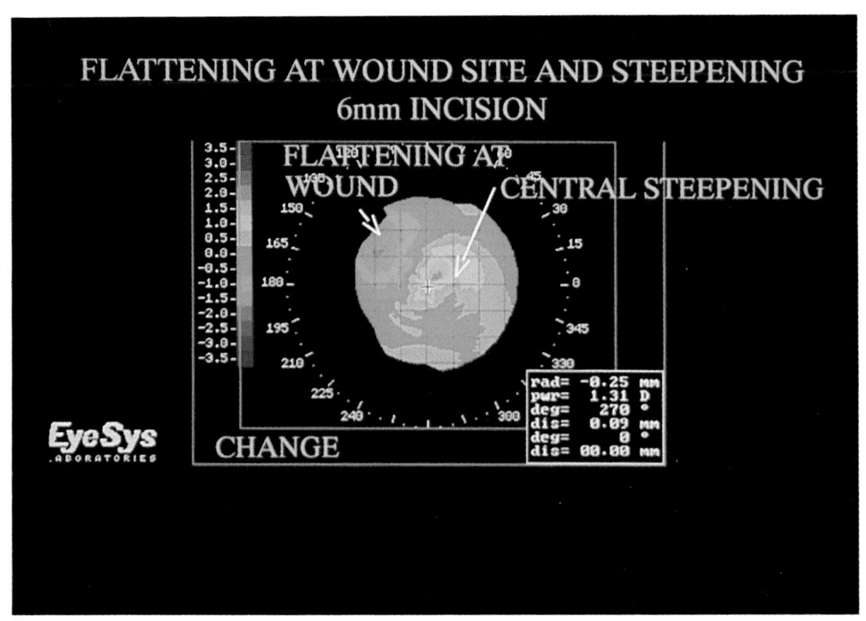

Figure 4.11A.

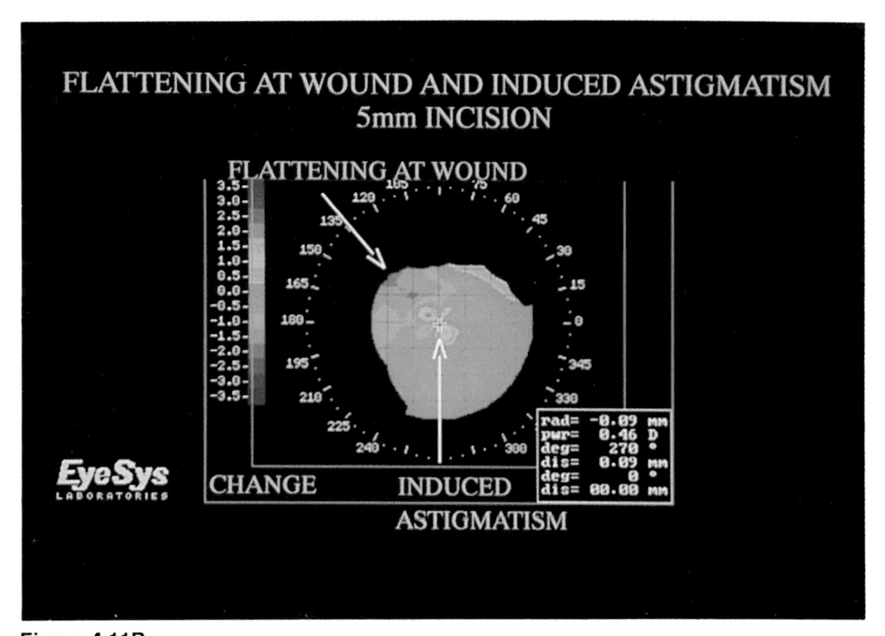

Figure 4.11B.

Figure 4.11: Corneal topography change maps with mixed pattern of peripheral flattening at the wound site with central steepening (A) or induced astigmatism (B).

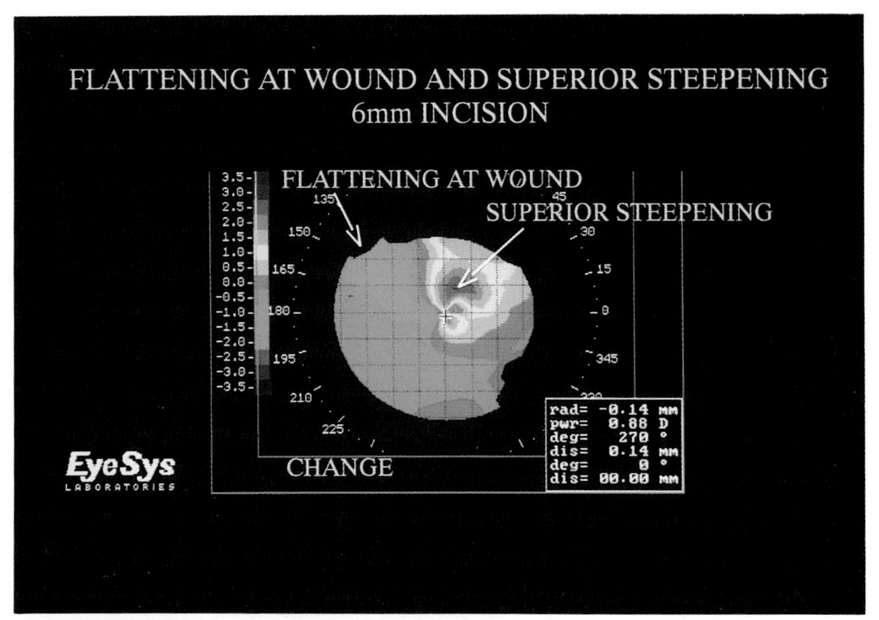

Figure 4.12A.

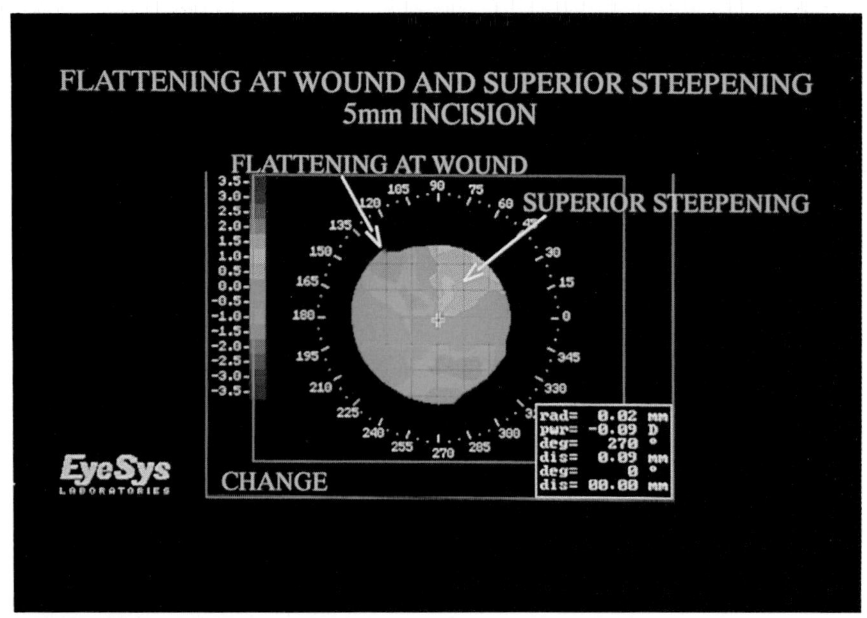

Figure 4.12B.

Figure 4.12: (A, B) Corneal topography change maps in cases of concurrent flattening at the wound site and steepening in the superior peripheral cornea.

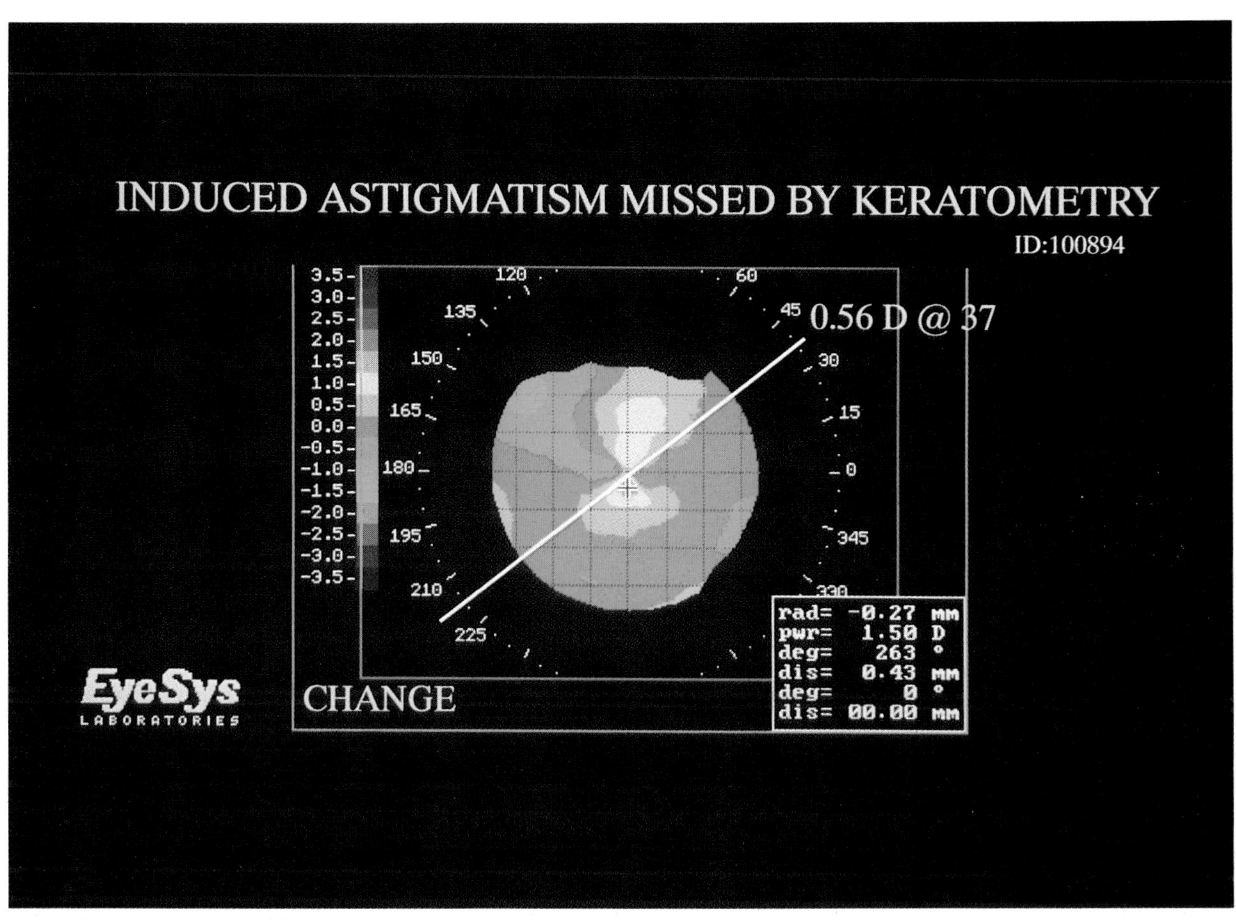

Figure 4.13: Corneal topography change map in a case where amount and meridian of induced astigmatism do not agree between topography and keratometry. White line indicates steep meridian of astigmatism.

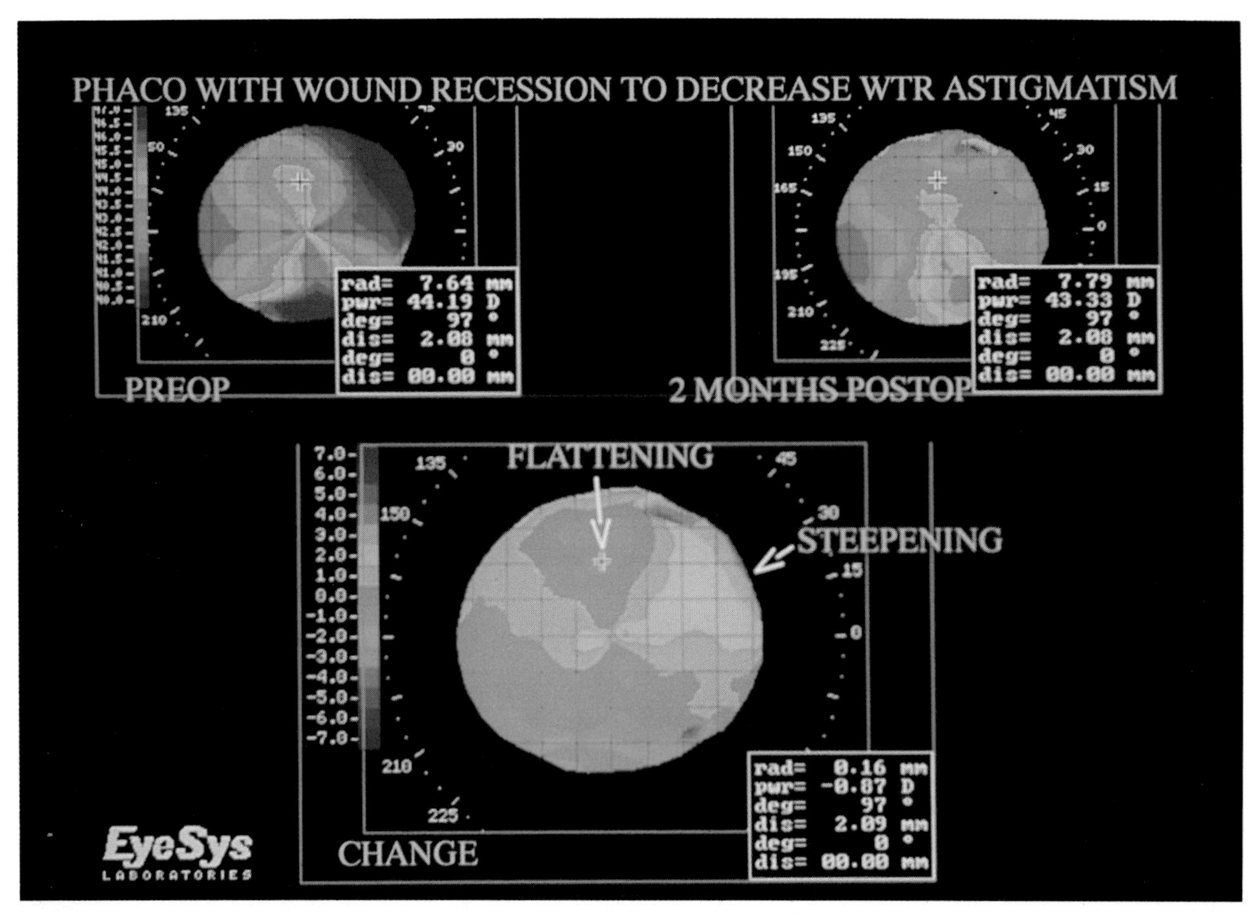

Figure 4.14: Preoperative, 3 month postoperative, and change or delta map of case receiving phacoemulsification and 1 mm scleral flap recession to decrease the patient's with-the-rule astigmatism (courtesy Douglas Koch, MD).

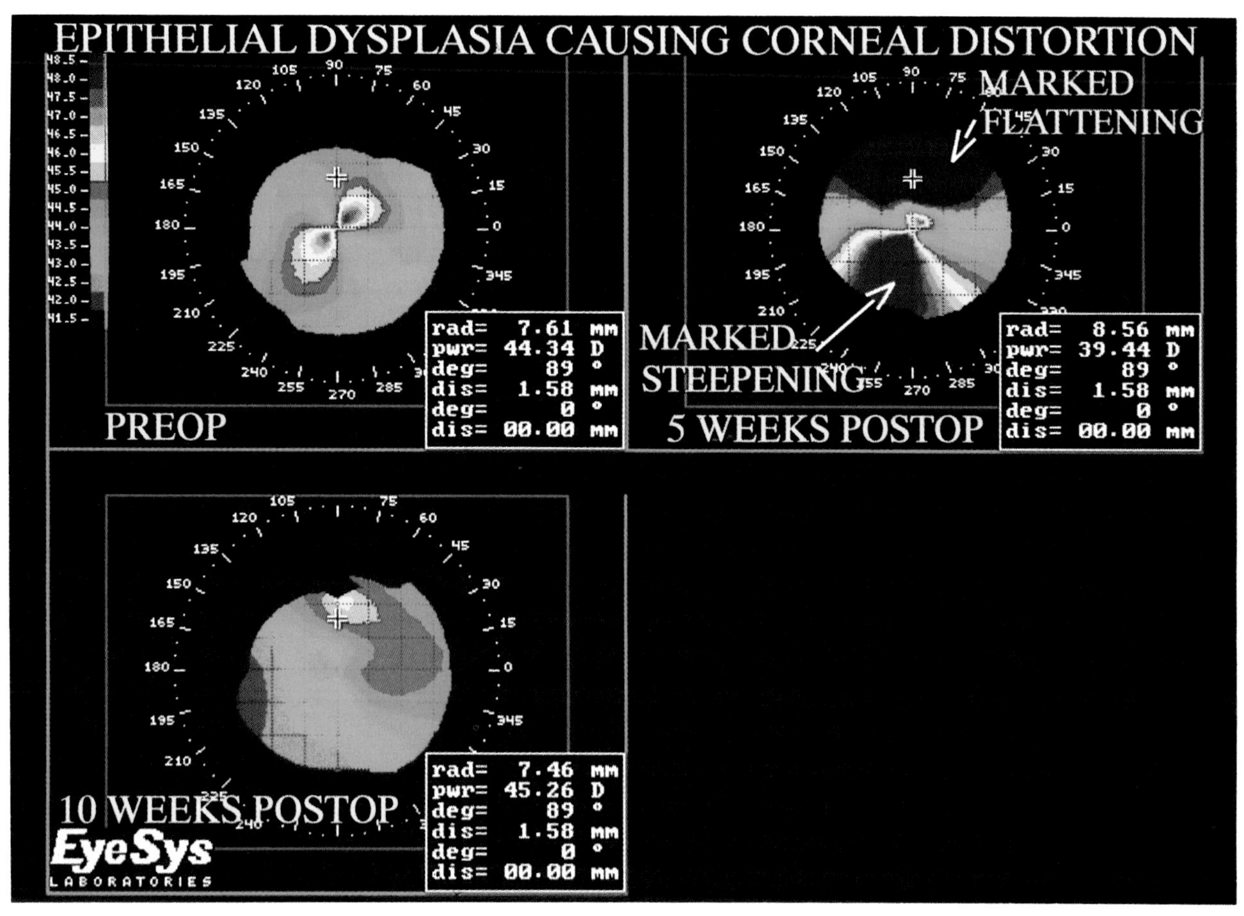

Figure 4.15A.

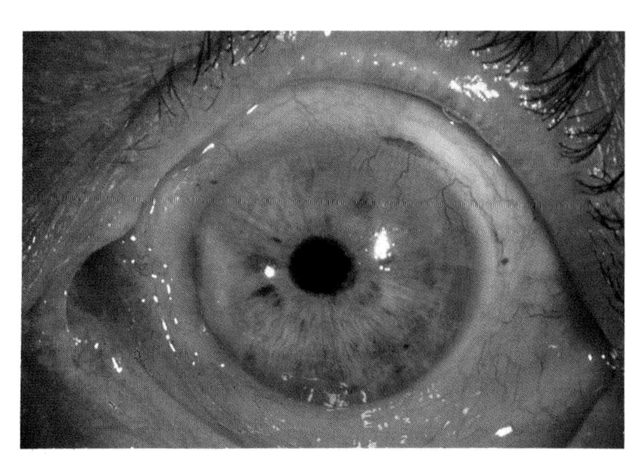

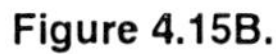

Figure 4.15B.

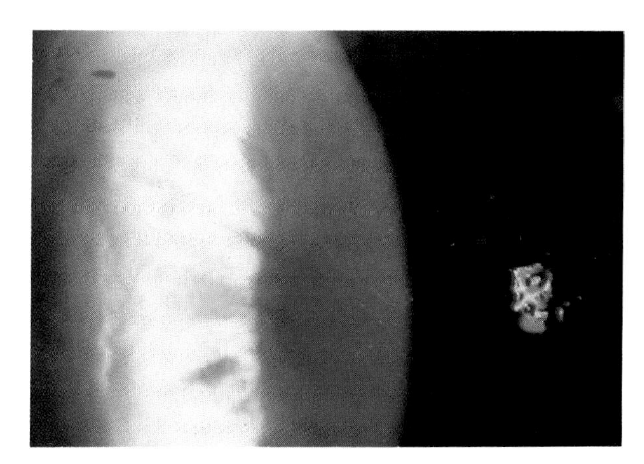

Figure 4.15C.

Figure 4.15: Patient who developed epithelial dysplasia following cataract extraction. (A) Preoperative, 5 week postoperative, and 10 week postoperative corneal topography. (B) Appearance of the cornea at 5 weeks postoperatively. (C) Close-up of the cornea demonstrating the line of epithelial dysplasia extending almost to the visual axis (courtesy Douglas Koch, MD).

Conclusions

Corneal topography permits the very precise visualization of surgical effect in cataract patients. Some apparent paradoxes in postoperative visual rehabilitation may be resolved with reference to topographic data. For example, patients may have poor postoperative visual acuity in spite of apparently normal clinical examinations and keratometric readings. This and other chapters have demonstrated that keratometry does not always adequately describe surgically induced effects. Furthermore, topography may allow the clinician to monitor the effect of surgical interventions and at times detect and characterize postoperative complications involving the cornea.

Reference

1. Martin RG, Sanders DR, Miller JD, et al: Effect of cataract wound incision size on acute changes in corneal topography. *J Cataract Refract Surg* in press.

5

DONALD R. SANDERS, MD, PhD

Evaluating Refractive Surgical or Laser Procedures

While the specific use of corneal topography in evaluating outcome of incisional refractive cases (radial and astigmatic keratotomy) (Chapter 6) and excimer laser photorefractive keratectomy (Chapter 7) are discussed elsewhere, there are two areas of evaluation that are common to both types of procedures and will be discussed here: preoperative screening for pathology and centering of corneal surgical procedures.

Preoperative Screening

Patient astigmatism may be an important consideration in the treatment of refractive surgery patients. As described in detail in Chapter 3, the regularity, symmetry and pattern of astigmatism cannot be determined by keratometry and indeed keratometric findings may be misleading. Therefore, if treatment of astigmatism is being considered, corneal topography may be essential.

Irregular or grossly distorted corneas can usually be detected by slit lamp examination and possibly by simple observation of keratometer mires. However, more subtle changes, as in early keratoconus, may be virtually undetectable by any means other than corneal topography.

Maguire and Bourne[1] studied nine eyes in seven patients with no slit lamp evidence of keratoconus. Five of the patients had keratoconus in the other eye just as the patient presented in Chapter 2 (Figure 2.1). The other two patients (four eyes) had mild spectacle blur with 20/30 or better vision and no clinical evidence of keratoconus in either eye. Six of the seven eyes that were documented with keratoconus by corneal topography had no, or very subtle, distortion of the keratometer mires. The two patients with no keratoconus clinically evident in either eye were most disturbing. They were young 2 to 3 D myopes and three of their four eyes had keratoconus by topography. These cases would have been considered excellent candidates for radial keratotomy or excimer laser photoablation in the absence of the corneal topography examination. If a surgeon is doing a significant number of refractive surgical techniques, corneal topography would be an invaluable screening tool to avoid an unhappy patient and to avoid the surgeon being blamed for a previously undiagnosed preexisting pathological condition.

Centering of Corneal Surgical Procedures

Centration on Center of Pupil

Decentration of refractive corneal procedures can result in blurred images, glare, ghost images, poor visual acuity or poor contrast sensitivity.[2,3] Various methods of centering surgical corneal refractive procedures have been described.[4,5] Walsh and Guyton[3] and Uozato and Guyton[2] have pointed out that currently used centering surgical procedures emphasize centering about the visual axis of the eye, which in many cases is not defined properly. They and Maloney[6] believe that the optimum method for centering surgical (and excimer laser) refractive procedures utilizes the line of sight and the entrance pupil and not the visual axis. Proper centering requires the patient to fixate on a point that is coaxial with the surgeon's sighting eye and the cornea is marked at the point in line with the center of the patient's entrance pupil, ignoring the corneal light reflex. Besides the optical arguments for using the entrance pupil, the Stiles-Crawford effect demonstrates with normal pupils that light passing through the center of the pupil is more effective in stimulating the photoreceptors than light passing through the peripheral pupil because photoreceptors are aimed toward or oriented to the center of the pupil. Studies on eccentric pupils[7,8] have demonstrated that photoreceptors also actively orient themselves toward the center of an eccentric pupil. These findings, therefore, suggest that the pupil and not the visual axis remains the proper optical reference for centering corneal refractive procedures. Errors of from 0.5 to 0.8 mm were found using current methods of procedure centration. These errors arose from the use of the corneal light reflex as the sighting and marking point instead of the center of the pupil, or from inadvertent monocular sighting in techniques requiring binocular sighting.

Centration of Topographical Maps

How does the recommended centering of refractive procedures fit in with the centration of corneal topographic maps? With the EyeSys corneal topography unit, the patient fixates coaxial to the videocamera image as recommended by Guyton and colleagues and Maloney. However, the center of the map is not coincident with the center of the pupil.

The center of the corneal topography map is referred to as the videokeratographic (VK) axis, or alternatively as the corneal vertex or vertex normal. Vertex normal can be more exactly defined as the line from the fixation point that intersects the corneal surface at right angles; the point of intersection on the cornea itself is called the corneal vertex. A light ray from the fixation point that travels down the vertex normal is reflected back on itself so the vertex normal must pass through the center of the first Purkinje image of the fixation target. The corneal vertex does not usually coincide with the geometric center nor does it necessarily coincide with the visual axis, but it does provide a reproducible point on the corneal surface.

In normal eyes the entrance pupil is not centered around the corneal vertex; the first Purkinje image of a fixation light usually lies nasal to the center of the entrance pupil.[9] In cases with distorted corneas or eccentric pupils there may be a great disparity between the center of the ring images and the center of the entrance pupil.

A major criticism of videokeratoscopes which center along the VK axis has been their failure in the past to provide information regarding the pupil center. Recently, however, new image enhancement and recognition software has been developed to detect and outline the patient's pupil and to mark the pupil center. This process was not trivial since corneoscopic ring images tend to mask the pupil margins. A very sophisticated computer algorithm was required to "subtract" the corneoscopic ring image from the photo and find the underlying pupil. With this new pupil recognition software, the corneal topography map can now be used to determine if corneal refractive procedures have been properly centered.

Figures 5.1A,B demonstrate corneal topographical maps in two cases with some disparity between the center of the ring images (VK axis) and the pupil center. The first two values in the cursor box in the lower right corner of the screen supply curvature information in radius of curvature (millimeters) and power in diopters, respectively, for the cornea at the location of the mouse cursor (large +). The third and fourth values from the top describe the position of the cursor relative to the center of the rings (VK axis). In these cases the mouse cursor is directly over VK axis so that the first degrees and distance are equal to 0. This data is provided as direction in degrees and distance in millimeters from the center of the rings to the cursor position.

When the pupil is located during eye image processing, the position of the mouse cursor (in this case located at the VK axis) relative to the pupil center will also be provided as direction in degrees and distance in millimeters, respectively, in the last two rows of the cursor box. Here we see in Figure 5.1A that the corneal vertex is 0.43 mm away from the center of the pupil in the direction of the 353° axis and in Figure 5.1B.

The corneal vertex is also 0.43 mm away from the center of the pupil but in the direction of the 329° axis. Figure 5.1B is a postoperative RK case. Note that in this case, pupil center is closer to the center of the flattened central zone indicating better centration than would be concluded if the VK axis rather than pupil center were used to determine centration.

Figure 5.2 demonstrates a case where the VK axis, pupil center, and center of the excimer laser ablation are all coincident.

Figure 5.3 demonstrates a slightly eccentric excimer laser ablation. The mouse cursor has been placed at the center of the ablative zone where the corneal power is 34.75 D. The center of the ablative zone is 0.9 mm toward the 180° axis relative to the VK axis and 0.78 mm toward the 193° axis relative to the center of the pupil as documented by the printout in the cursor box in the lower right hand corner of the figure.

Figure 5.4 demonstrates a symptomatic, markedly decentered excimer laser photorefractive keratectomy. The mouse cursor is centered in the ablative zone and demonstrates a corneal power of 42.96 D. The last two numbers in the cursor box indicate that the ablative zone is decentered 1.26 mm toward the 29° axis relative to the center of the pupil.

By looking at the corneal topography maps of their post-treatment refractive surgery cases, surgeons can observe and hopefully correct any consistent problems in technique resulting in decentration. See Chapter 10 for a more complete discussion of the alignment of videokeratoscopes with regard to the major reference points and axes of the eye (line of sight, pupillary axis, visual axis, and VK axis).

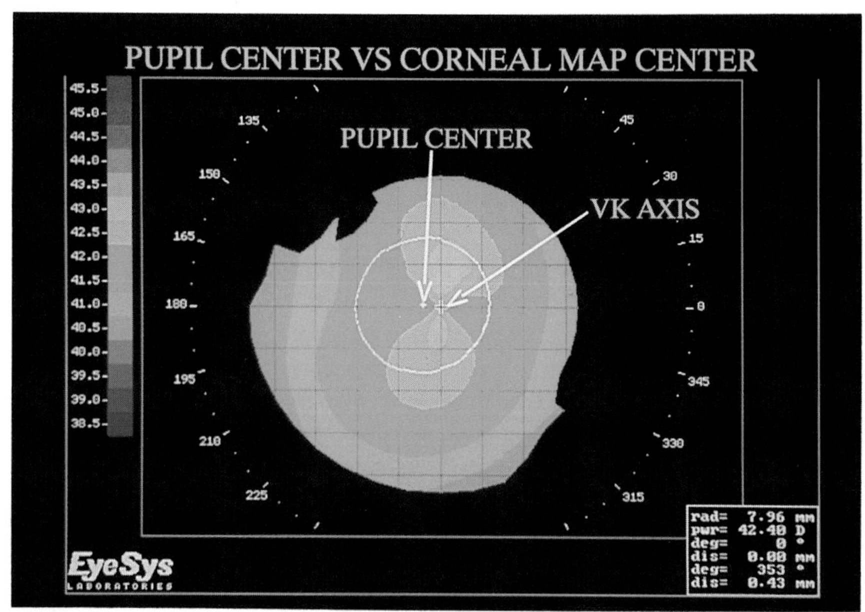

Figure 5.1A.

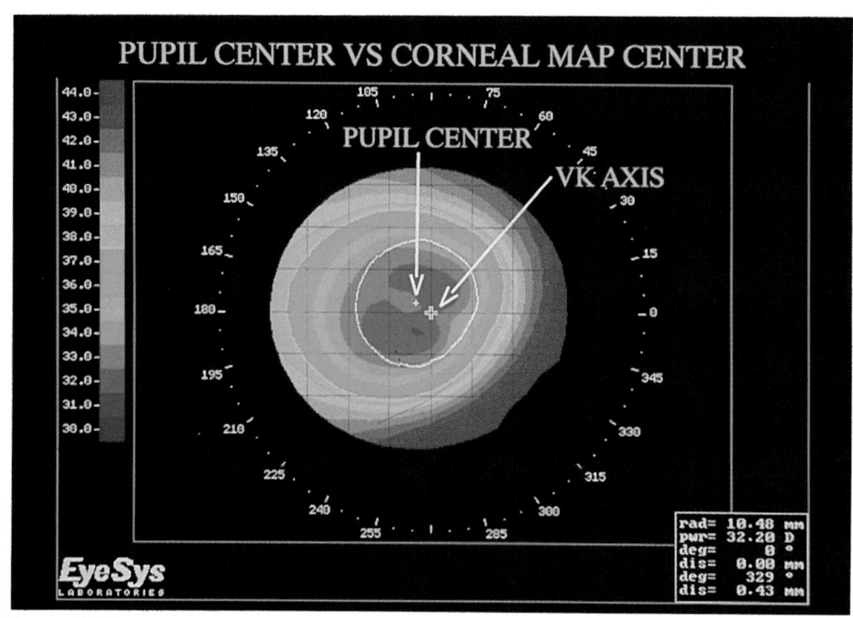

Figure 5.1B.

Figure 5.1: Corneal topographical maps of the right eyes of two cases where the corneal vertex is nasal to the pupil center. (A) Normal unoperated eye. (B) Postoperative radial keratotomy case.

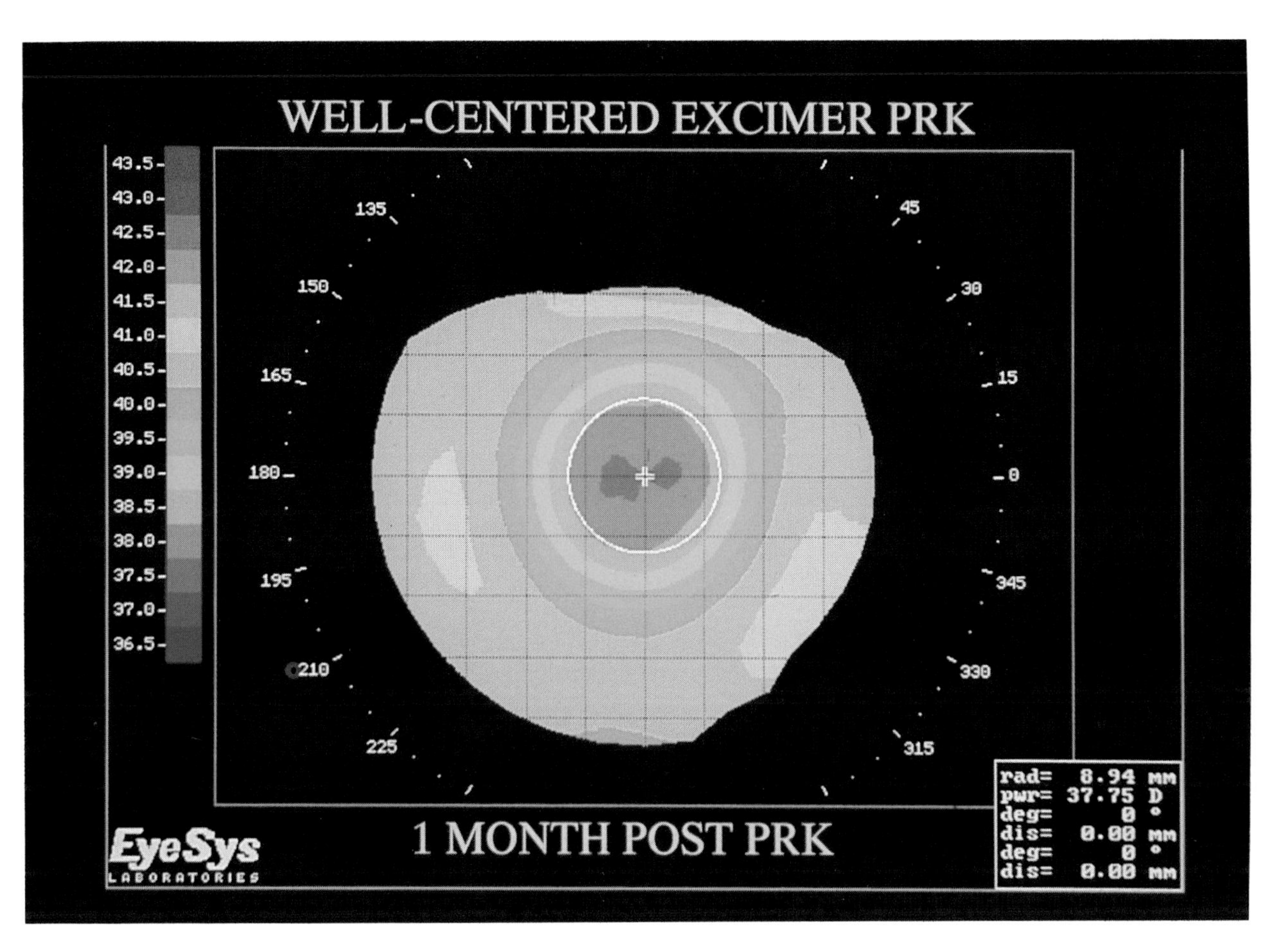

Figure 5.2: Post-treatment excimer laser photorefractive keratectomy. The cursor box in the lower right indicates that the pupil center and corneal vertex are coincident. Observation of the topographical map indicates excellent centration of white pupil outline within the ablative zone.

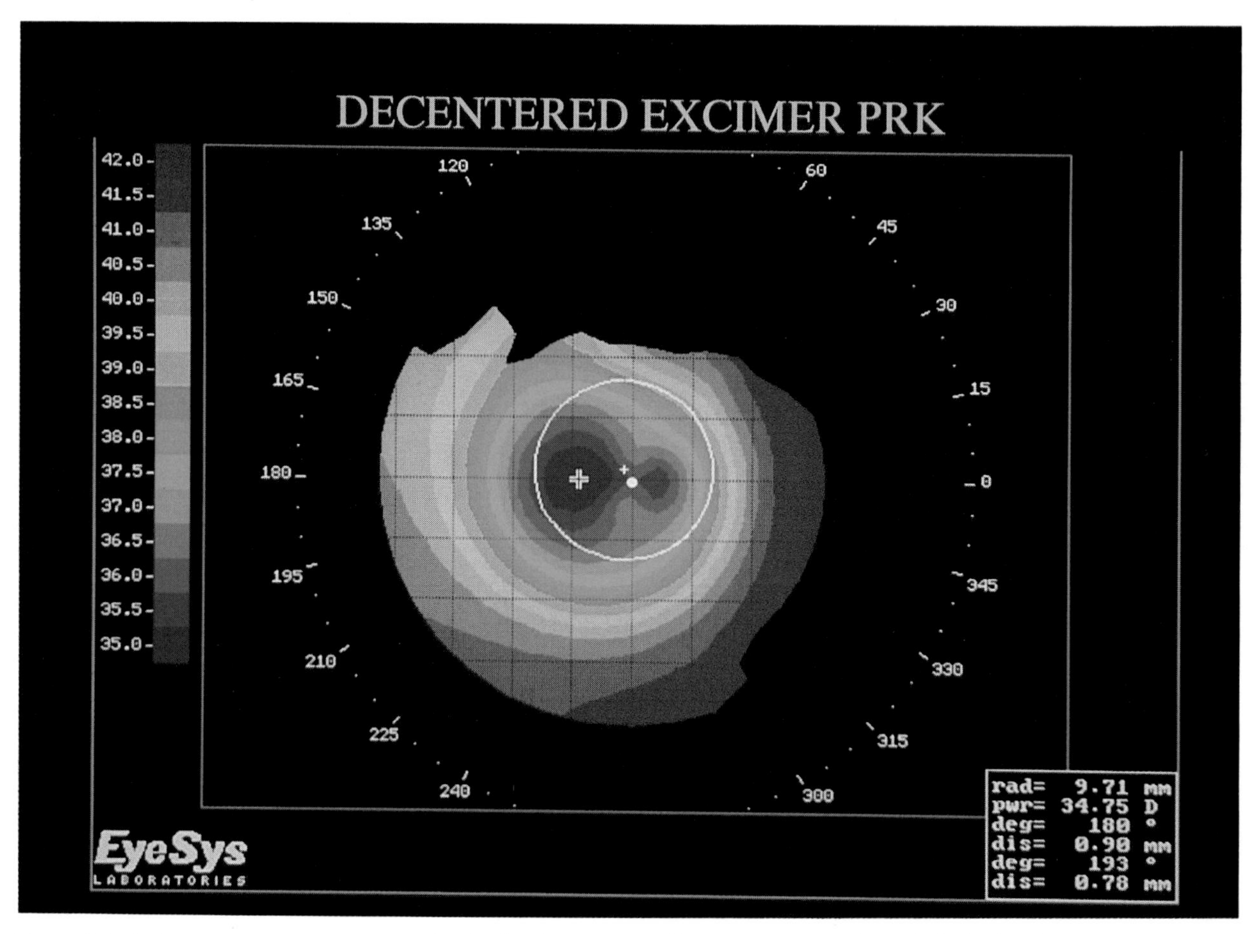

Figure 5.3: A decentered excimer laser photorefractive keratectomy. The mouse cursor (large "+") is placed at the center of the photoablative zone and the small "+" marks the pupil center. The first two degree and distance numbers in the cursor box (lower right) quantitate the degree of decentration of ablation relative to the VK axis (small white circle). The last two numbers in the cursor box quantitate the degree of decentration of the ablation relative to the pupil center.

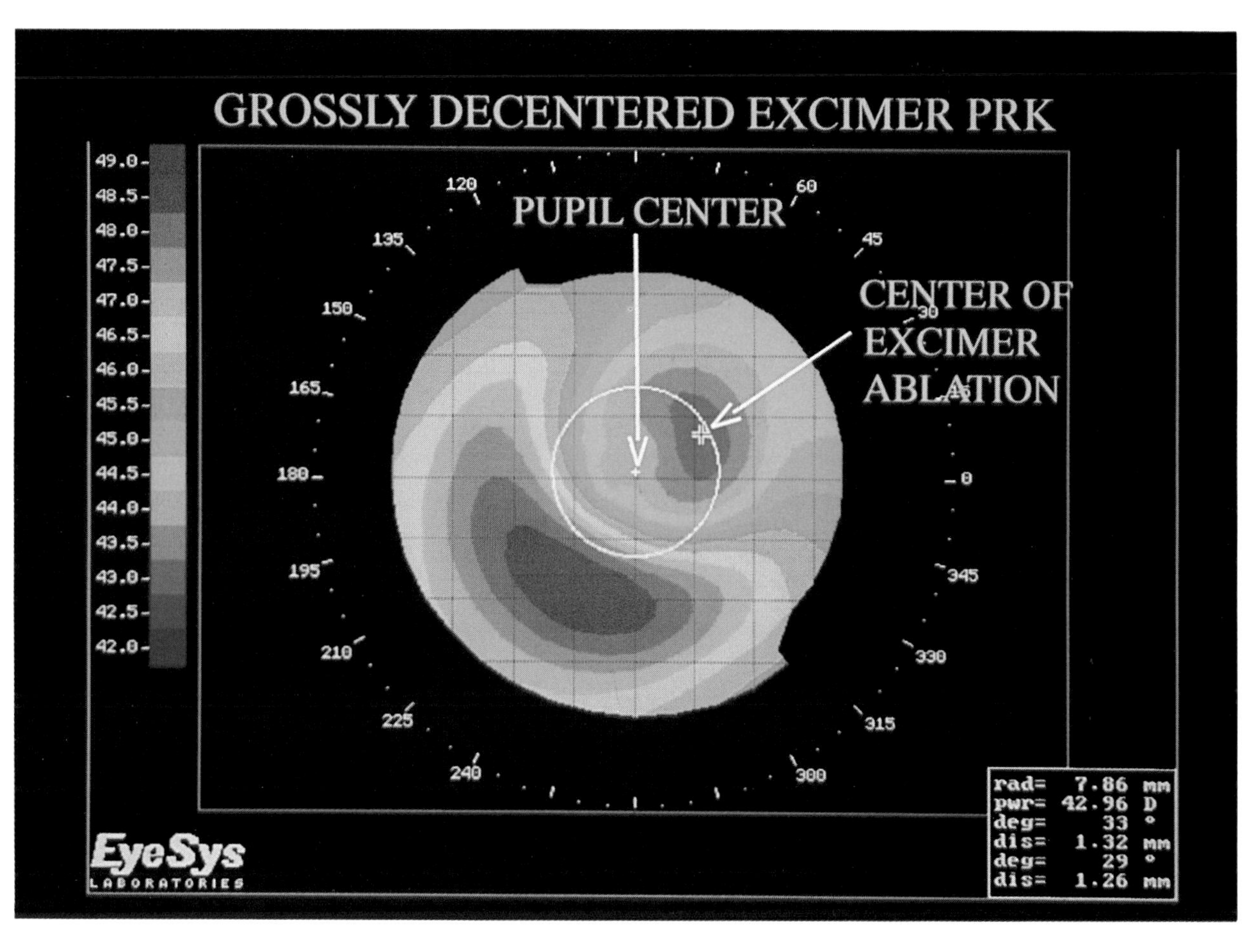

Figure 5.4: A decentered excimer laser photorefractive keratectomy. The mouse cursor (large "+") is placed at the center of the photoablative zone and the small "+" marks the pupil center. See Figure 5.3 for explanation of degree and distance numbers in cursor box (lower right).

References

1. Maguire LJ, Bourne WM: Corneal topography of early keratoconus. *Am J Ophthalmol* 108:107-112, 1989.
2. Uozato H, Guyton DL: Centering corneal surgical procedures. *Am J Ophthalmol* 103:264-275, 1987.
3. Walsh PM, Guyton DL: Comparison of two methods of marking the visual axis on the cornea during radial keratotomy. *Am J Ophthalmol* 97:660, 1984.
4. Steinberg EB, Waring GO, III: Comparison of two methods of marking the visual axis on the cornea during radial keratotomy. *Am J Ophthalmol* 96:605, 1983.
5. Thornton SP: Surgical armamentarium. In Sanders DR, Hofmann RF, Salz JJ (eds.): *Refractive Corneal Surgery*. Thorofare, New Jersey, Slack Inc., 1986, p. 134.
6. Maloney RK: Corneal topography and optical zone location in photorefractive keratectomy. *Refract Corneal Surgery* 6:363-371, 1990.
7. Enoch JM, Laties AM: An analysis of retinal receptor orientation. II. Prediction for psychophysical tests. *Invest Ophthalmol Vis Sci* 10:959, 1971.
8. Bonds AB, MacLeod DIA: A displaced Stiles-Crawford effect associated with an eccentric pupil. *Invest Ophthalmol Vis Sci* 17:754, 1978.
9. Uozato H, Makino H, Saishin M, Nakao S: Measurement of the visual axis using a laser beam. In: Breinin GM, Siegal IM (eds.): *Advances in Diagnostic Visual Optics*. Berlin, Springer-Verlag, 1983, p. 22.

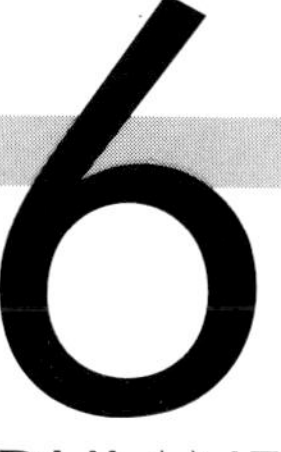

DAVID DULANEY, MD
SPENCER P. THORNTON, MD
ROBERT G. MARTIN, MD

Corneal Topography in Refractive Surgical Procedures

The results of refractive surgery for myopia and astigmatism are not as predictable as clinicians or patients would like. While many patients are highly satisfied with the correction achieved by surgery, a substantial minority experience undercorrection, overcorrection, and/or some degree of corneal and visual distortion. The use of corneal topography provides the potential to improve the predictability of refractive procedures, as well as being a useful tool in monitoring and evaluating results.

Radial Keratotomy (RK)

Figures 6.1A, B show the right and left eyes of a patient with 3 D of myopia bilaterally. The image in the upper left corner of each slide is preoperative. The corneas have a typical prolate appearance, being steeper centrally. The image in the upper right corner of both figures was made 1 week postoperatively. As expected, the central cornea in both eyes is now flatter than the periphery, which is referred to as an oblate-shaped cornea. This result is consistent with what we know about the mechanism of action of the RK procedure, in which the periphery steepens and bows out while the center flattens. Surgery resulted in refractions of +0.25 D in the right eye and −0.25 D in the left eye at 1 week. In the change images (bottom images), the darkest blue in the center of the corneas indicates 3 to 3.6 D of flattening. This flattening is fairly symmetrical and well centralized around the videokeratographic (VK) axis, indicating a successful RK. Note that the pupil was localized in the postoperative image in the left eye (Figure 6.1B, upper right), and in this case the center of the pupil is coincident to the corneal vertex. Notice also that while the postoperative flattened zone is not completely symmetrical, especially in the right eye (Figure 6.1A, upper right), the surgically induced change is (bottom). This result is probably due to the corneal asymmetry in

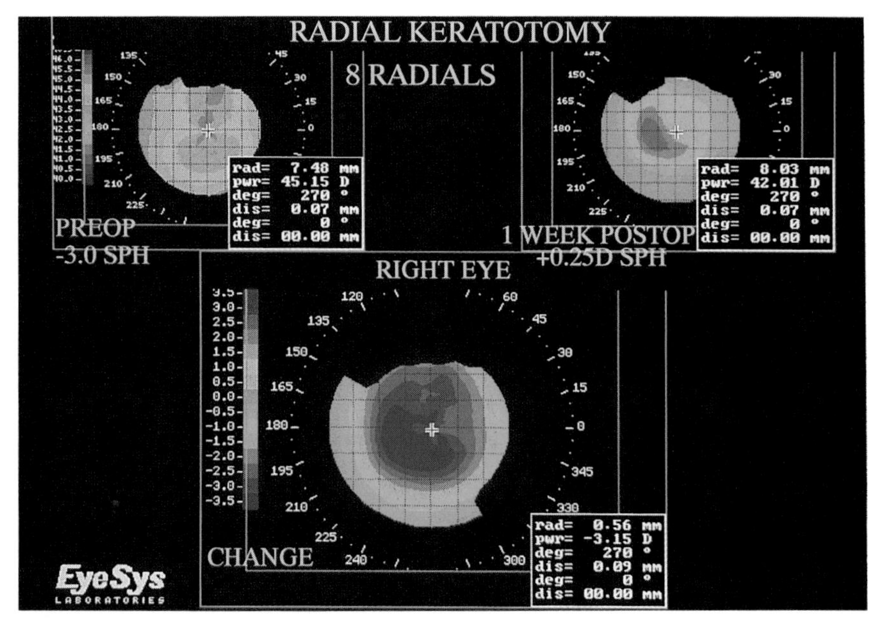

Figure 6.1A.

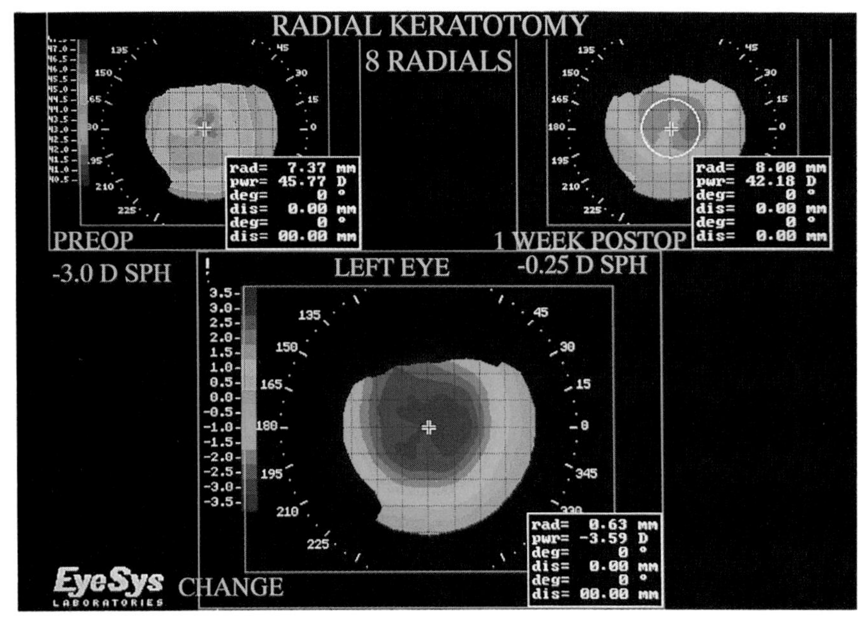

Figure 6.1B.

Figure 6.1: Preoperative, 1 week postoperative and change or delta maps of the right (A) and left (B) eyes of a patient with 3 D of myopia bilaterally. Note the large area of symmetrical flattening of 3 to 3.6 D shown in the change maps (bottom).

power that can be observed preoperatively.

Figures 6.2A, B are the right and left eyes of an RK case with 7 D of myopia bilaterally, plus 1 D of refractive astigmatism in the left eye. He received eight radial incisions in each eye plus a short T-cut in the left eye. Note the obvious central flattening in both eyes, indicated by blue in the postoperative and change images. In the right eye, the flattening is very symmetrical and well centered, as expected from simple radial keratotomy. In the left eye, the flattening is again well centered, but somewhat less symmetrical, possibly because of the T-cut used in addition to the radial incisions. Note that the scale of the change graphs (bottom) is in 1 D steps as compared to 0.5 D steps for Figure 6.1. This scaling is used in order to better visualize the greater degree of corneal flattening in this case.

Figures 6.3A, B show a very successful bilateral case, in spite of substantial preoperative myopia. This patient had more than 10 D of myopia and 1.5 D of with-the-rule astigmatism in the right eye, and 11.5 D of myopia and 2.5 D of astigmatism in the left eye. The preoperative images show the astigmatism clearly. At 1 week after surgery, this patient had −2.75 D of myopia with no residual astigmatism in the right eye, and −6.25 D +1.50 D in the left eye. The result in the right eye is excellent and the left eye is also very much improved. The patient experienced substantial central flattening with good correction of the astigmatism. The asymmetry of the blue area in the change images, especially in the left eye, indicates that the greatest flattening occurred in the regions of greatest preoperative steepness.

Figures 6.4A, B show another bilateral RK case with moderate myopia and astigmatism. In the right eye, the astigmatism is clearly steeper inferiorly, while in the left eye it is more symmetrical. The patient received eight radial incisions and a T-cut in each eye. He has no residual astigmatism in his right eye, as shown in the postoperative image. Notice how the blue area in the bottom change image, representing 2.5 to 3.5 D of change, can be virtually superimposed on the corresponding steep area represented by orange in the preoperative image. The results were nearly as good in his left eye. Again notice how the change image corresponds to the location of the shape of the preoperative astigmatism.

Figure 6.5 shows the right and left eyes of a patient who has undergone bilateral RK. In this particular case, the patient sees well with the right eye but is complaining of visual distortion and discomfort using the left eye. The pattern of flattening in the left eye appears to be heart-shaped. From the scale it is apparent that each color encompasses a half-diopter interval. Figure 6.6 shows a zoom image of the central cornea. Keep in mind that each square on the grid outline is 1 mm by 1 mm. Within the central 2 mm optical zone, there is a range of 4 D of power represented. Within a 4 mm optical zone, there is a 5 D range. Thus the most probable cause for the patient's visual complaints is this multifocal central cornea. Only the corneal topographical mapping would suggest a possible surgical solution to this problem: a single or double T-cut only done superiorly, or possibly deepening or redoing the superior radial cut.

Astigmatic Keratotomy (AK)

As seen in Figures 6.2 through 6.4, transverse (T) incisions can be successfully combined with radial keratotomy to correct astigmatism. One major value of corneal topography in this situation would be to detect asymmetric astigmatism which might benefit from asymmetric surgery.

Figure 6.7 demonstrates a case where most of the astigmatic power is present superiorly in the cornea. A four-incision RK with asymmetric arcuate T-incisions (35° of arc superiorly and only 25° of arc inferiorly)

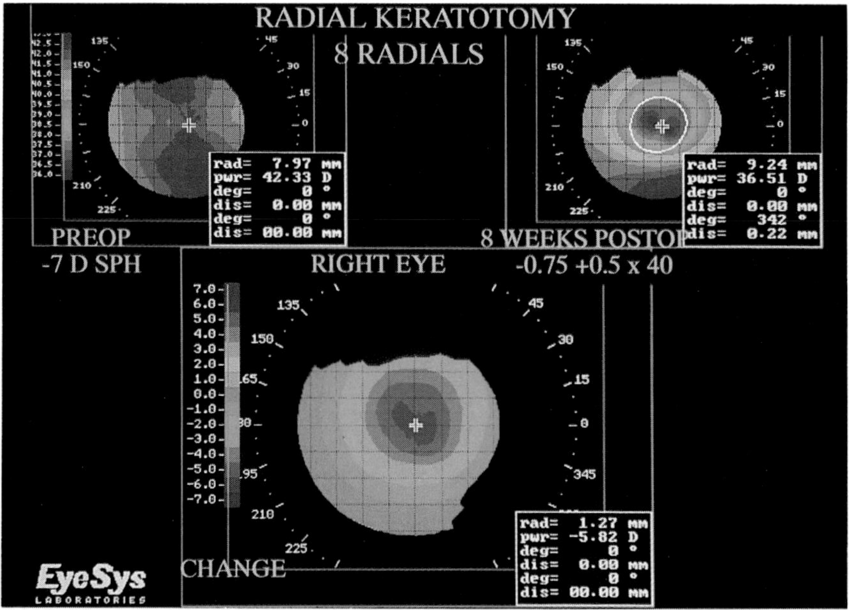

Figure 6.2A.

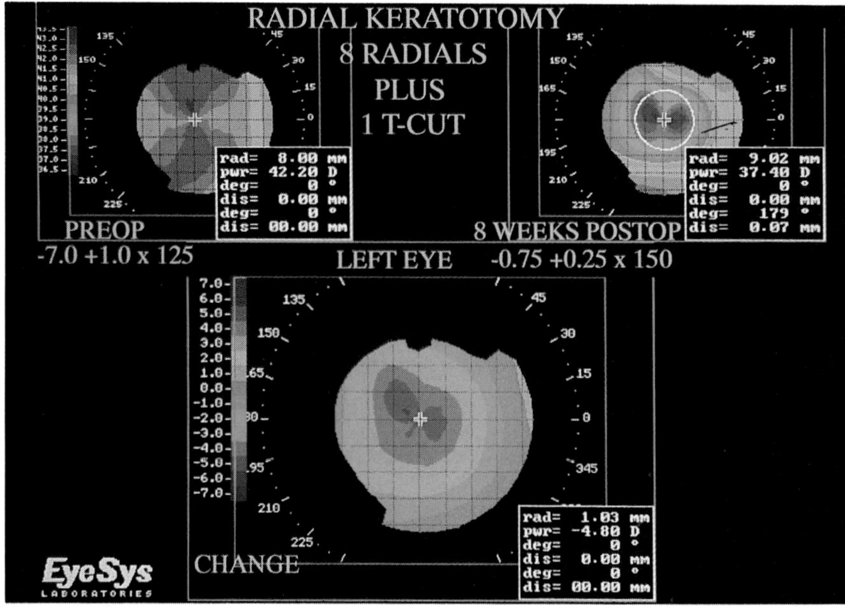

Figure 6.2B.

Figure 6.2: Preoperative, 6 week postoperative and change or delta maps of the right (A) and left (B) eyes of a patient with 7 D of myopia bilaterally.

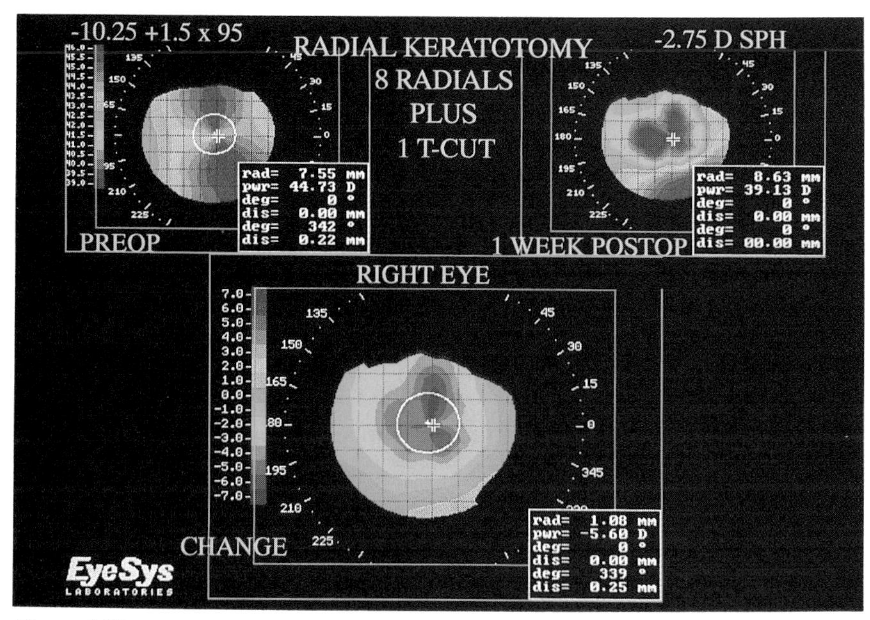

Figure 6.3A.

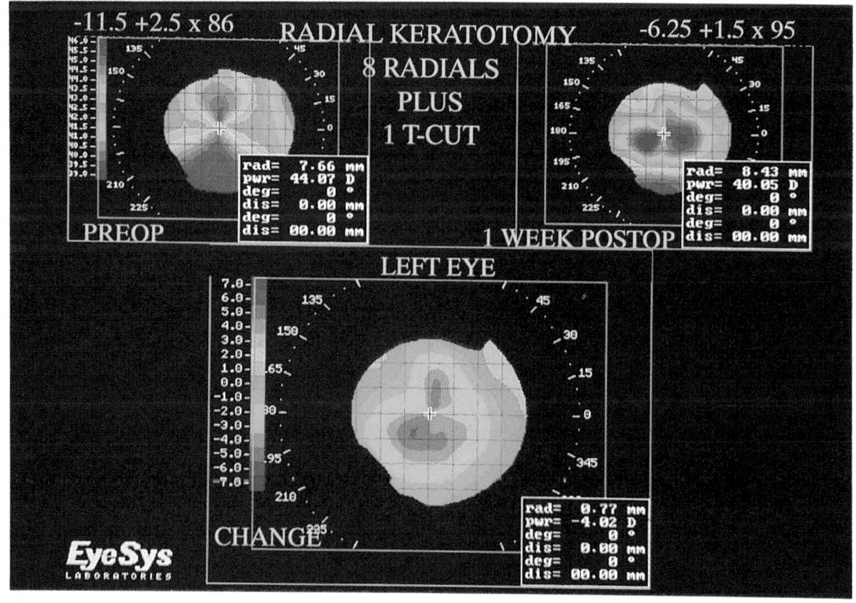

Figure 6.3B.

Figure 6.3: Preoperative, 1 week postoperative and change or delta maps of the right (A) and left (B) eyes of a patient with very high (>10 D) myopia with astigmatism.

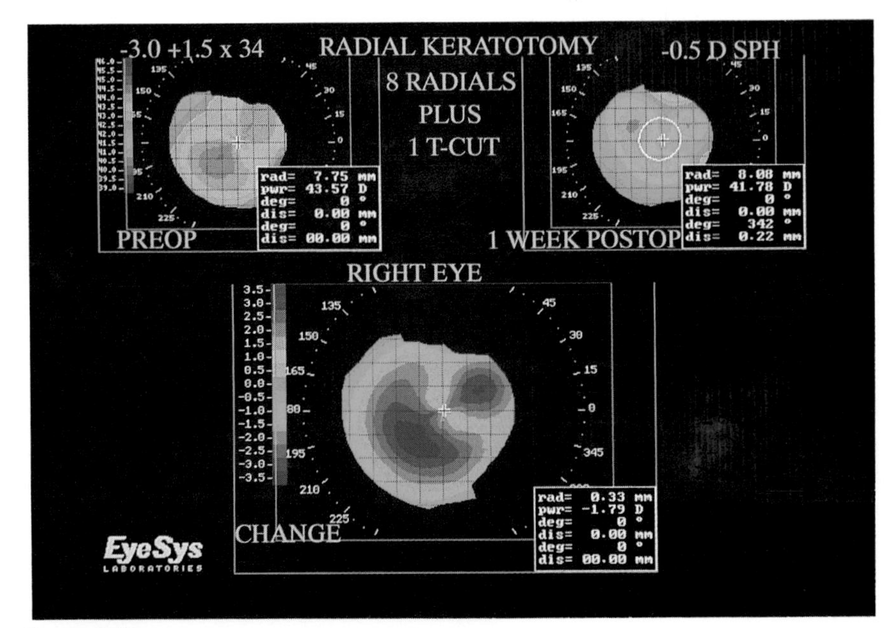

Figure 6.4A.

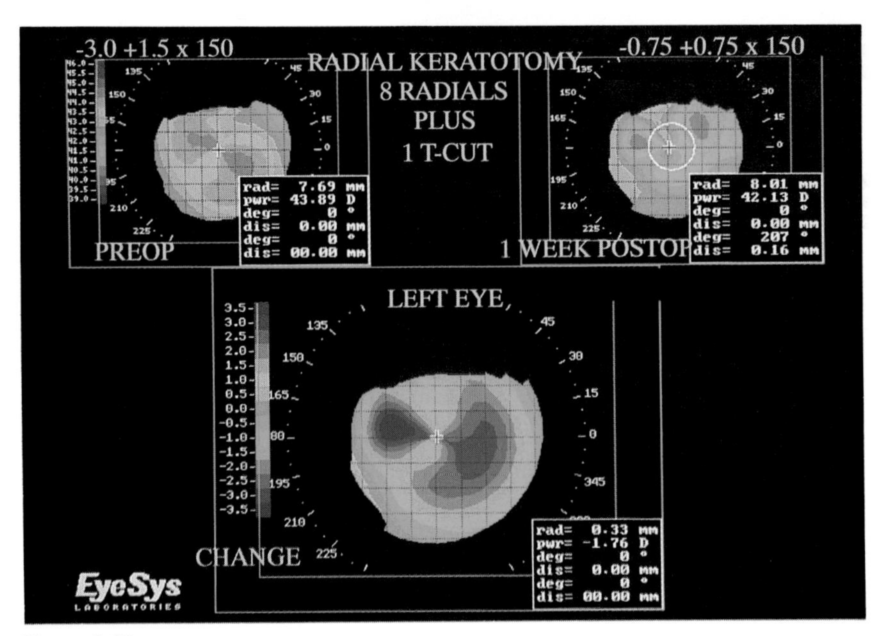

Figure 6.4B.

Figure 6.4: Preoperative, 1 week postoperative and change or delta maps of the right (A) and left (B) eyes of a patient with moderate myopia and astigmatism preoperatively. T-incisions resulted in a marked decrease in astigmatism postoperatively.

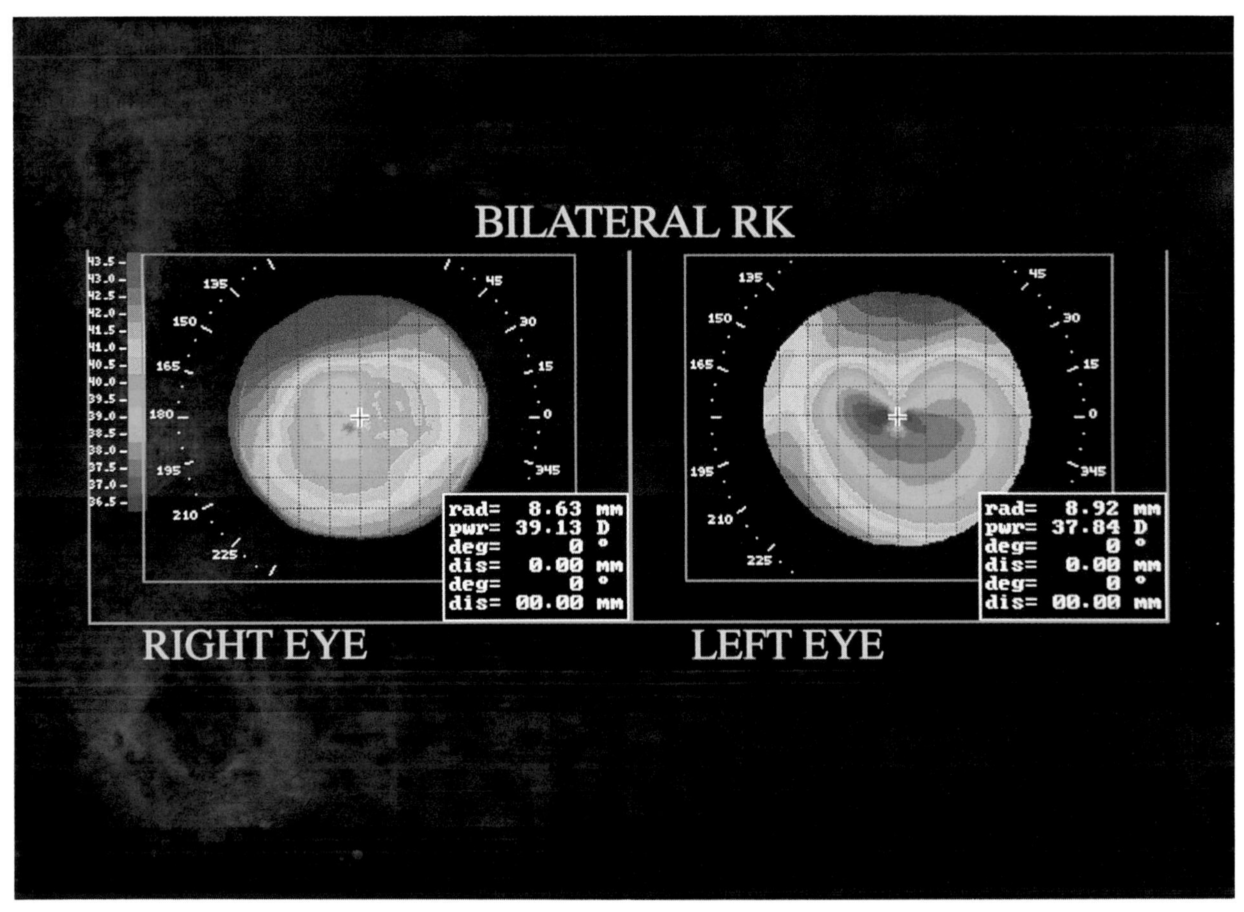

Figure 6.5: Late postoperative corneal topography maps of a patient who underwent bilateral RK. Patient complains of visual distortion and discomfort using the left eye.

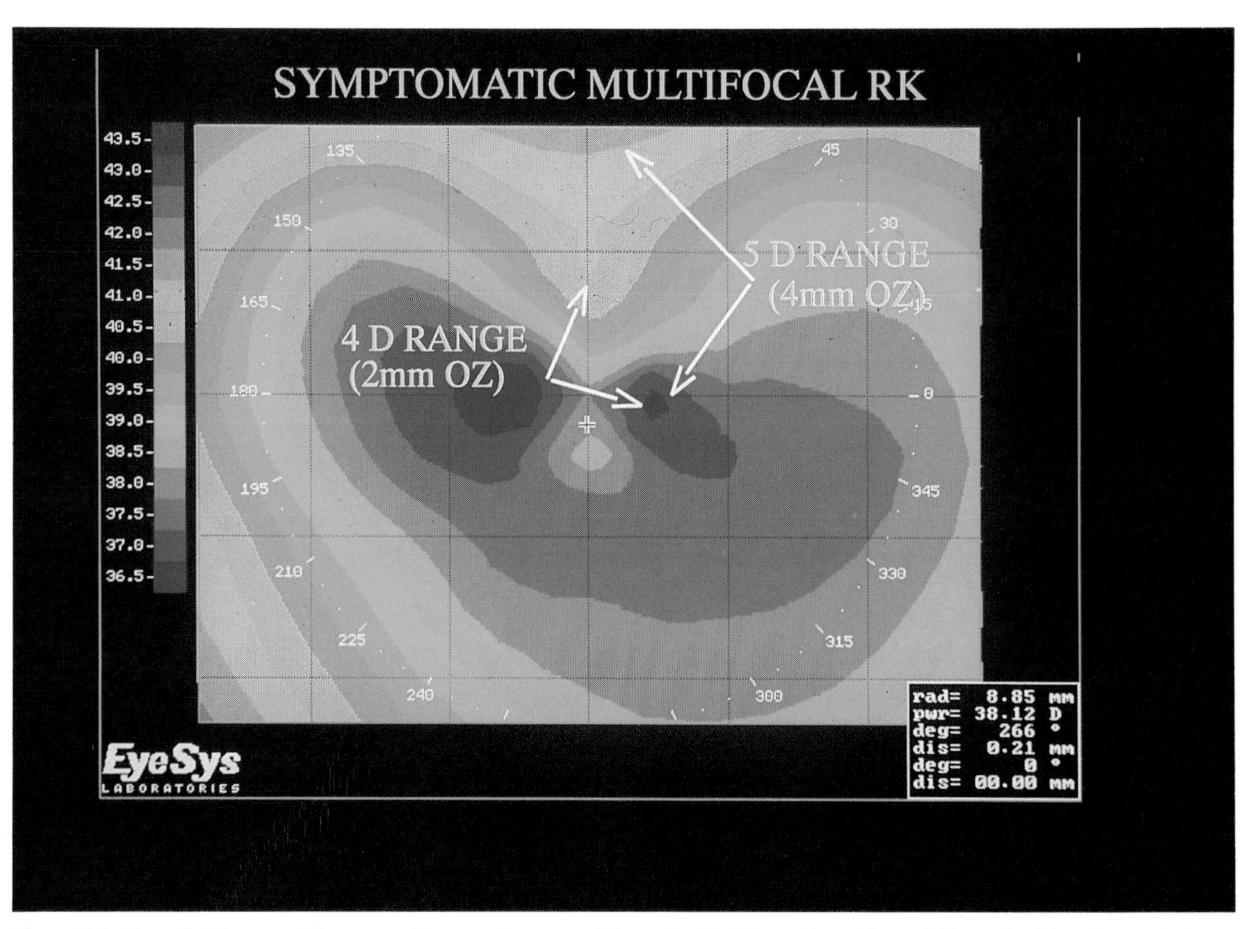

Figure 6.6: Magnified image of the corneal topography map of the patient's left eye from Figure 6.5 emphasizing the central area demonstrating a multifocal central cornea, probably causing the patient's visual symptoms.

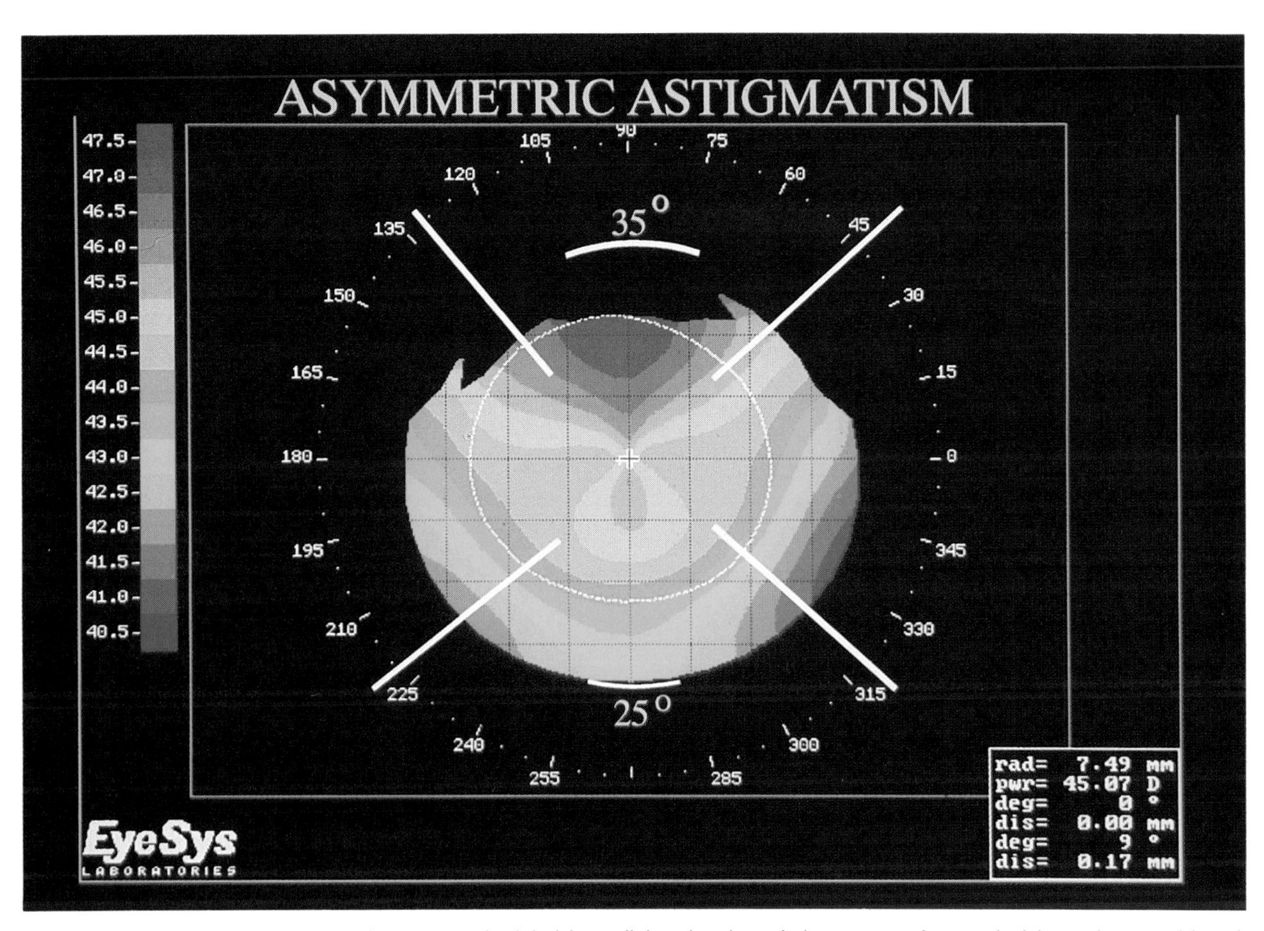

Figure 6.7: Asymmetric astigmatism in a case scheduled for radial and astigmatic keratotomy. Arcuate incisions of unequal length were chosen to treat the asymmetric astigmatism in addition to four radial incisions.

was performed. Figure 6.8 demonstrates a fairly symmetrical flattening postoperatively. One of the authors (SPT) has routinely begun designing asymmetric surgical plans in such cases (Figures 6.9A, B) with good result.

Astigmatic Keratotomy and Cataract Surgery

With the advent of truly small-incision cataract surgery utilizing foldable IOLs and sutureless surgery, significant surgically induced astigmatism has been largely eliminated. The surgeon can now concentrate on treating a patient's preexisting astigmatism without being concerned with large iatrogenic changes. In a recent survey of American Society of Cataract and Refractive Surgery (ASCRS) members, 8.7% of surgeons report using corneal relaxing incisions as an adjunct to cataract surgery and 68% consider it a viable option even though they may not personally utilize it.

A number of studies on the efficacy of the procedure with cataract extraction have been reported[1-7]. In general the efficacy variable has been change in keratometric cylinder. As has been demonstrated in Chapter 3, keratometry may give incomplete information at best and at worst be misleading.

We will show through a number of illustrations how corneal topography provides much more information and gives the surgeon a greater feel for the effect of the surgical procedure upon the cornea.

Figures 6.10A, B show a patient who underwent sutureless cataract surgery and corneal relaxing incisions to treat a little over 4 D of preoperative corneal astigmatism by keratometry. Three weeks following small incision sutureless surgery, the cornea does not demonstrate a normal topographic configuration as shown in the postoperative topographical map in Figure 6.10A. There is only 20/40 best-corrected visual acuity which is probably explained by the corneal distortion as shown in Figure 6.10B. All we know from keratometry is that the astigmatism has decreased by 2.5 D. The change graph at the bottom of Figure 6.10A shows that the deep blue areas of corneal flattening are in the steep meridian of the preoperative astigmatism and in the axis of the corneal relaxing incisions.

Figure 6.11 shows a patient who received a pair of arcuate incisions at the time of cataract surgery. The location of the incisions is indicated on the preoperative image. While not a classic bow-tie or butterfly pattern, the patient had 2.75 D of against-the-rule astigmatism preoperatively, shown by the red areas in the upper left image. At 1 day postoperatively, shown in the upper right image, the patient's astigmatism was greatly reduced. The lower image shows the change induced by surgery. Green areas represent no change. The deep blue areas represent flattening in approximately the axis of the preoperative astigmatism. Conventional keratometry indicated residual astigmatism of 1.25 D at 110°, nearly 90° away from the original astigmatism. Obviously keratometry does not accurately reflect what happened to this eye as a result of corneal relaxing surgery. One cannot always predict the visual acuity based on appearance of the corneal topographic map. At 1 day postoperatively, this patient's uncorrected visual acuity was 20/30.

Figure 6.12 shows a patient with asymmetrical with-the-rule astigmatism preoperatively, steeper superiorly than inferiorly (upper left image). The patient received a pair of straight transverse incisions at axis 90° at the 7 mm optical zone. The 2-week postoperative image on the upper right clearly indicates a decrease (note the lack of yellow) and redirection of the patient's astigmatism. The change image (bottom) shows how this result occurred. The patient experienced steepening (yellow) at approximately 10°, and flattening at approximately 110°, greater superiorly than inferiorly.

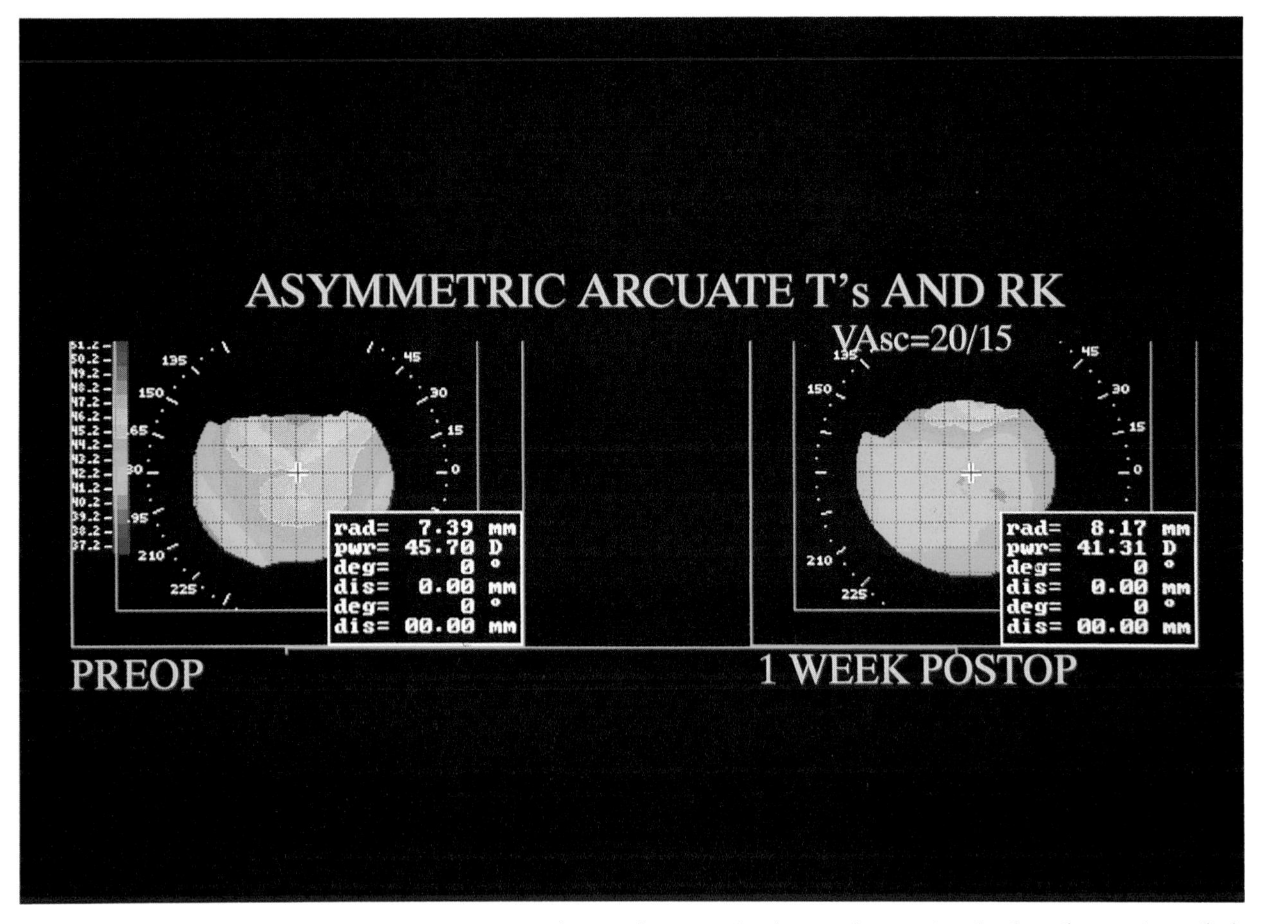

Figure 6.8: Preoperative and 1 day postoperative corneal maps demonstrating improved symmetry of astigmatism postoperatively due to the use of asymmetric astigmatism surgery.

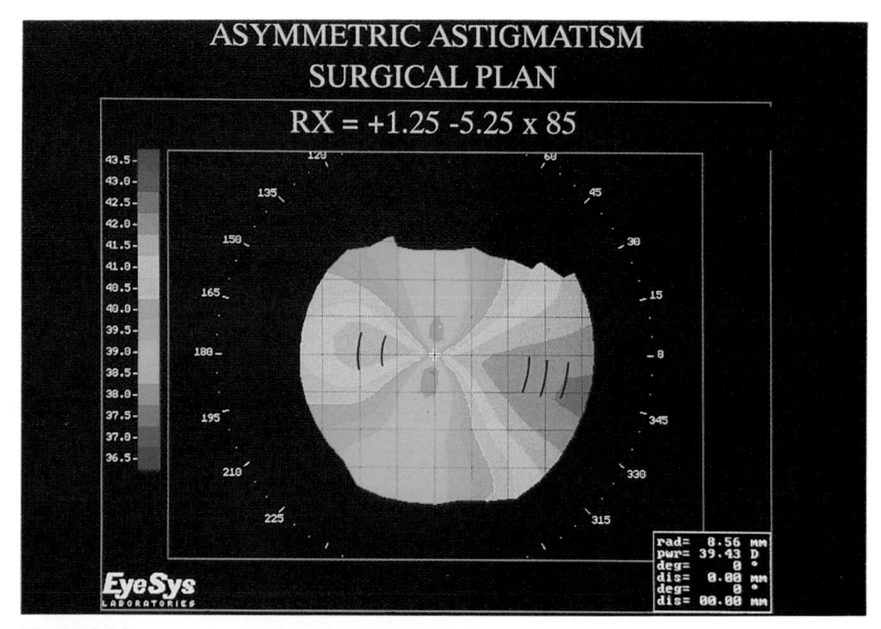

Figure 6.9A.

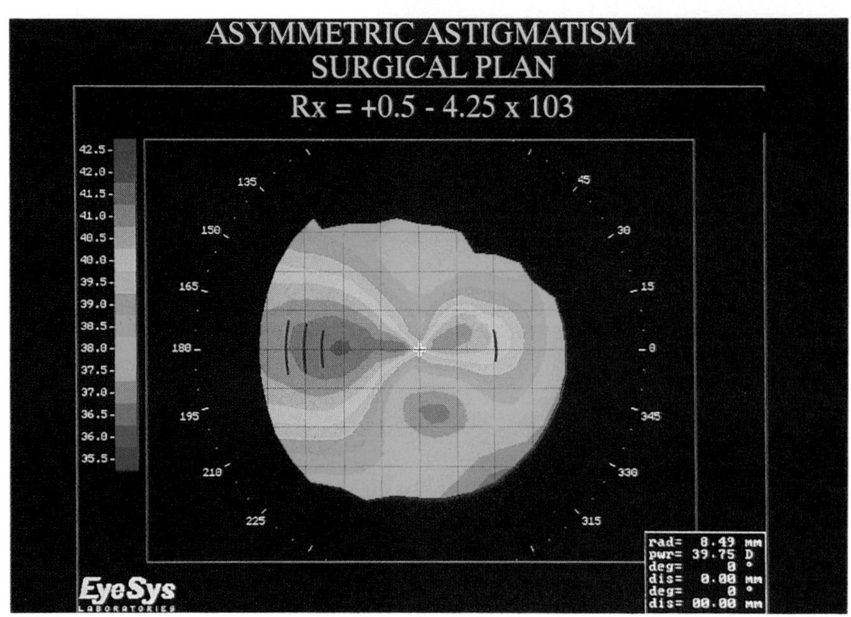

Figure 6.9B.

Figure 6.9: (A,B) Preoperative cases of asymmetrical astigmatism with more arcuate incisions planned in the area of greater corneal steepening.

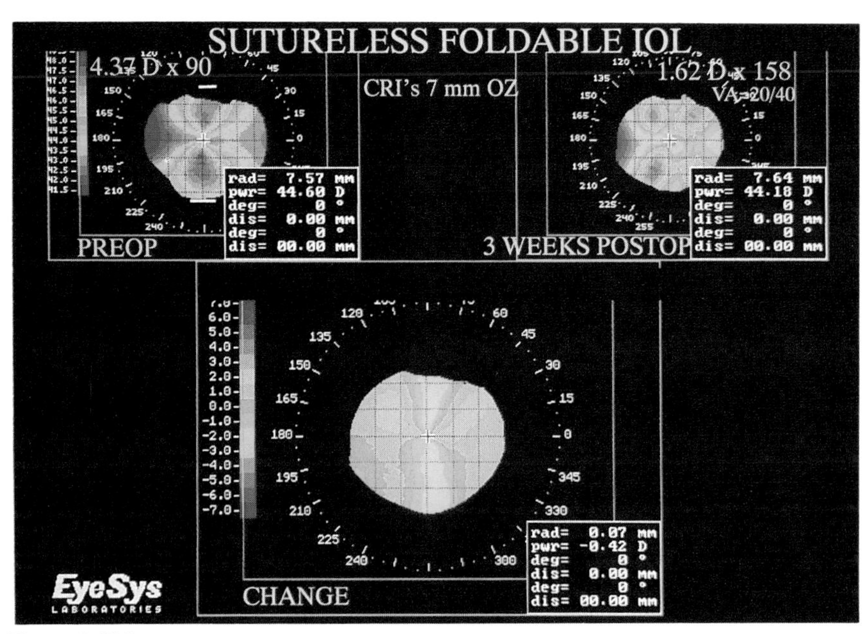

Figure 6.10A.

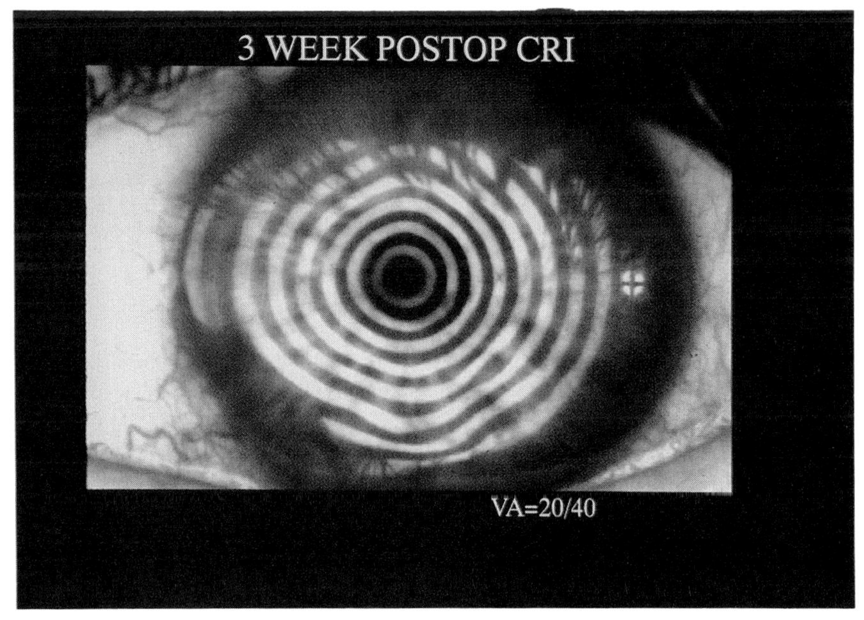

Figure 6.10B.

Figure 6.10: Patient who underwent sutureless cataract surgery and corneal relaxing incisions for 4.0 D of corneal astigmatism. (A) Preoperative, 3 week postoperative and change or delta map. The postoperative corneal map demonstrates disruption of the astigmatic pattern while the change map demonstrates surgically induced flattening in the meridian of preoperative corneal steepness. (B) Corneoscopic view demonstrates corneal distortion in the areas of the T-incisions at 12 o'clock and 6 o'clock.

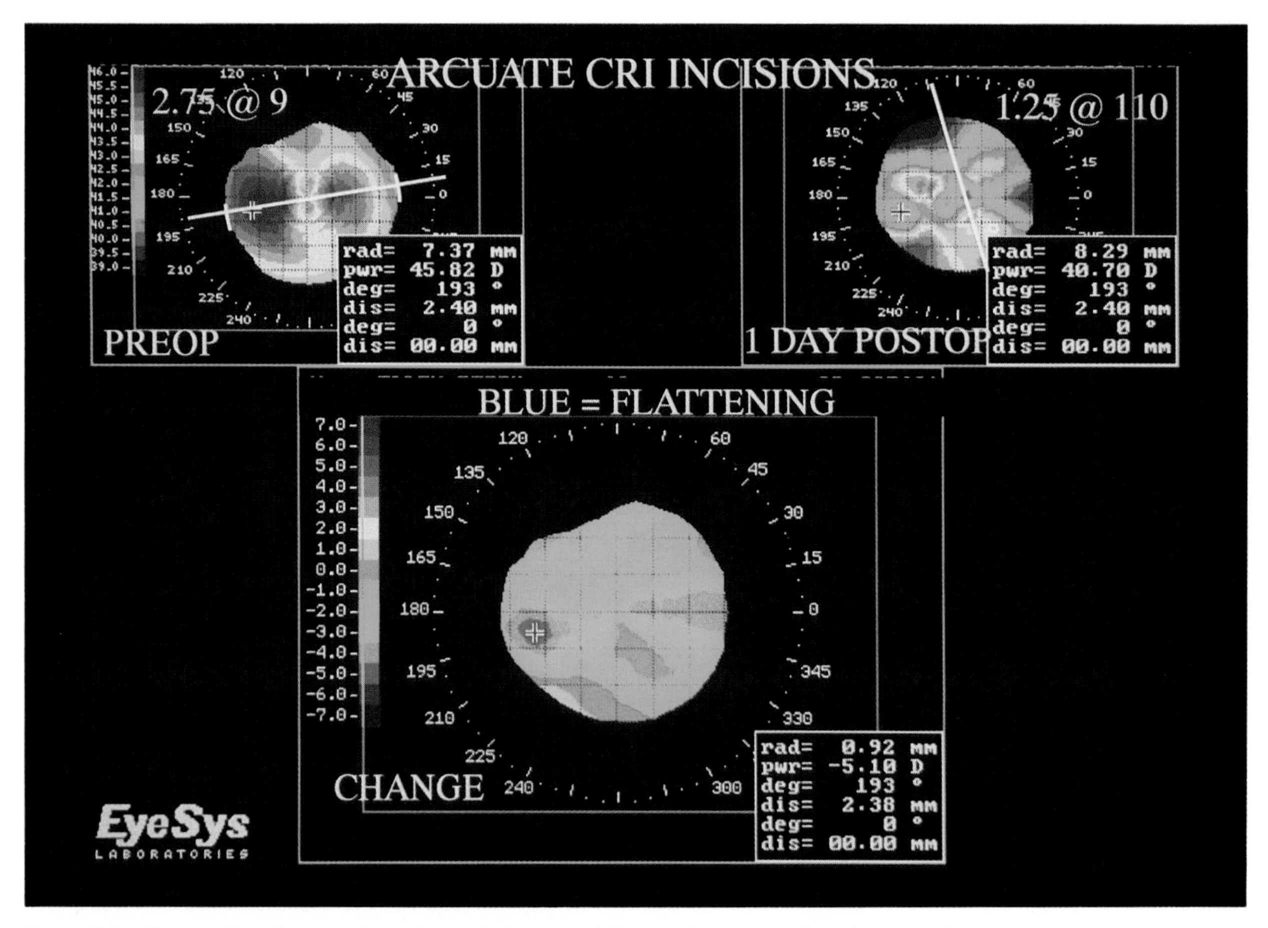

Figure 6.11: Preoperative, 1 day postoperative and change or delta map in a case undergoing sutureless cataract surgery and arcuate T-incisions. The change graph indicates flattening in approximately the steep meridian of the pre-existing astigmatism, although the pre- and postoperative patterns are somewhat unusual and difficult to interpret.

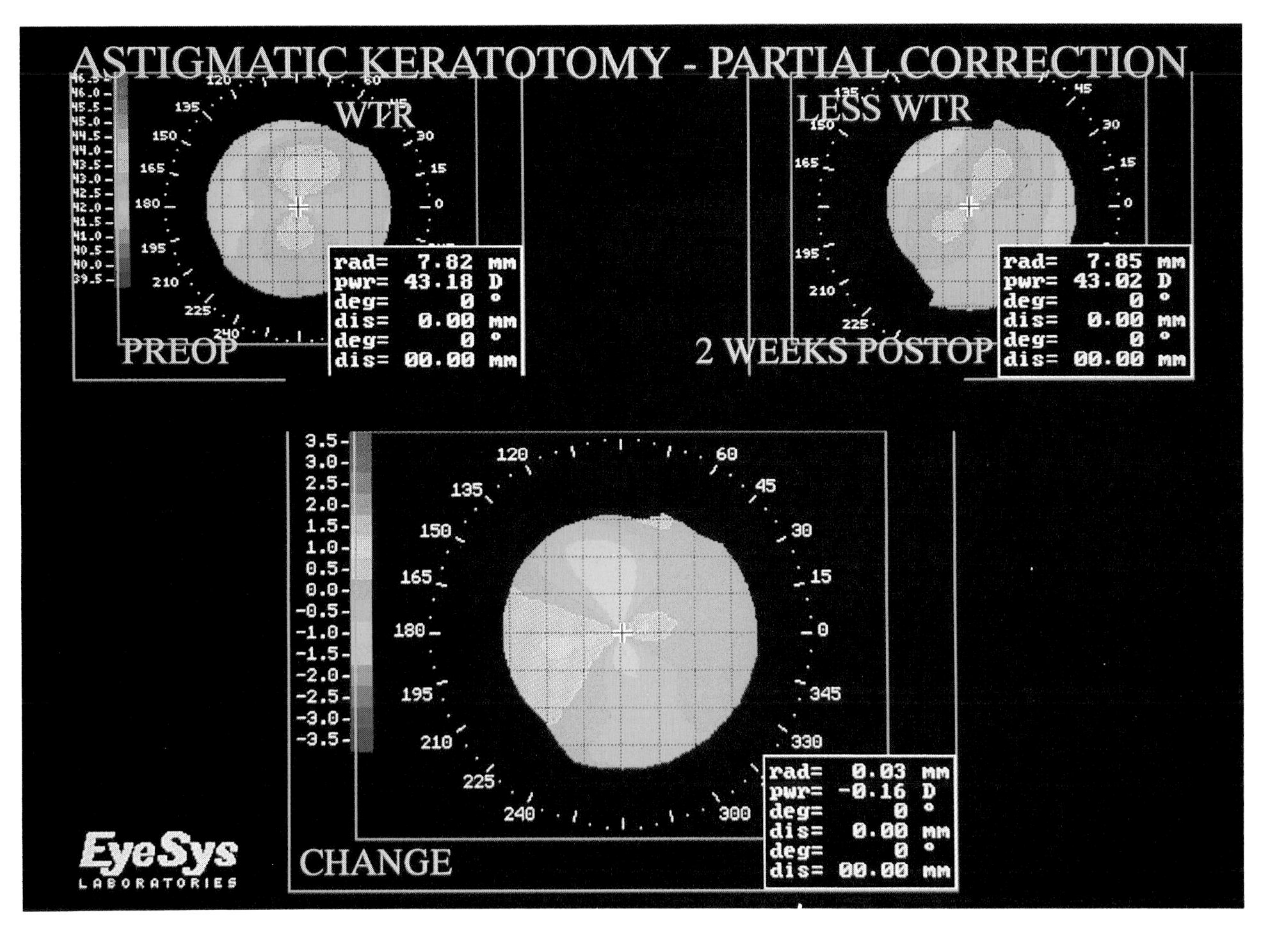

Figure 6.12: Preoperative, 2 week postoperative and change or delta map of a patient who underwent sutureless cataract surgery and astigmatic keratotomy.

Figure 6.13 shows a case of overcorrection. Preoperatively, the patient had against-the-rule astigmatism with steeper portions of the cornea oriented horizontally. At 2 weeks postoperatively, shown in the upper right image, the patient had substantial with-the-rule astigmatism, indicated in red. The change image clearly shows substantial steepening at 90° and substantial flattening at 180°, indicating induced with-the-rule astigmatism.

Figure 6.14A shows an unusual result of astigmatic keratotomy. Preoperatively, the patient had 1 D of with-the-rule astigmatism measured keratometrically, although the topographic image fails to show a classic bow-tie type of astigmatism pattern. The patient received a pair of T-cuts 1.25 mm in length at the 7 mm optical zone at axis 85° as an adjunct to 5.5 mm incision sutureless cataract surgery, which resulted in substantial superior steepening that extends almost to the center of the pupil. Figure 6.14B shows another similar case, but with against-the-rule astigmatism and T-cuts at 180°. At 3 weeks postoperatively, this pattern of superior steepening is again apparent. The keratometry readings for both patients demonstrate a good result, but the topography reveals a somewhat different picture. It is possible that in these cases the astigmatic keratotomy failed to have any effect and the changes seen were a result of the cataract surgery itself.

Figure 6.15 shows an even more dramatic case of atypical response to corneal relaxing surgery. Keratometry indicated 1.75 D of astigmatism at 180°, and the patient received a pair of T-cuts at the 7 mm optical zone on the 180° axis. However, the preoperative corneal topography image shows that the patient had oblique astigmatism. At 2 weeks postoperatively, keratometry indicated only 0.25 D of residual astigmatism, but the T-cuts at the horizontal axis resulted in an extremely irregular distortion of the cornea, as shown in the postoperative topographic image. Red areas in the change image represent 3.5 D of steepening nasally and deep blue areas indicate 3.5 D of flattening temporally. Since the keratometer averages two points 180° on either side of the optical axis, it averaged the very steep cornea portion and very flat portion of the cornea and found little or no astigmatism in the cornea.

Figure 6.16A demonstrates the power of corneal relaxing incisions in corneal transplant cases. This case had over 11 D of against-the-rule astigmatism preoperatively, and by 4 weeks postoperatively demonstrated 5 D of with-the-rule astigmatism. This 16 D shift is so gross that it is obvious on the corneoscopic pictures shown in Figures 6.16B, C.

Keratomileusis

Topography is also useful in monitoring the results of keratomileusis. Figures 6.17A, B each show the right and left eyes of a bilateral 20 D correction keratomileusis case. In Figure 6.17A the colors are scaled for 1.5 D intervals, showing the transition to the markedly flat 25 to 26 D power central corneas. By changing the scale to 0.5 D color intervals and concentrating only on the low end of the scale (Figure 6.17B), more detail of the corneal power distribution of the central cornea becomes apparent.

Epikeratophakia

Corneal topography plays a vital role in all phases of the management of patients undergoing epikeratophakia. For myopic epikeratophakia, computer-generated topographic images are important tools for assessing the baseline corneal topography of the eye, particularly to check for the presence of asymmetric astigmatism or occult topographic disorders such as early keratoconus. For epi-

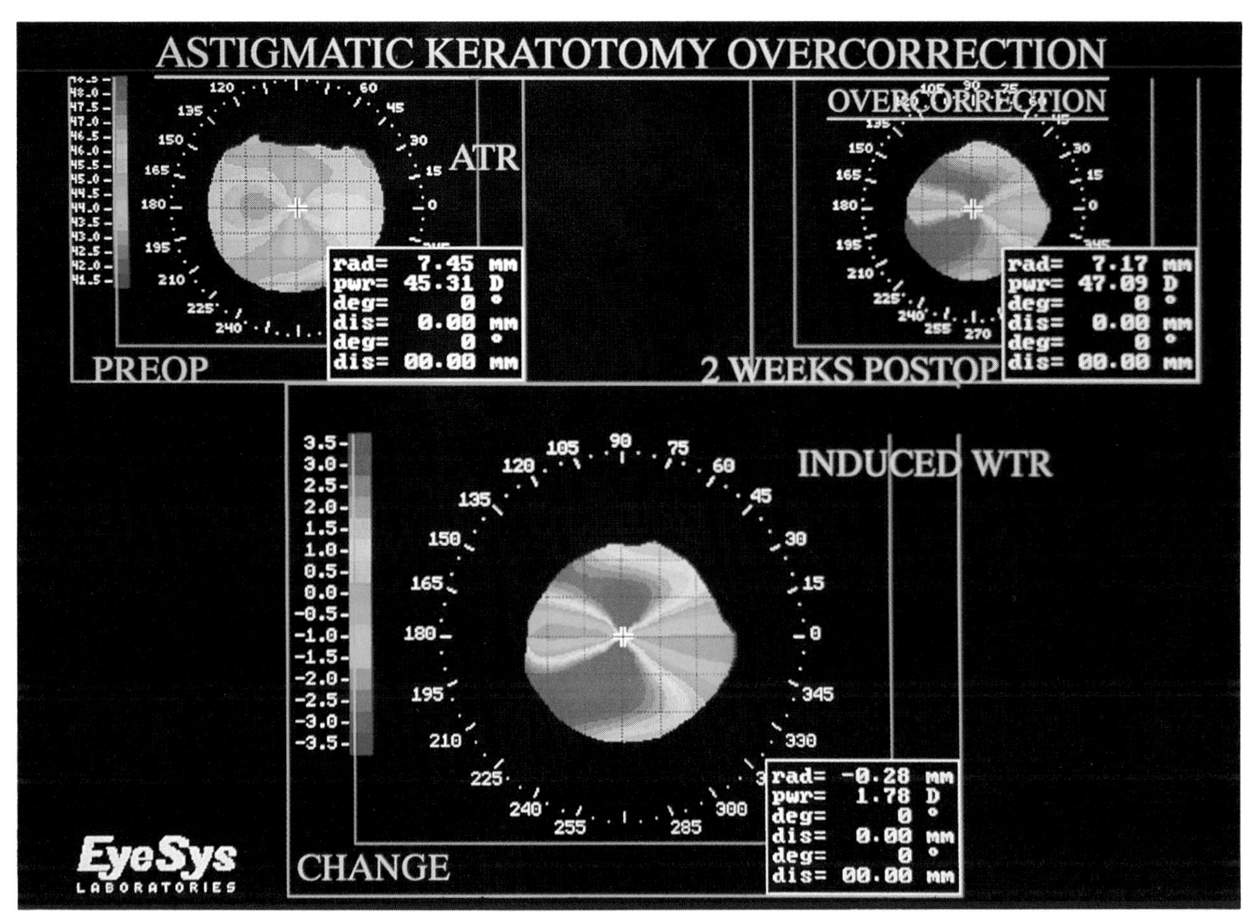

Figure 6.13: Preoperative, 2 week postoperative and delta or change map of a patient who underwent sutureless cataract surgery and astigmatic keratotomy. Patient had a marked overcorrection going from against-the-rule astigmatism to with-the-rule astigmatism.

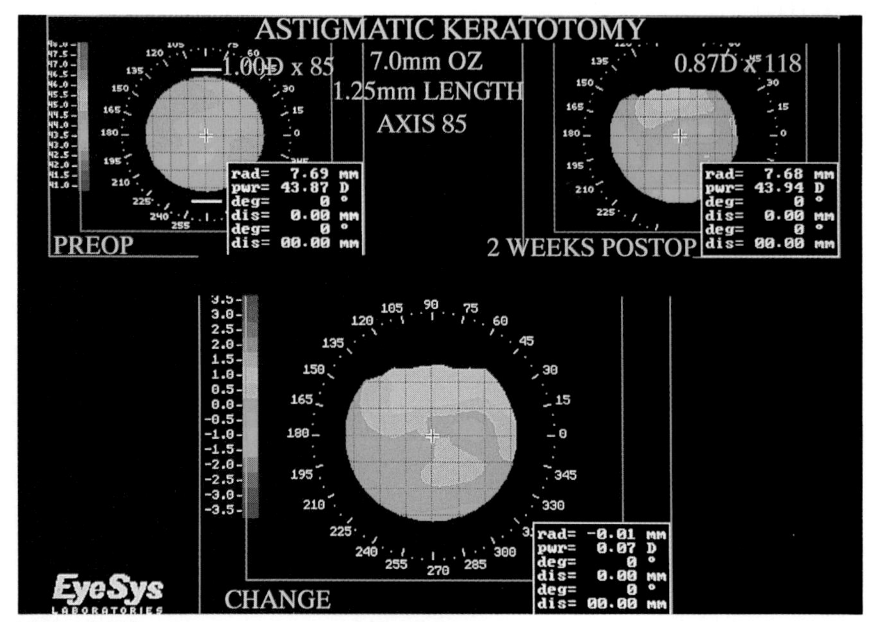

Figure 6.14A.

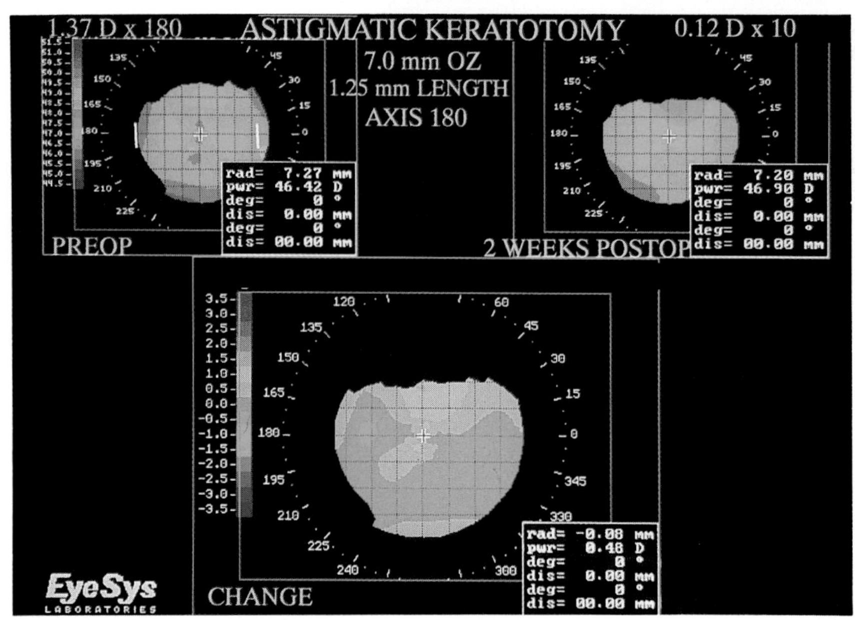

Figure 6.14B.

Figure 6.14: Unusual superior steepening in cases undergoing sutureless cataract surgery and astigmatic keratotomy. The fact that one case had T-cuts placed at 90° (A) and the other had T-cuts placed at 180° (B) suggests that this phenomenon is related to the sutureless surgery and not the T-incisions.

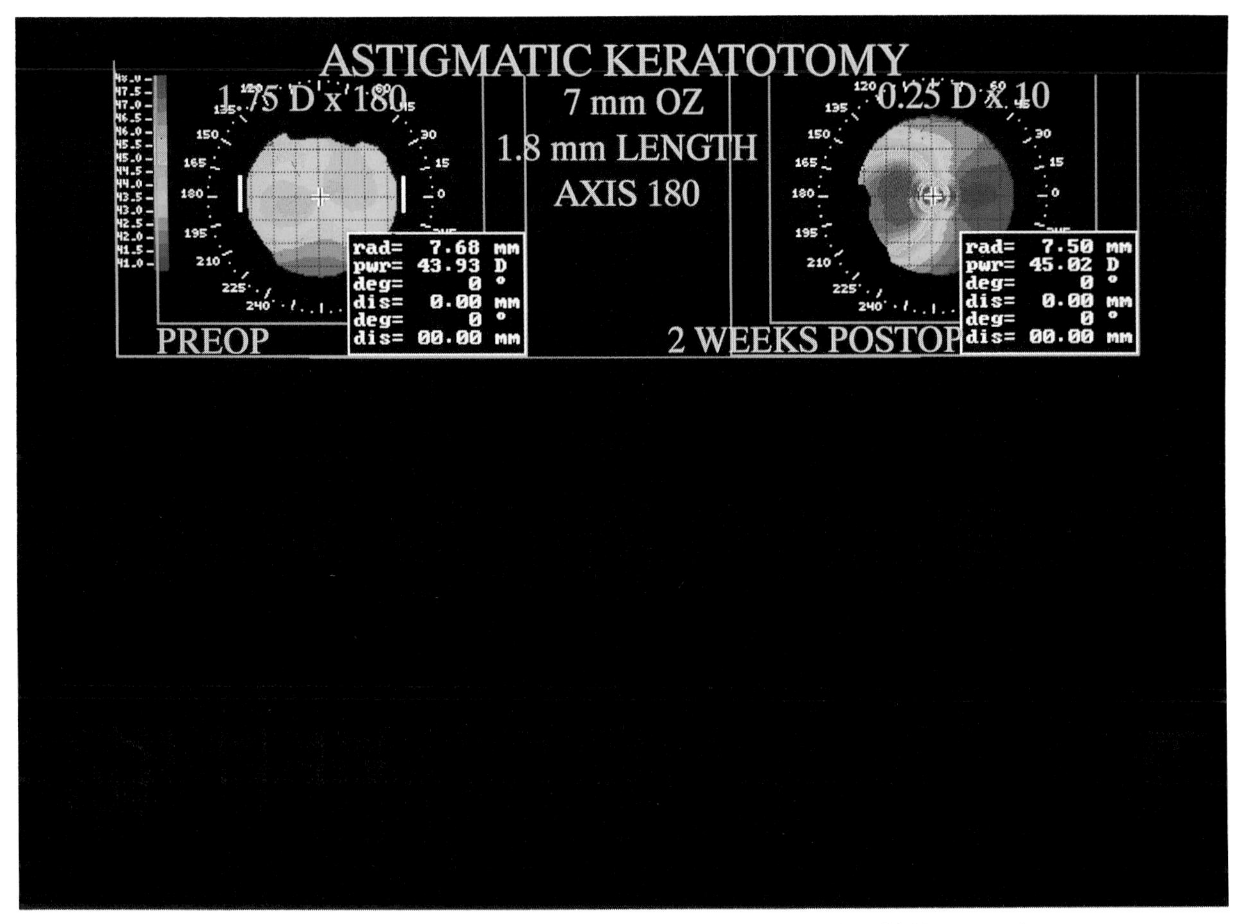

Figure 6.15: Preoperative and 2 week postoperative topography maps in a case with a highly unusual response to surgery. Keratometry failed to detect the marked distortion due to surgery and indicated an excellent astigmatic result.

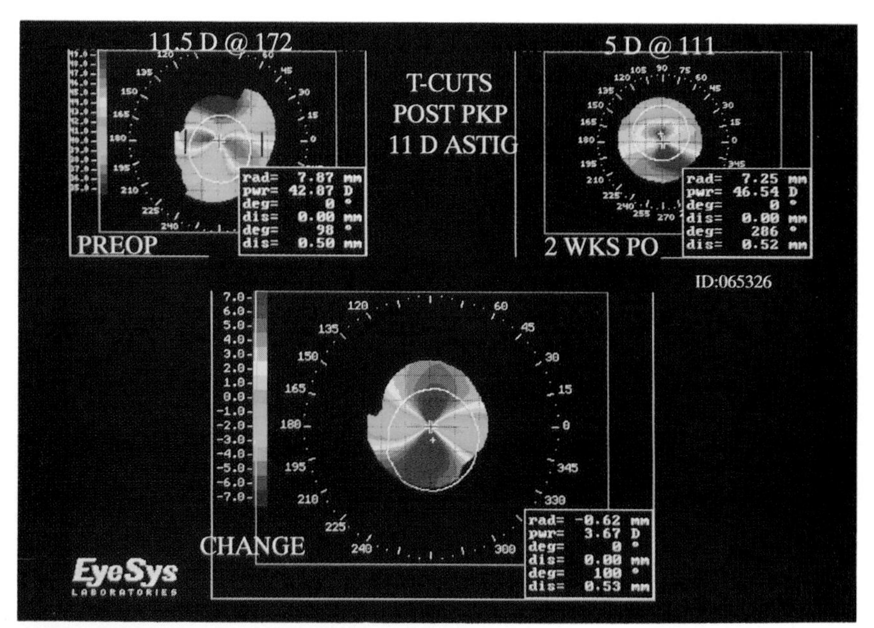

Figure 6.16A.

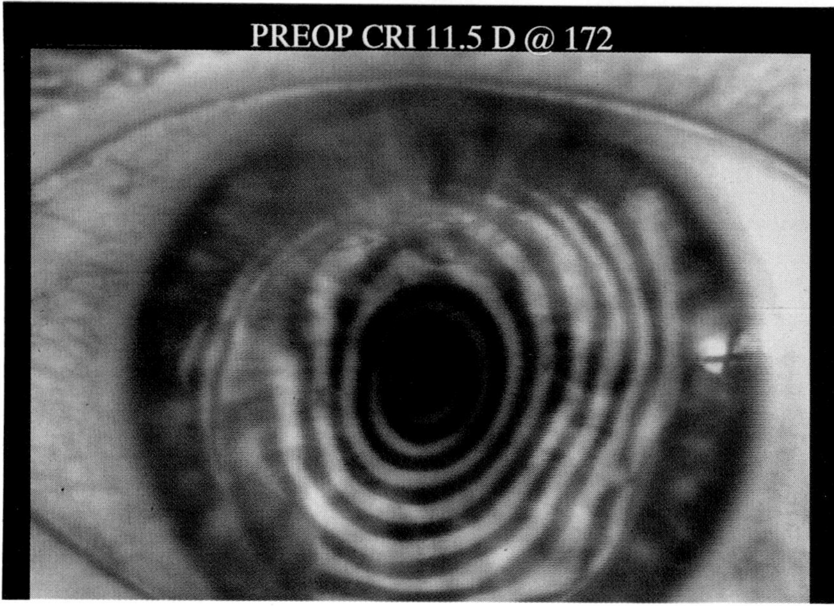

Figure 6.16B.

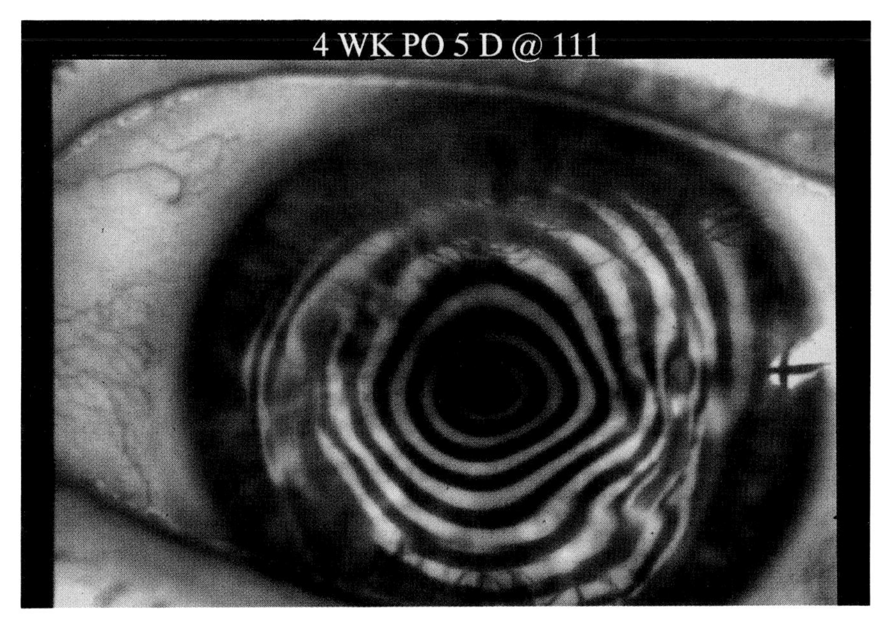

Figure 6.16C.

Figure 6.16: Case with marked overcorrection which received corneal relaxing incisions following corneal transplantation. (A) Preoperative, 1 week postoperative and change or delta map demonstrating the marked overcorrection. (B) Preoperative corneoscopy demonstrating large degree of against-the-rule astigmatism. (C) Postoperative corneoscopy demonstrating corneal distortion due to the T-incisions and with-the-rule astigmatism.

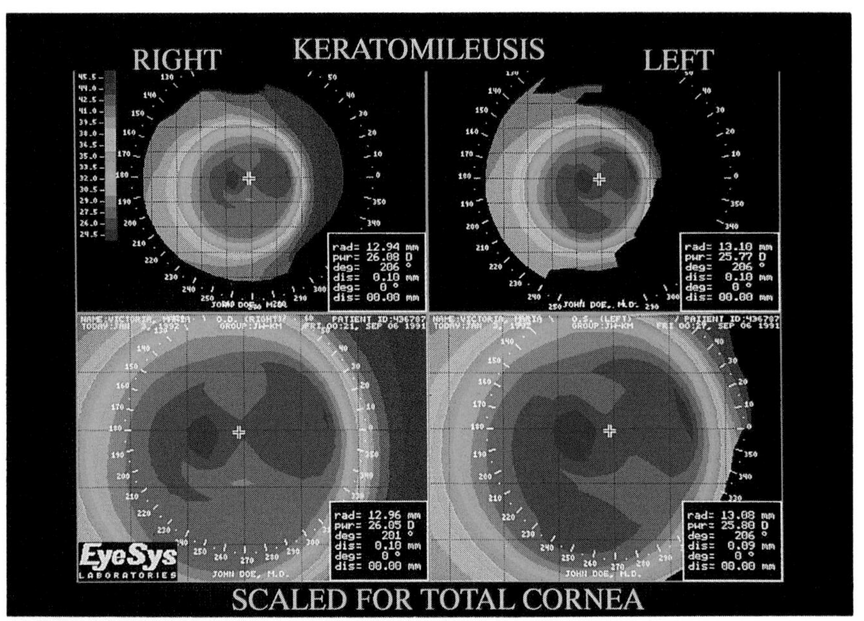

Figure 6.17A.

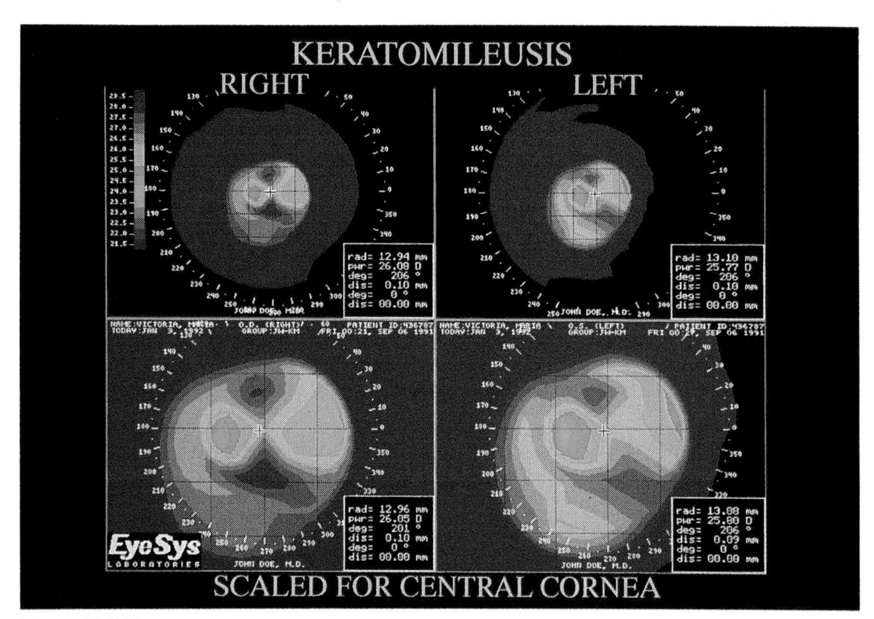

Figure 6.17B.

Figure 6.17: Right and left eyes of patient undergoing bilateral keratomileusis. Bottom images are magnified images of the central cornea. (A) Scale is chosen in 1.5 D intervals to emphasize the whole range of corneal change and to demonstrate the marked difference between central and peripheral cornea. (B) Scale is chosen in 0.5 D intervals only in the extreme flat portion to accentuate the central corneal power distribution.

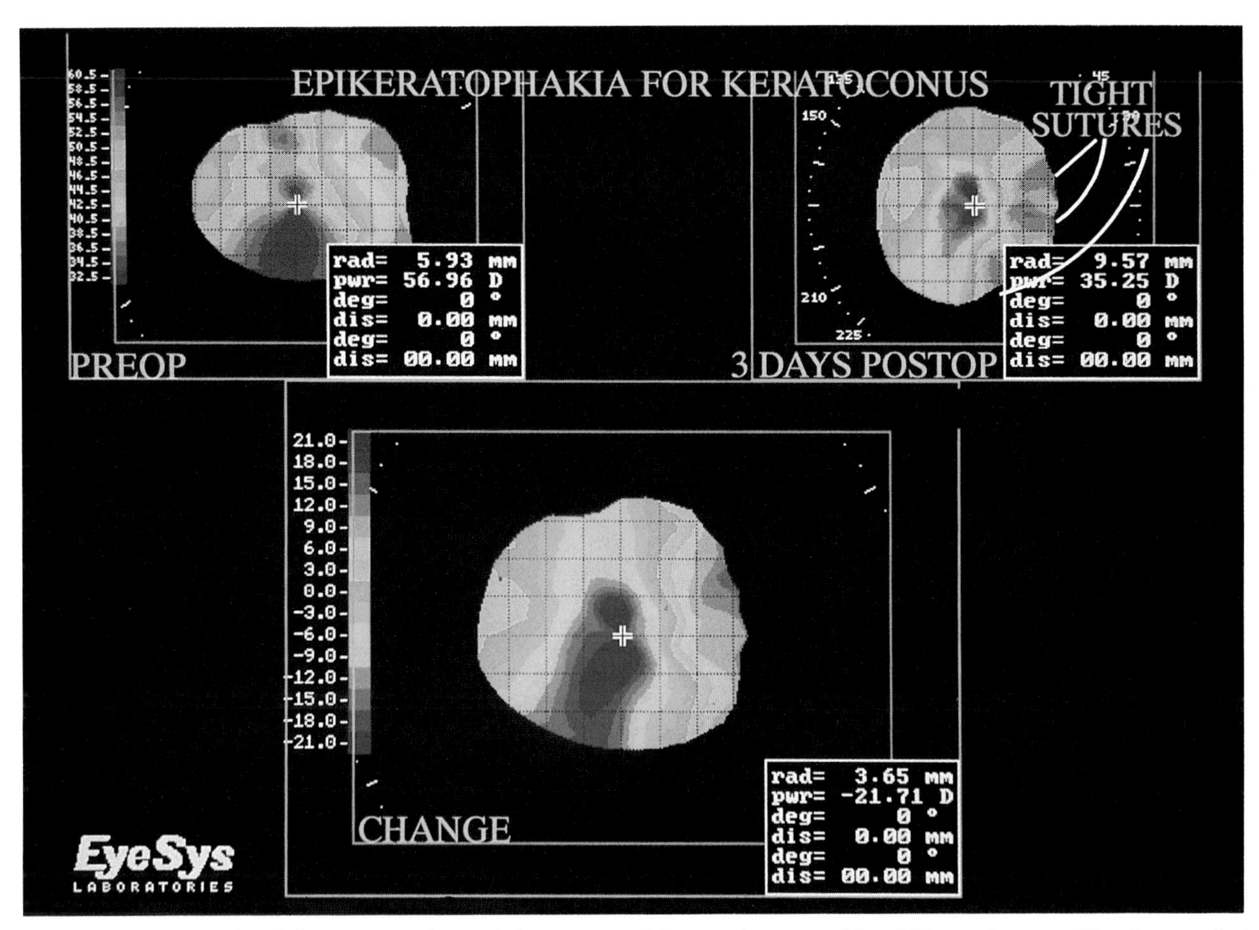

Figure 6.18: Preoperative, 3 day postoperative and change corneal topography maps of the right eye of a case of keratoconus that received a planar epikeratophakia. Tight sutures were responsible for the nasal steepening observed. Later removal of these sutures evened out the topographic picture (courtesy Dr. S. Ganem, Paris, France).

keratophakia for keratoconus, preoperative topography is extremely useful for analyzing the type of cone (Figure 6.18), since the success rate of epikeratophakia tends to be higher in corneas with small central cones.

Topography is also a key component in the postoperative follow-up and management of epikeratophakia patients. It can assist in selective suture removal (Figure 6.19), and is essential in the evaluation of the centration, size, and uniformity of the optical zone (Figures 6.20 and 6.21). It is also useful in managing any complications should they occur (Figure 6.22).

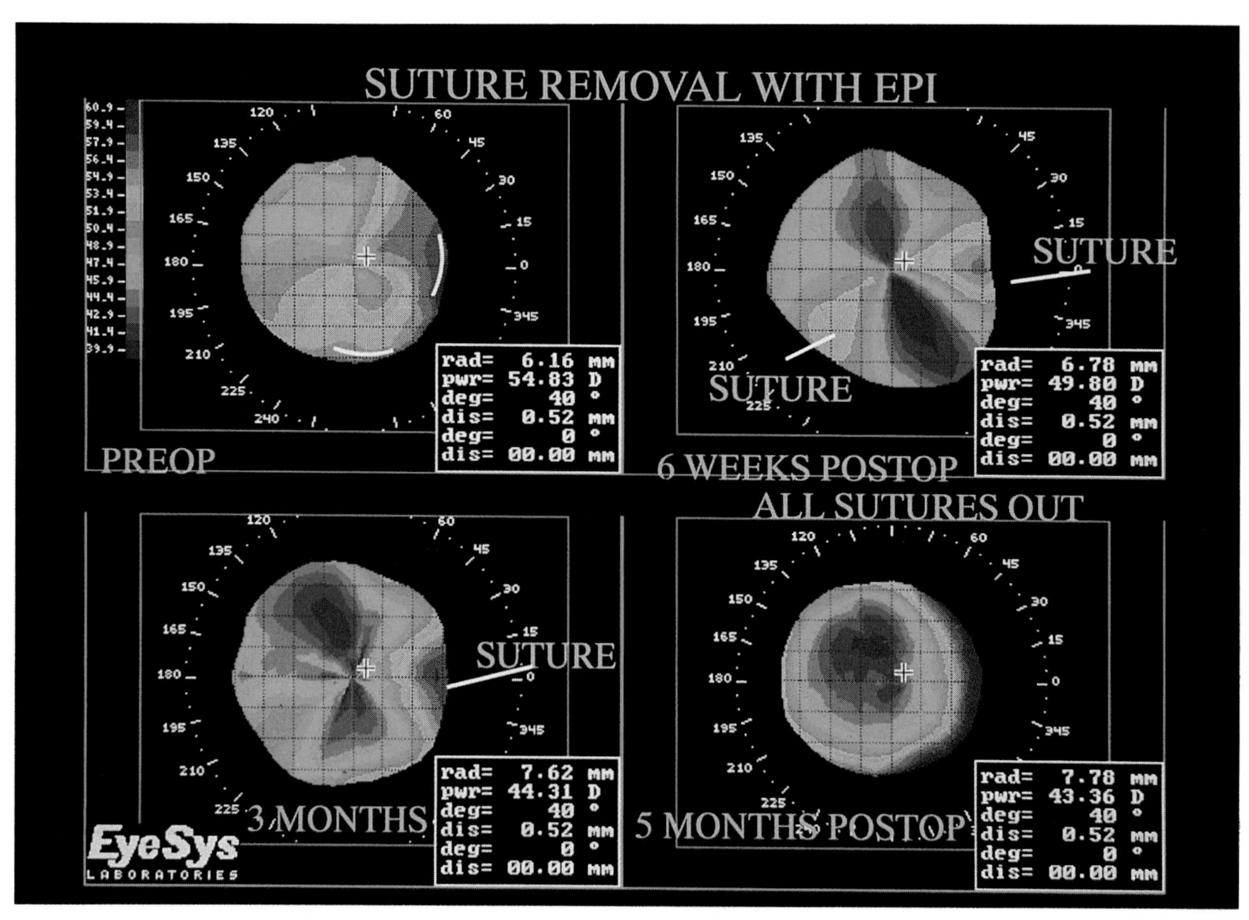

Figure 6.19: Upper left, right cornea of 24-year-old female who had undergone penetrating keratoplasty 2 years previously for herpetic corneal scarring. Refraction was −13.00 +5.75 × 30, with VAcc of 20/200. With a contact lens, she could see 20/80, but she was contact lens intolerant. Arcuate 45° incisions were placed just inside the graft-host junction along the two steep semimeridians, and a myopic epikeratophakia was placed over the entire graft. Upper right, at 6 weeks postoperatively, there is moderate astigmatism at 5° and 230° due to the presence of interrupted sutures. Lower left, 3 months postoperatively, following removal of all but the 3 o'clock sutures, much of the astigmatism has been resolved. Lower right, 5 months postoperatively, all sutures are out. Keratometric astigmatism is 1.75 D, and refraction is −2.00 +1.50 × 25 with VAcc of 20/25. Note the mild temporal centration of the optical zone, paralleling the location of the flat region preoperatively (Courtesy Douglas Koch, MD).

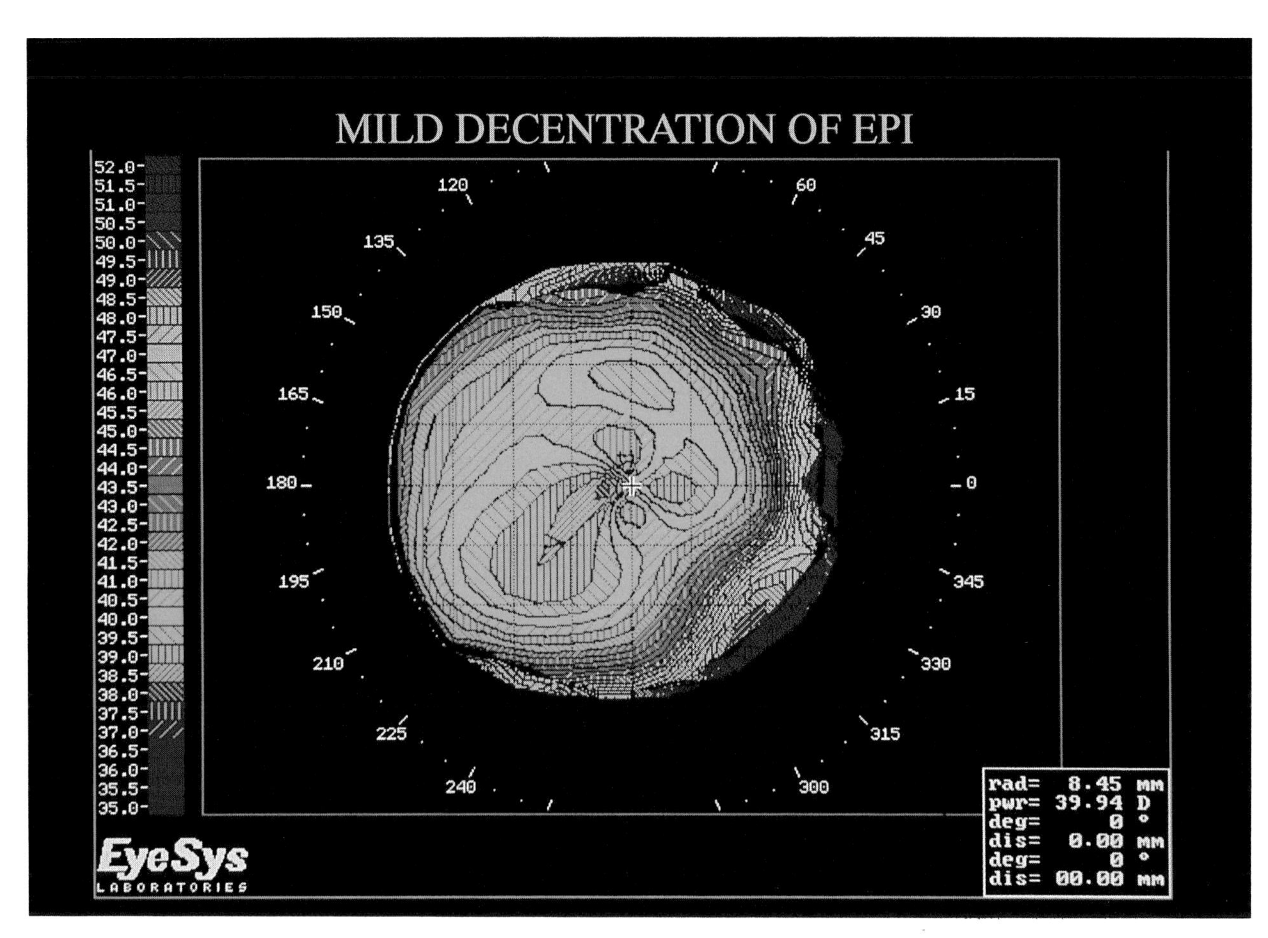

Figure 6.20: Topographic map (absolute scale) of right cornea 4 years following myopic epikeratophakia. Preoperative refraction was −16.00 +4.75 X 120 with VAcc of 20/40, and postoperative refraction was −0.50 +1.75 X 120 with VAcc of 20/40. Note the mild (approximately 1 mm) temporal decentration and the variable zones of power in the central cornea.

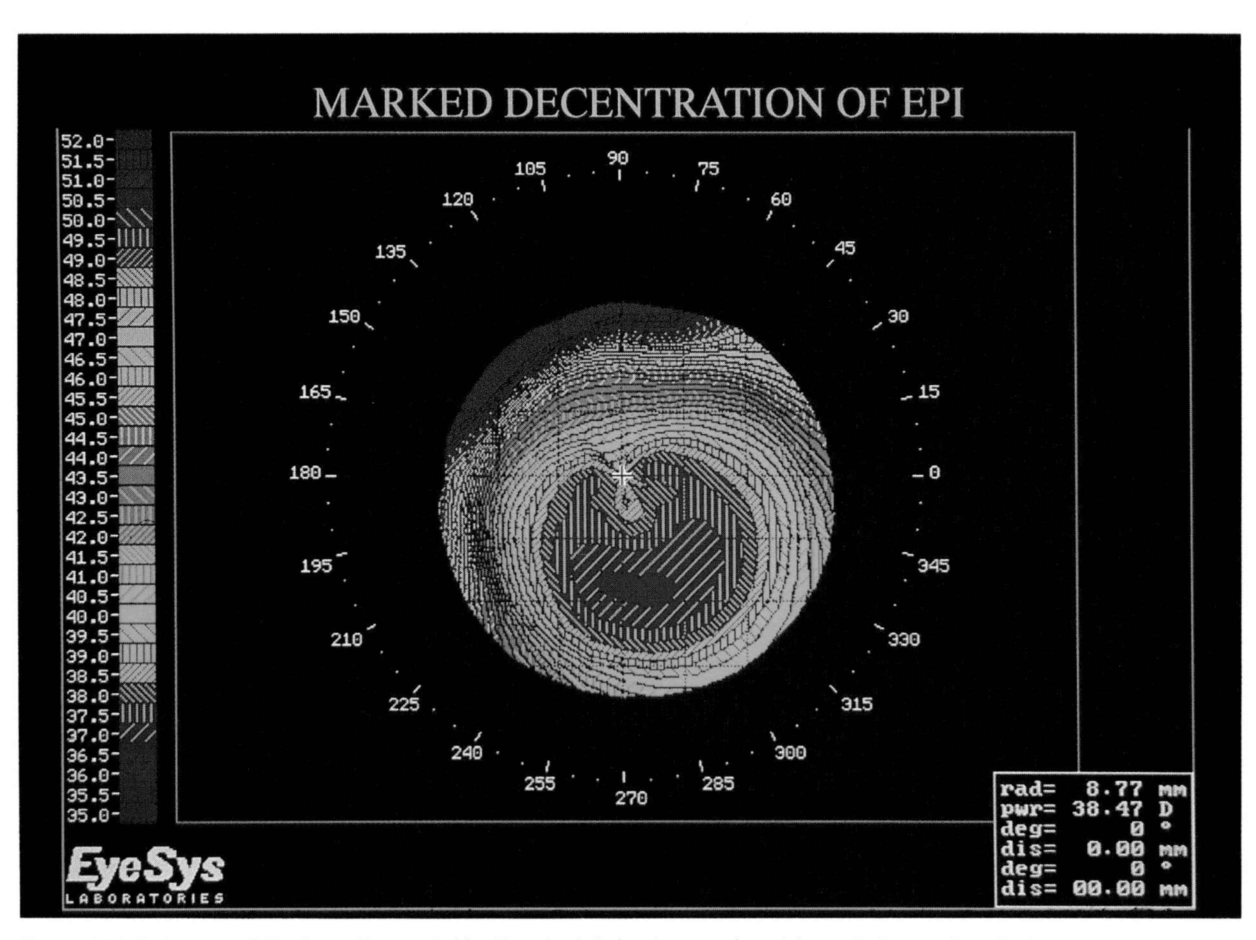

Figure 6.21: Left cornea following epikeratophakia. Note the inferior decentration of the optical zone. Despite best-corrected vision of 20/20 to 20/25, the patient complained of haloes, especially at night.

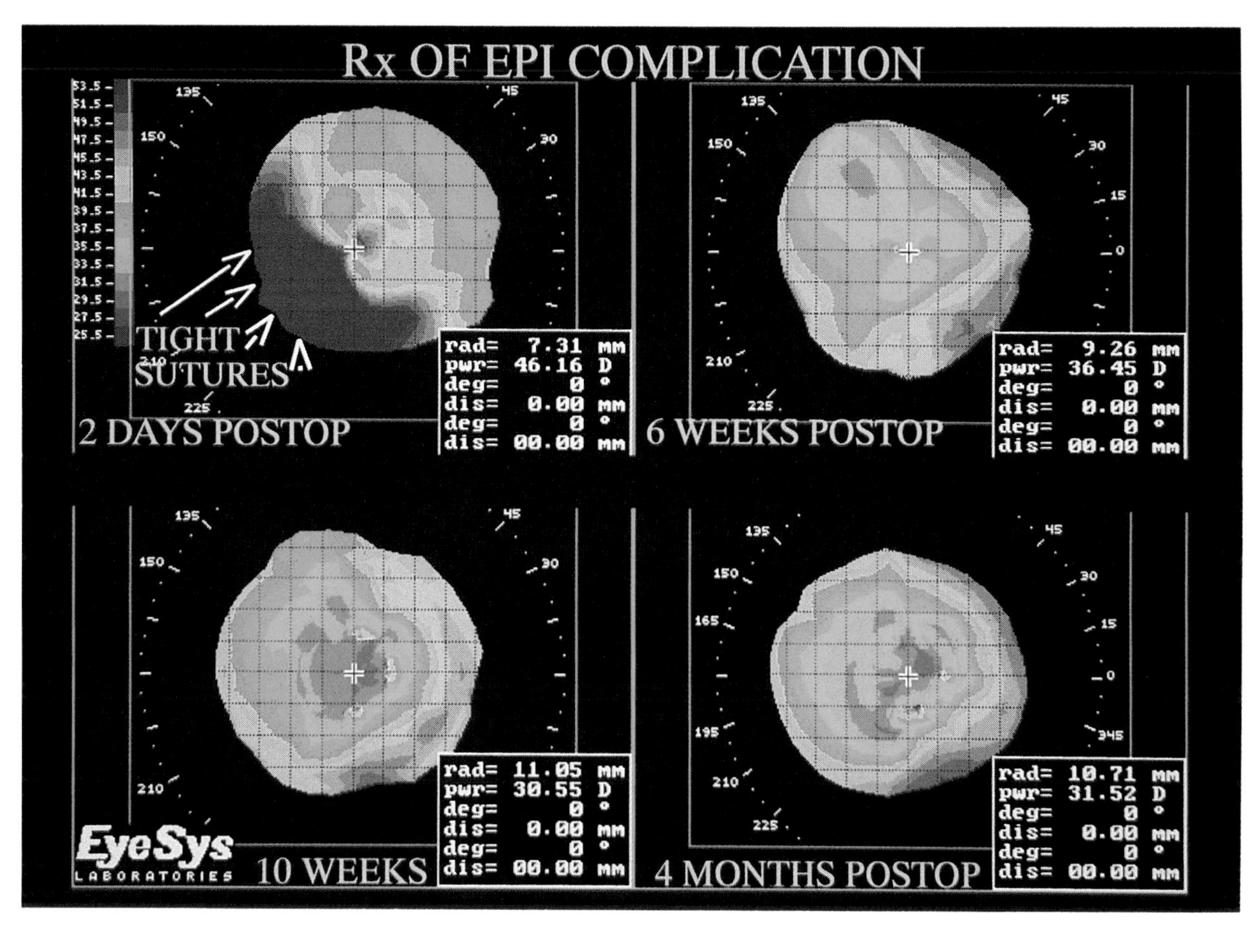

Figure 6.22: Upper left, immediate postoperative appearance after treatment of epithelial invasion of epikeratophakia graft-host interface. There is asymmetric astigmatism with a biphasic cornea due to four interrupted sutures at 190°, 200°, 210° and 220° responsible for the steep curvature of this hemimeridian. Upper right, 6 weeks postoperative. The optical zone is reappearing, but is decentered after cutting the sutures. Lower images, result after recentering the epikeratoplasty lens (courtesy Dr. S. Ganem, Paris, France).

Summary

The survey of the corneal topographic findings with the refractive procedures discussed above demonstrates the usefulness of videokeratography in understanding the effect of these procedures upon the cornea. It is clear that by relying upon keratometry alone the refractive surgeon is literally "flying blind."

All refractive surgeons have experienced the disappointment of apparently well-planned refractive surgery that produced negligible, incomplete or unexpected results. The consideration of corneal topographic data in the planning of surgery may improve the predictability of results, and may begin to explain the occasional treatment failure.

References

1. Thornton SP, Sanders DR: Graded nonintersecting transverse incisions for correction of idiopathic astigmatism. *J Cataract Refract Surg* 13:27-31, 1987.
2. Osher RH: Paired transverse relaxing keratotomy: A combined technique for reducing astigmatism. *J Cataract Refract Surg* 15:32-37, 1989.
3. Davison JA: Transverse astigmatic keratotomy combined with phacoemulsification and intraocular lens implantation. *J Cataract Refract Surg* 15:38-44, 1989.
4. Maloney WF, Grindle L, Sanders DR, et al: Astigmatism control for the cataract surgeon: A comprehensive review of surgically tailored astigmatism reduction (STAR). *J Cataract Refract Surg* 15:45-54, 1989.
5. Shepherd JR: Correction of preexisting astigmatism at the time of small incision cataract surgery. *J Cataract Refract Surg* 15:55-57, 1989.
6. Agapitos PJ, Lindstrom RL, Williams PA, et al: Analysis of astigmatic keratotomy. *J Cataract Refract Surg* 15:13-18, 1989.
7. Maloney WF, Sanders DR, Pearcy DE: Astigmatic keratotomy to correct preexisting astigmatism in cataract patients. *J Cataract Refract Surg* 16:297-304, 1990.

7

DANIEL S. DURRIE, MD
TIMOTHY B. CAVANAUGH, MD
MICHAEL VRABEC, MD

Corneal Topography With Excimer Laser Photorefractive Keratectomy

The use of corneal topography in the preoperative evaluation and in the centration of excimer laser photorefractive keratectomy (PRK) was discussed in Chapter 5. This chapter will focus on the relationship between corneal topography and the refractive effects of PRK.

Patterns of Healing

We have observed three patterns of healing of excimer laser PRK procedures, documented by slit lamp observation, that affect the rate and extent of refractive and corneal topographic changes. All patients described below received the same postoperative steroid treatment.

Type I

The first pattern, which we refer to as Type I healing, occurs in approximately 85% of cases. It is characterized by a progression of a fairly normal amount of healing corneal haze which peaks at about 3 months and then begins to resolve. It is best seen in a diffuse beam brought in from the side (Figures 7.1A-D) and can be masked with direct focal illumination (Figures 7.2A-D).

The topographic findings for the case shown in Figures 7.1 and 7.2 are shown in Figure 7.3. The attempted correction was -3 D, and the patient had a refraction of plano at all postoperative visits. Readings at the mouse cursor centered at vertex normal or the videokeratographic (VK) axis corroborate that the desired correction of approximately 3 D was obtained, although there appeared to be multifocal areas of the central cornea most obvious at 1 and 3 months. Type I healing is usually characterized by a hyperopic shift at 1 month post-treatment which typically regresses to the desired effect at 3 to 6 months. This refractive pattern is seen better in the next case (Figures 7.4A-D, 7.5, and 7.6) where central corneal power

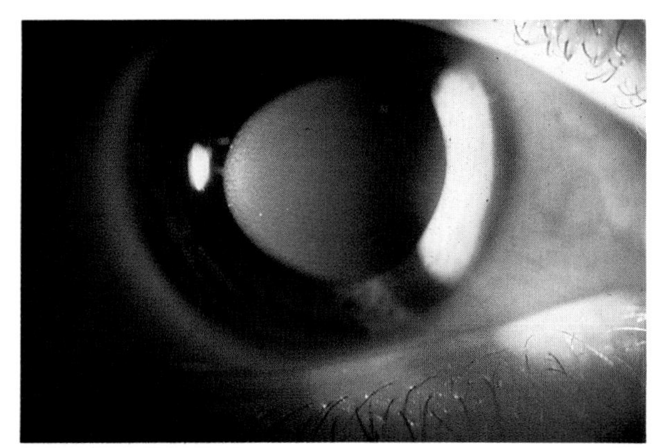

Figure 7.1A.

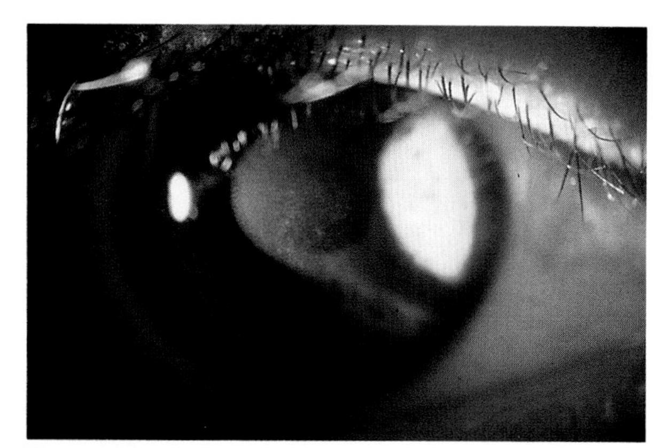

Figure 7.1B.

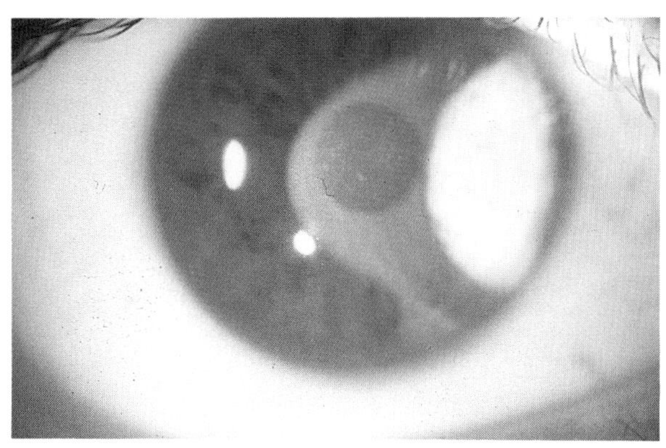

Figure 7.1C.

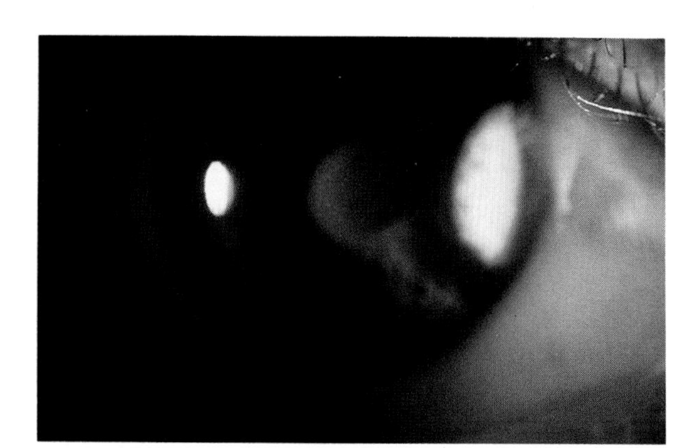

Figure 7.1D.

Figure 7.1: Appearance of Type I healing characterized by corneal haze which peaks at about 3 months. Illumination is provided by a diffuse beam coming in from the periphery. (A) Pre-PRK appearance, (B) 1 month post-PRK, (C) 3 months post-PRK, and (D) 6 months post-PRK.

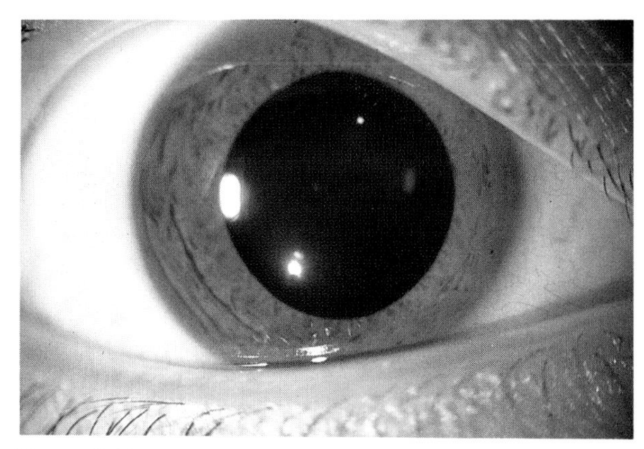

Figure 7.2A.

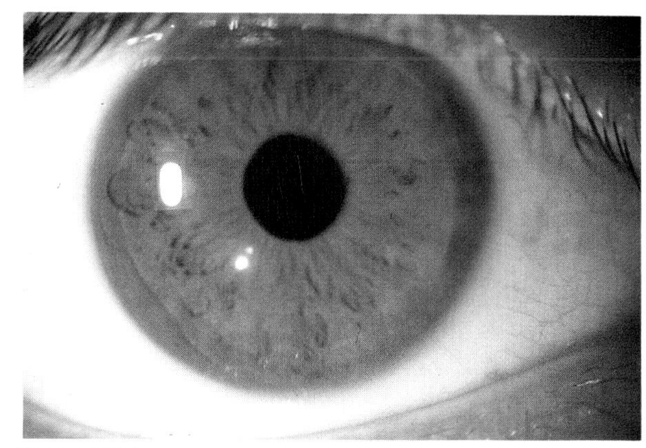

Figure 7.2B.

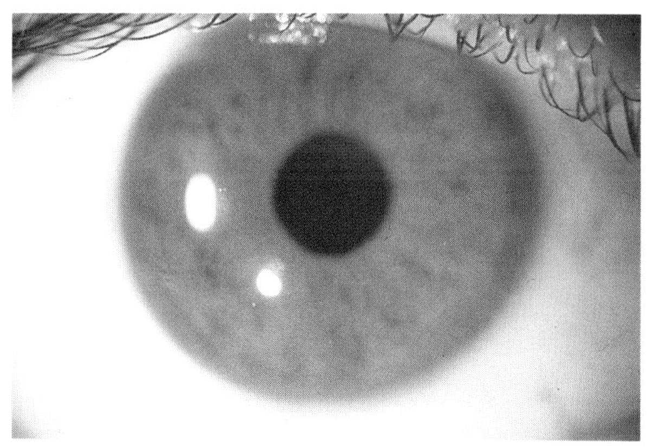

Figure 7.2C.

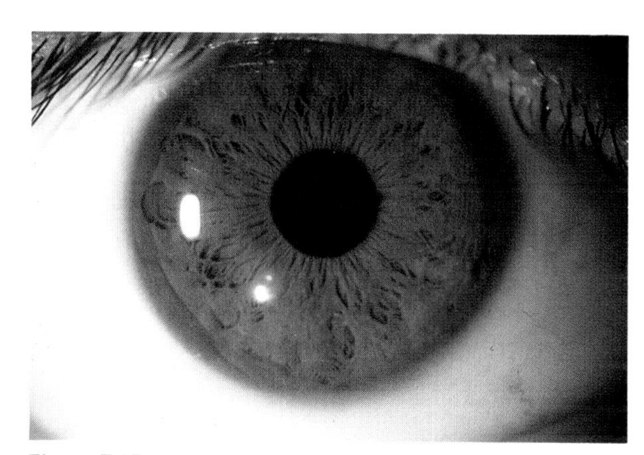

Figure 7.2D.

Figure 7.2: Same eye and time periods as Figure 7.1, but direct focal illumination masks the corneal haze. (A) Pre-PRK appearance, (B) 1 month post-PRK, (C) 3 months post-PRK, and (D) 6 months post-PRK.

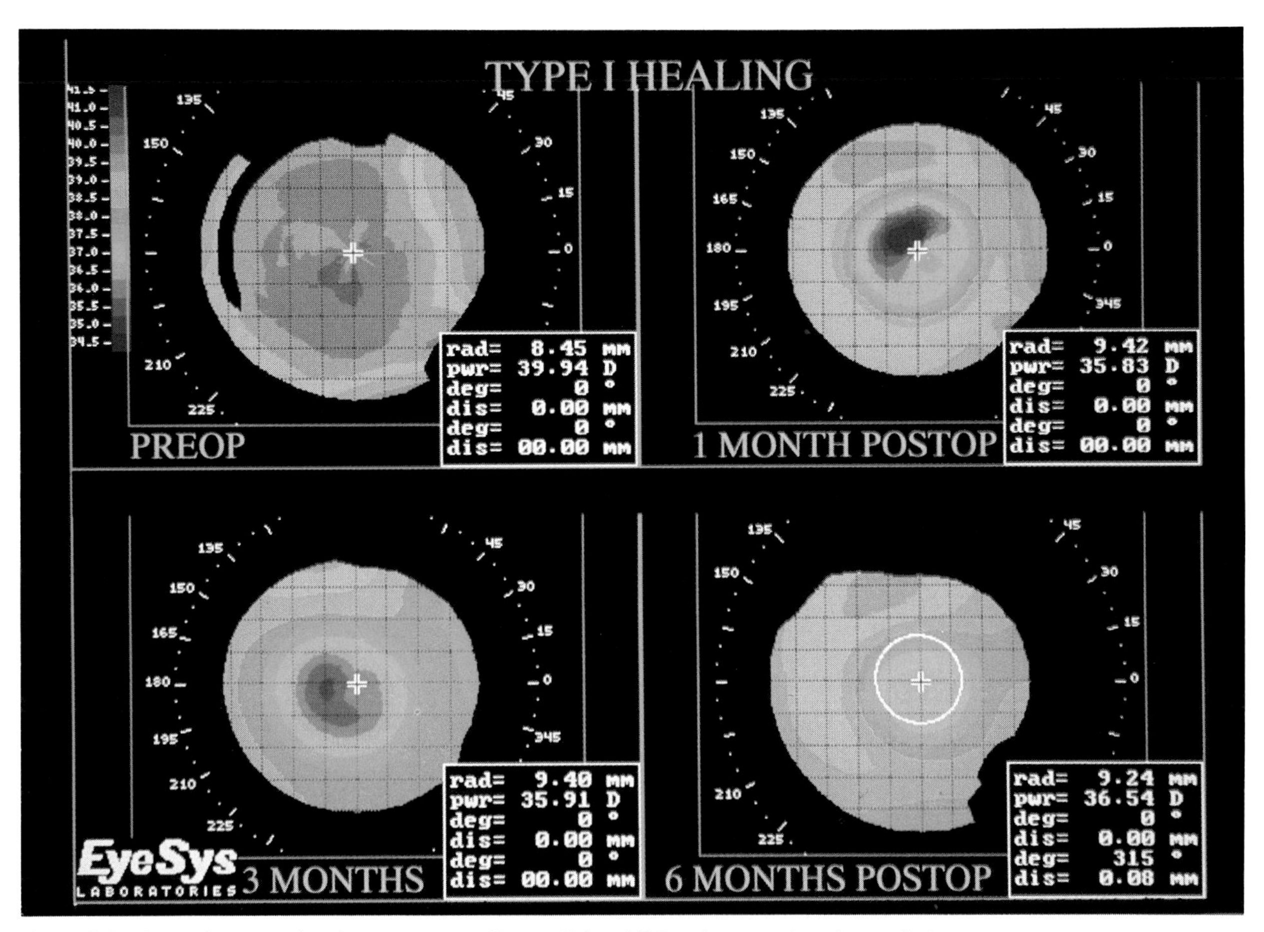

Figure 7.3: Corneal topography of same case as Figures 7.1 and 7.2 at the same four time periods.

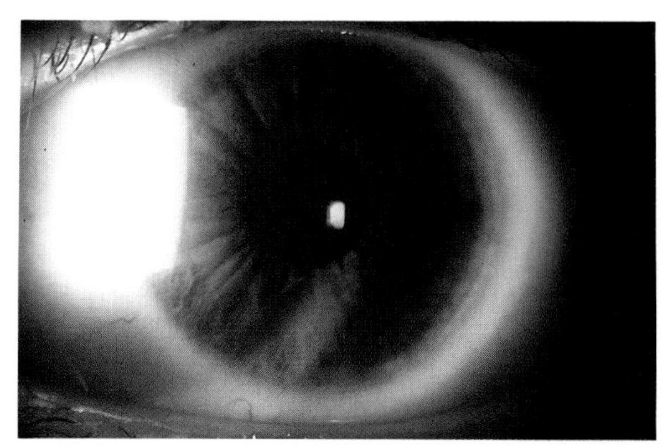
Figure 7.4A.

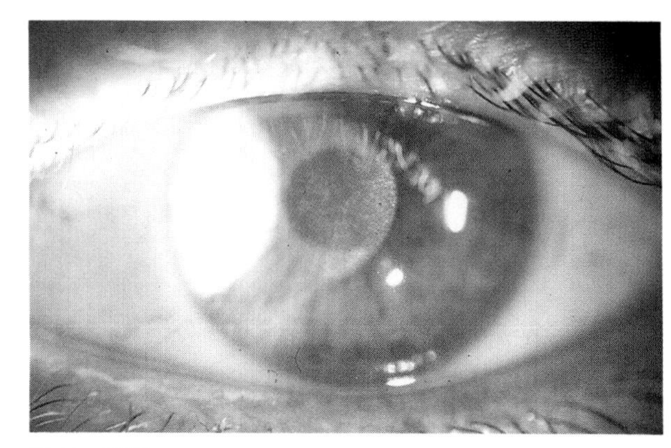
Figure 7.4B.

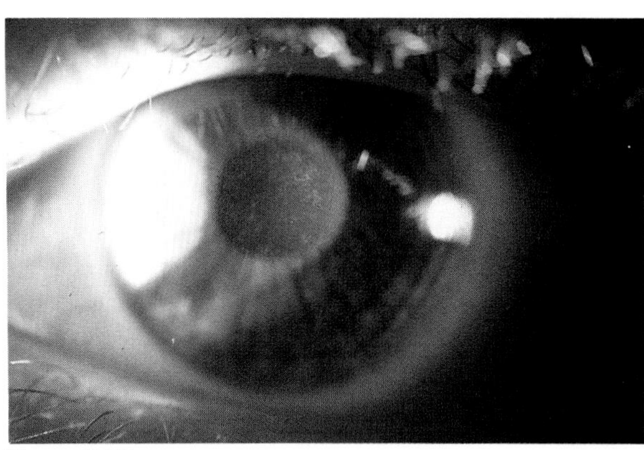
Figure 7.4C.

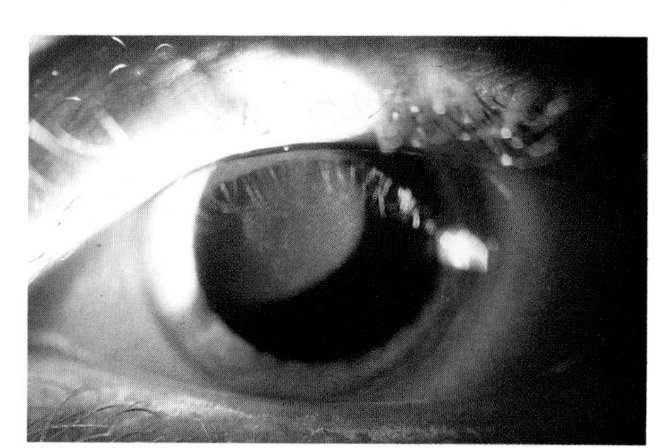
Figure 7.4D.

Figure 7.4: Appearance of Type I healing, diffuse peripheral illumination. (A) Pre-PRK, (B) 1 month post-PRK, (C) 3 months post-PRK, (D) 6 months post-PRK.

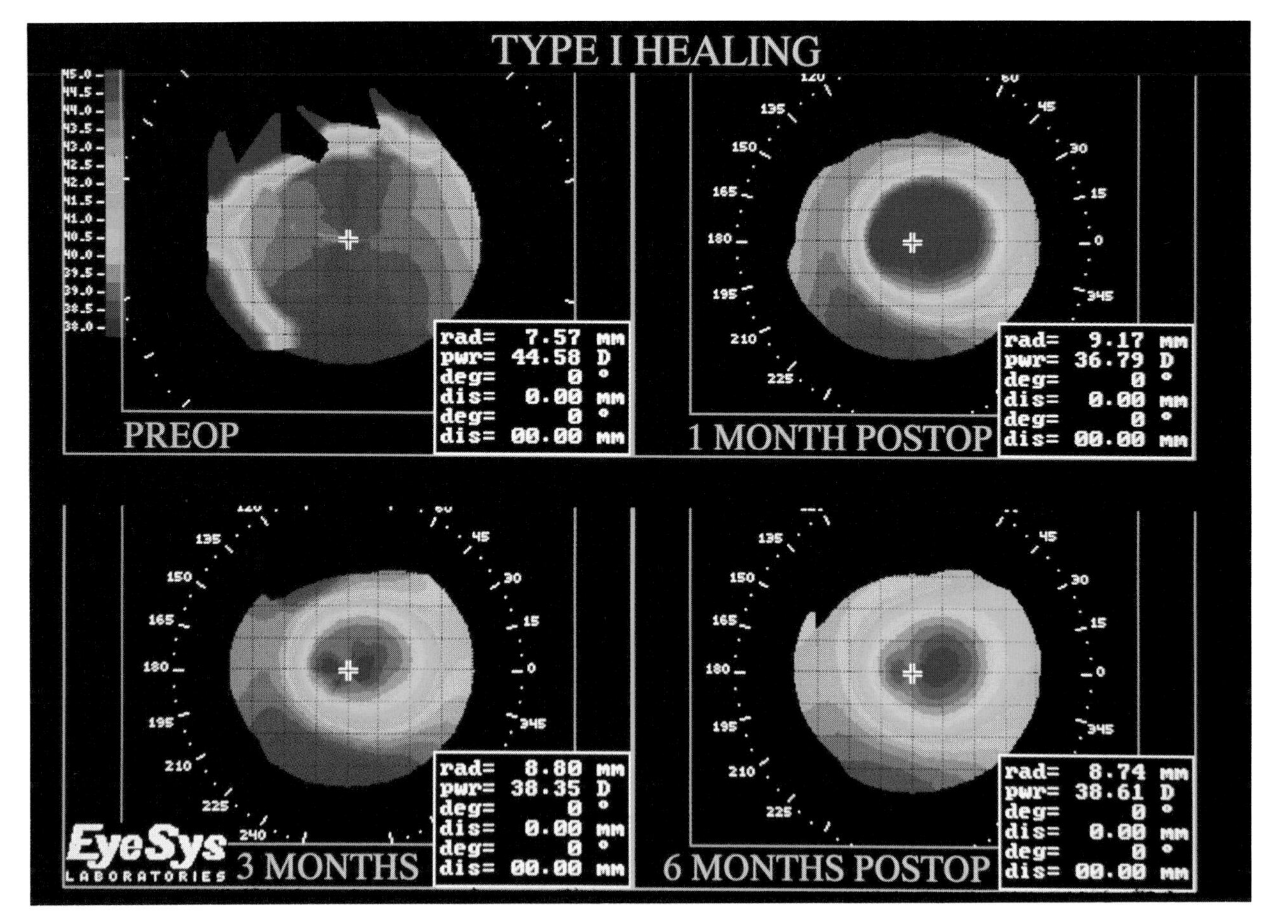

Figure 7.5: Corneal topography of same case as Figure 7.4 at same four time periods. Note that the excimer ablation is somewhat decentered relative to the videokeratographic axis. Irregular blue areas in the pre-treatment map are unedited artifacts.

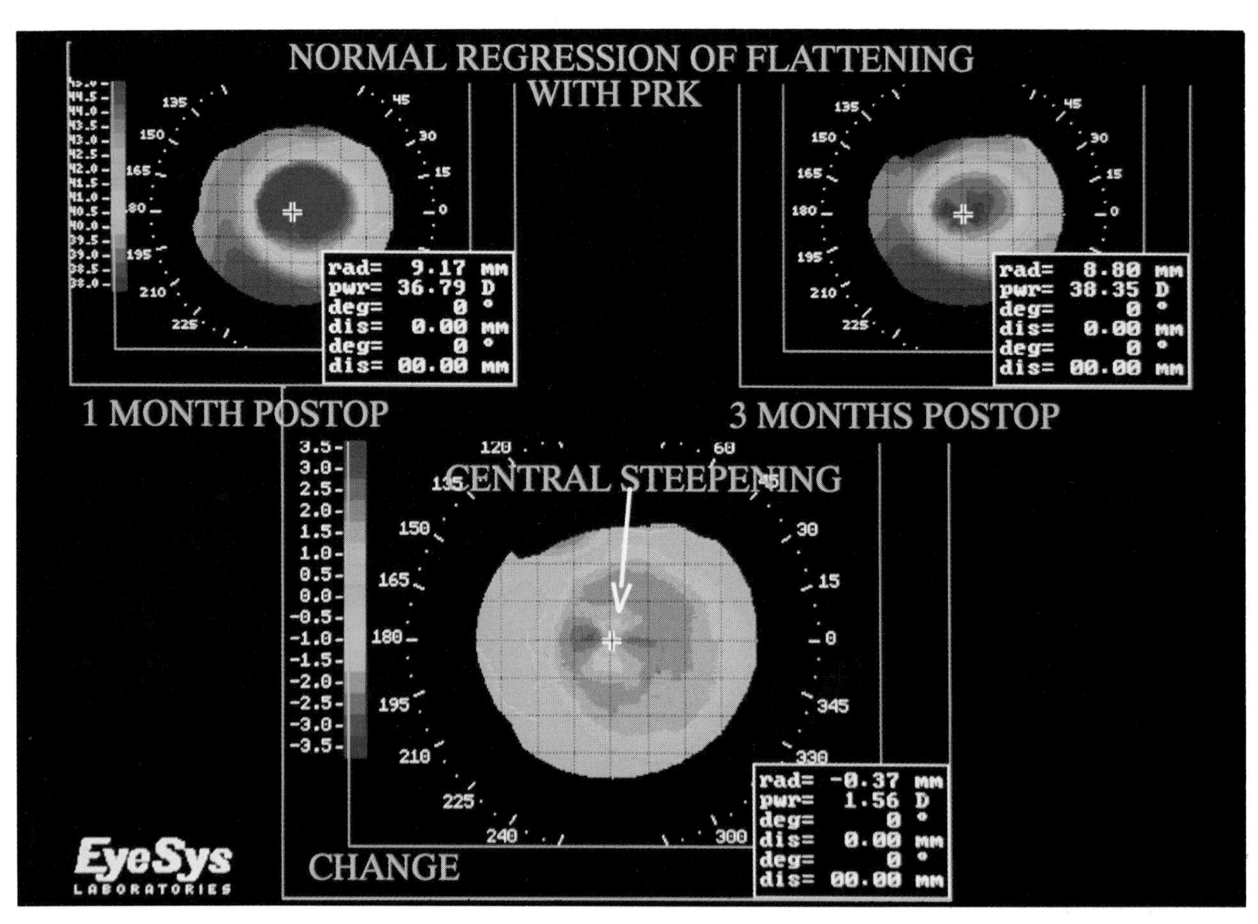

Figure 7.6: Normal regression of flattening effect between 1 month and 3 month post-PRK with Type I healing. This effect is best seen as steepening in the change graph (bottom).

is 36.79 D at 1 month which changes to 38.35 D at 3 months. The patient was 0.5 D hyperopic at 3 months and was plano with 20/16 uncorrected vision at 6 months.

Type II

The second pattern, or Type II healing, includes those patients that we refer to as slow healers; they constitute approximately 10% of cases and do not present a normal healing haze but remain relatively clear throughout the post-treatment period (Figures 7.7A-D). These cases typically are hyperopic at 1 month and retain their hyperopia, regressing much more slowly. The case shown in Figures 7.7 and 7.8 was 2 D overcorrected at 1 month and remained approximately 1 D overcorrected at 6 months. Figure 7.9 is a corneal topography study of another case with Type II healing. This case was 3 D overcorrected at 1 month and still had a residual overcorrection of 1.5 D at 3 months. Both cases had residual hyperopia at 3 to 6 months.

Type III

The third pattern of healing, or Type III, includes patients who appear to overreact, producing much more than normal haze and, in fact, frequently producing subepithelial fibrosis and scarring (Figure 7.10A-D). Such cases show significant regression of effect. Figure 7.11 demonstrates the corneal topographic changes with time which correlated very well with refractive outcome. The patient was 1.5 D hyperopic at the 1 month visit but by the 3 month visit he was 2.0 D myopic and at 6 months was 2.5 D myopic. This dramatic regression of effect is best seen with the change graph (Figure 7.12). Another case with Type III healing had significant corneal haze (Figures 7.13A-D, 7.14A-D) and almost total loss of correction by 6 months post excimer treatment (Figure 7.15). Interestingly, this case was retreated with the subepithelial fibrosis removed and experienced a much decreased haze response with the second treatment (Figures 7.16A-C, 7.17), which resulted in an excellent visual and refractive response: 20/25 uncorrected vision with a +0.50 − 0.75 × 25 correction and 20/16 uncorrected vision at 1 year post-retreatment.

In summary then, the normal Type I healing pattern has a trace corneal haze maximum at about 3 months which results in a stable predictable correction at the 3-6 month period. The Type II healing pattern has a clear cornea throughout the healing phase at six months and is usually overcorrected. The Type III pattern has increased haze and will usually be markedly undercorrected.

Excimer with Undercorrected RK

We have had some experience treating undercorrected radial keratotomy (RK) cases with the excimer. In the first case (Figures 7.18A, B), the post-RK pre-PRK topography (Figure 7.19 left) demonstrates that the cornea is flatter centrally with some residual astigmatism. The 1 month post-PRK appearance demonstrates a profound central flattening with a large flat zone. In another case (Figures 7.20A, B), topography reveals little evidence of effect from RK (Figure 7.21 left) and again an excellent effect from the PRK (Figure 7.21 right).

Excimer for Spherical Correction Does Not Correct Astigmatism

Our excimer laser as it is presently configured can only affect spherical correction. In Figure 7.22, the plus cylinder is present in axis 100 in a somewhat asymmet-

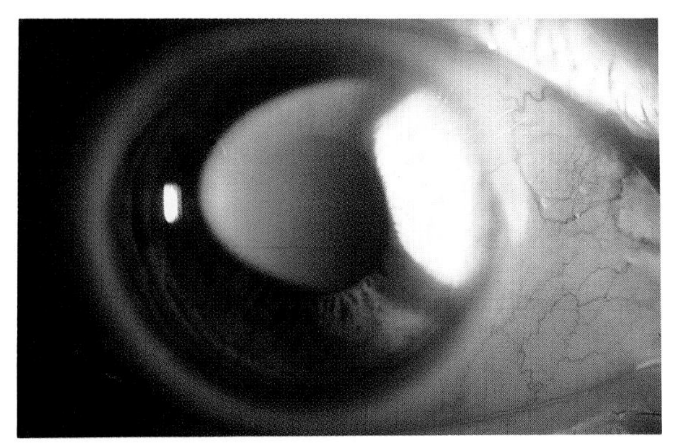

Figure 7.7A.

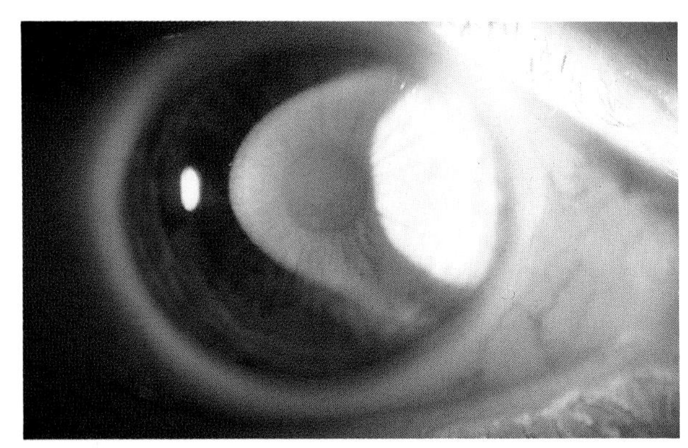

Figure 7.7B.

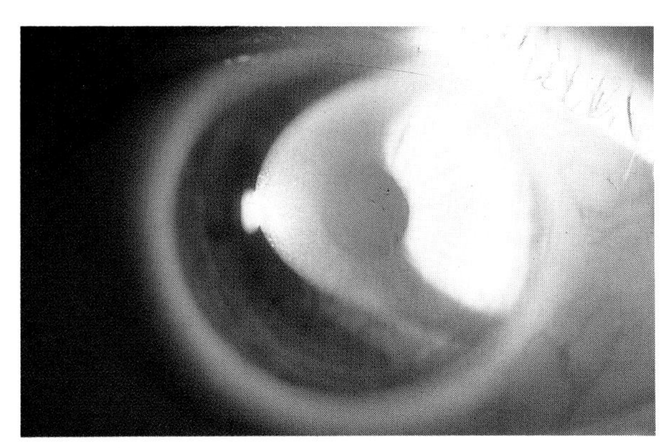

Figure 7.7C.

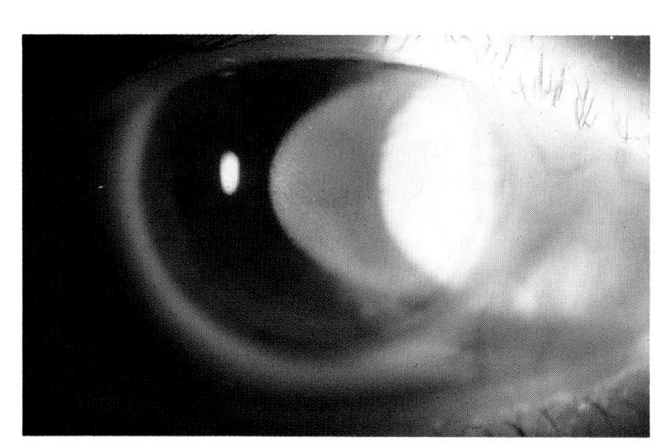

Figure 7.7D.

Figure 7.7: Appearance of Type II healing. (A) Pre-PRK, (B) 1 month post-PRK, (C) 3 months post-PRK, and (D) 6 months post-PRK.

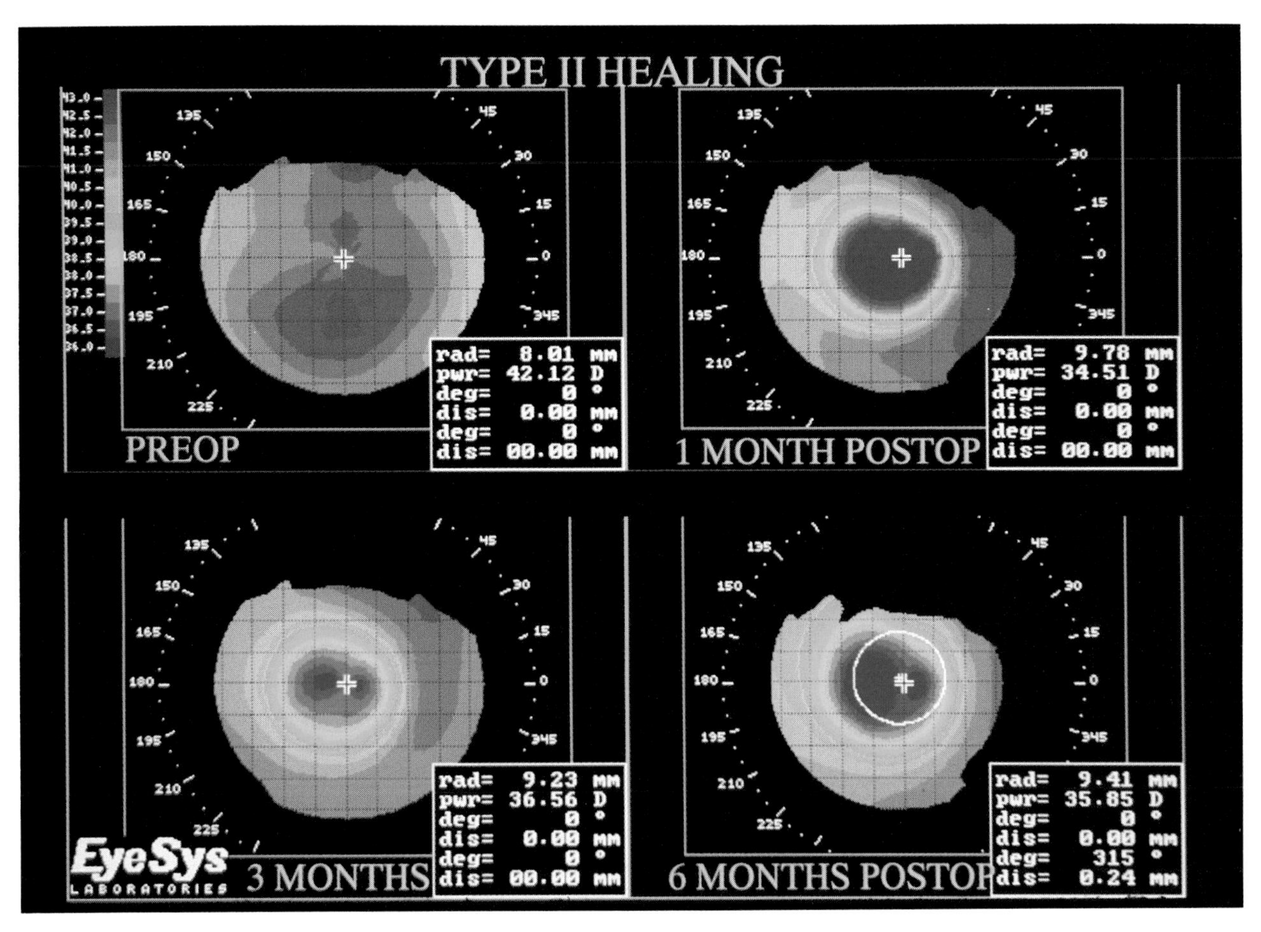

Figure 7.8: Corneal topography of same case as Figure 7.7 at same four time periods.

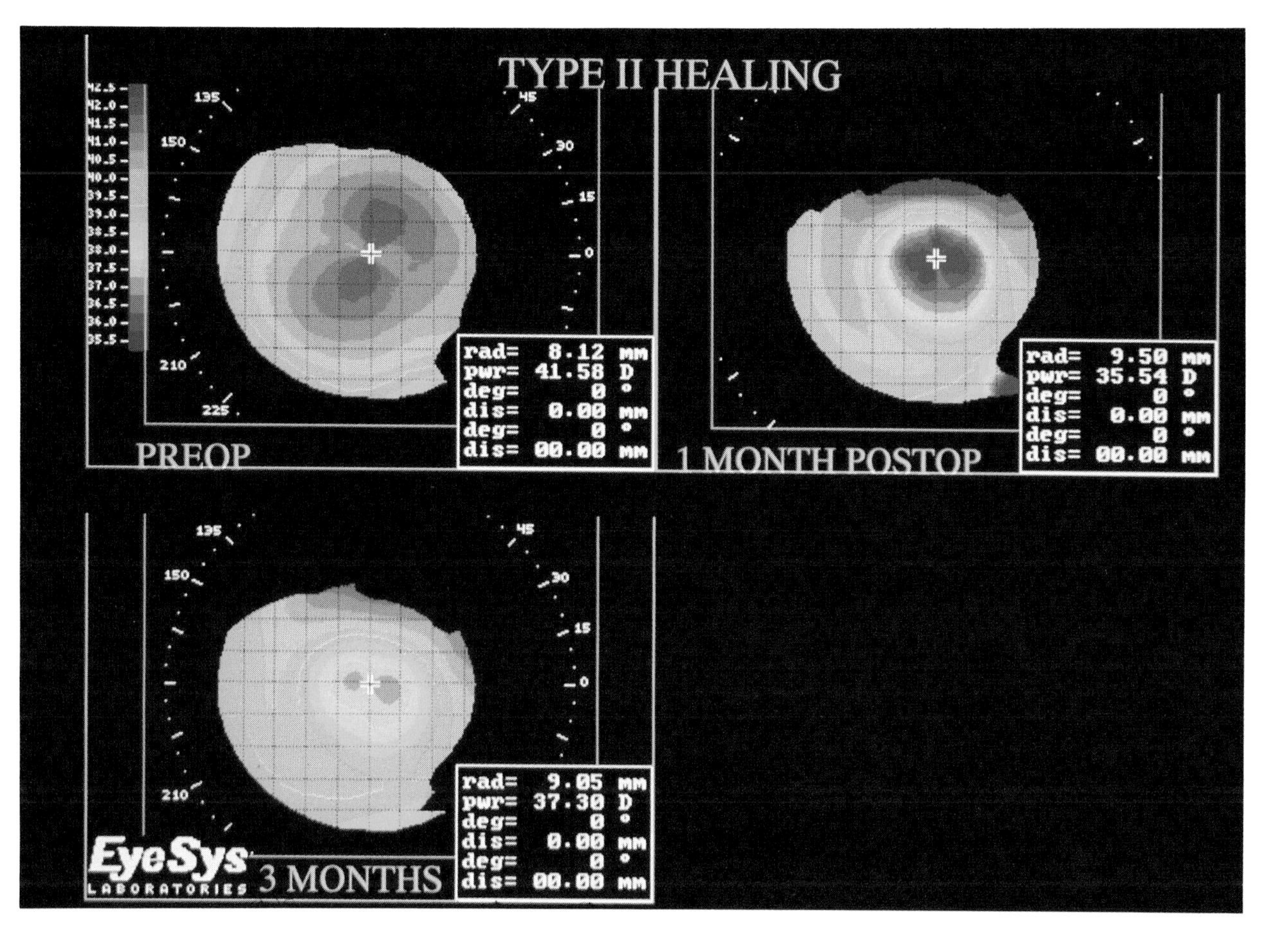

Figure 7.9: Corneal topography of case with Type II healing.

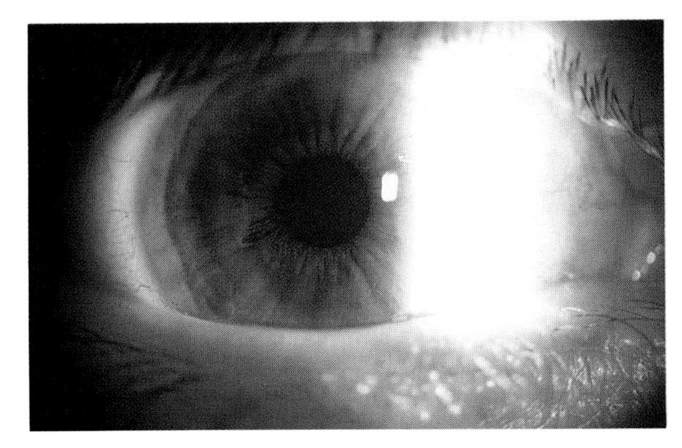

Figure 7.10A.

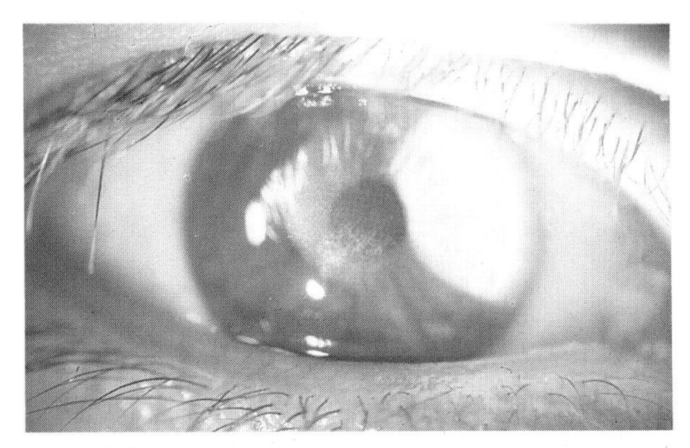

Figure 7.10B.

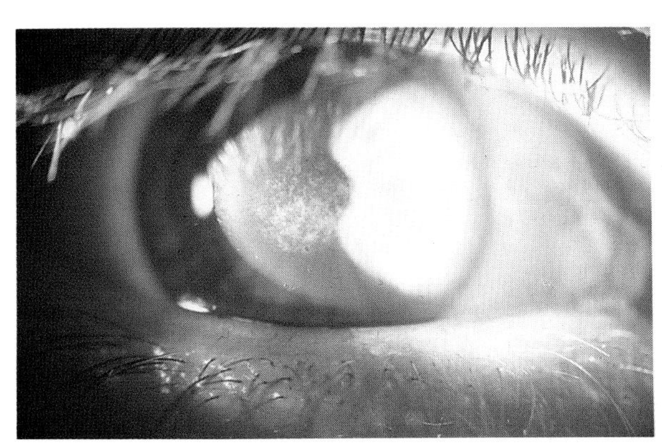

Figure 7.10C.

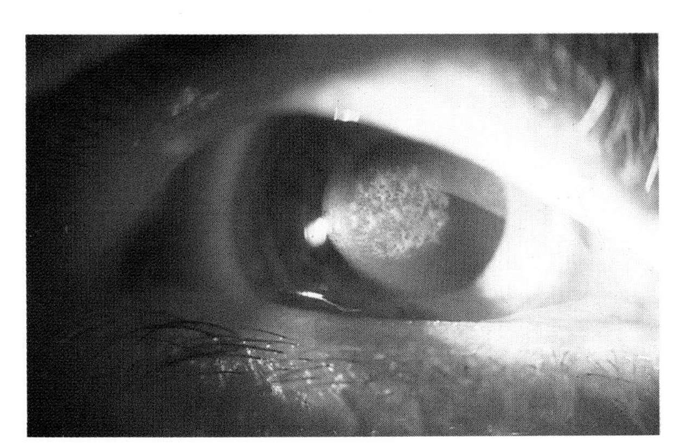

Figure 7.10D.

Figure 7.10: Appearance of Type III healing. (A) Pre-PRK, (B) 1 month post-PRK, (C) 3 months post-PRK, and (D) 6 months post-PRK.

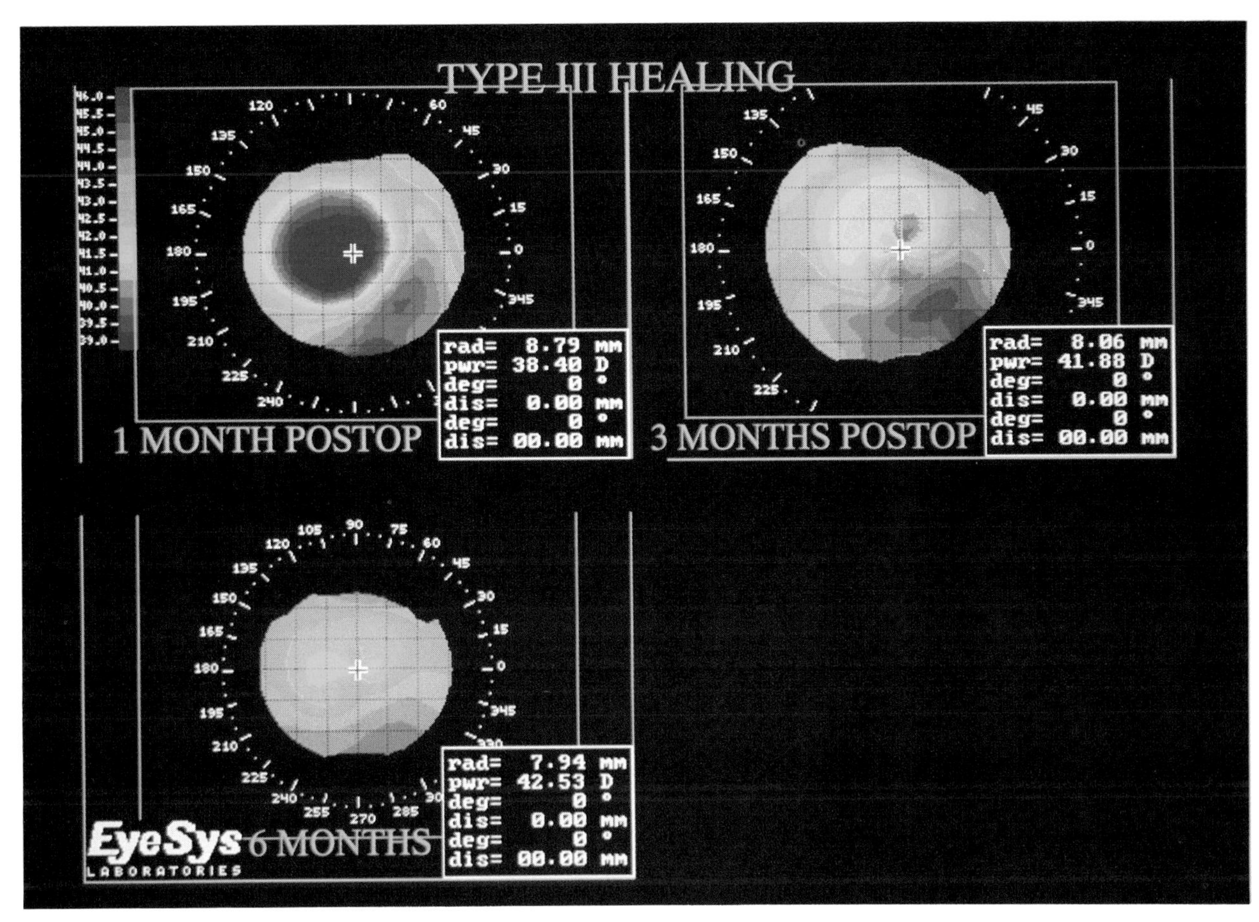

Figure 7.11: Corneal topography of same case as Figure 7.10. No pre-treatment topography was taken.

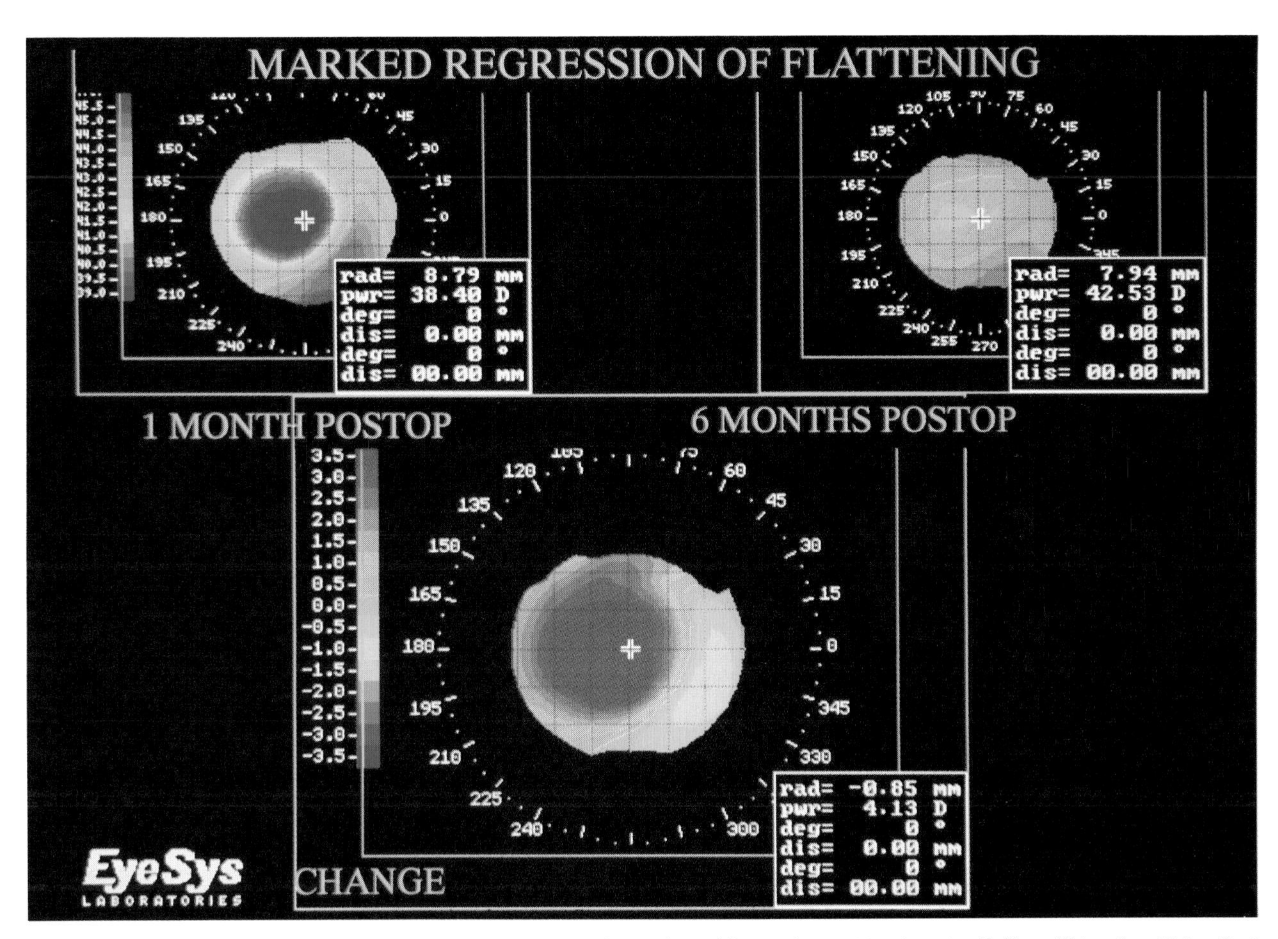

Figure 7.12: Marked regression of flattening effect between 1 month and 6 months post-treatment with Type III healing. This effect is best seen as steepening in the change graph (bottom).

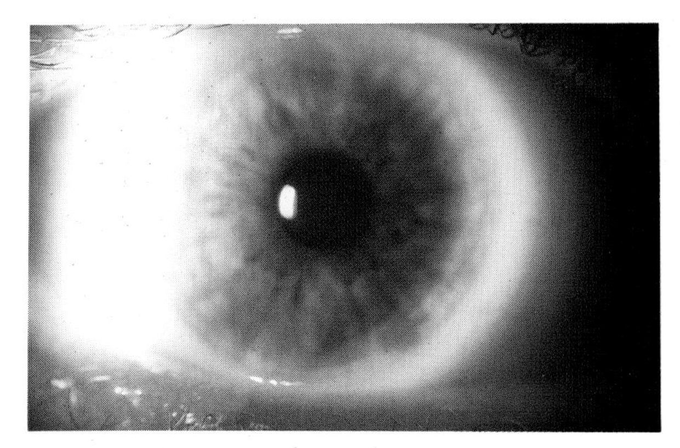

Figure 7.13A.

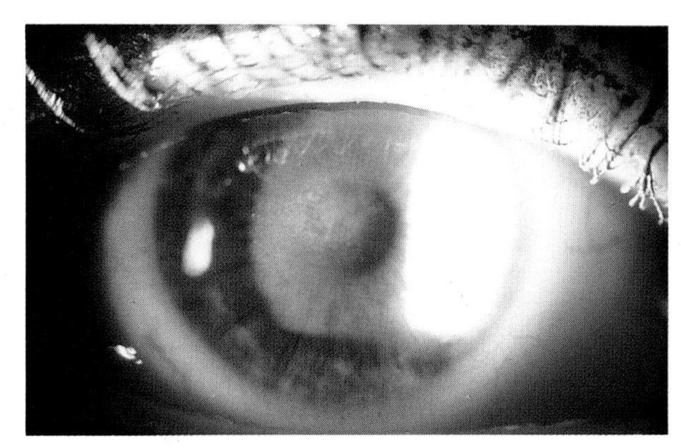

Figure 7.13B.

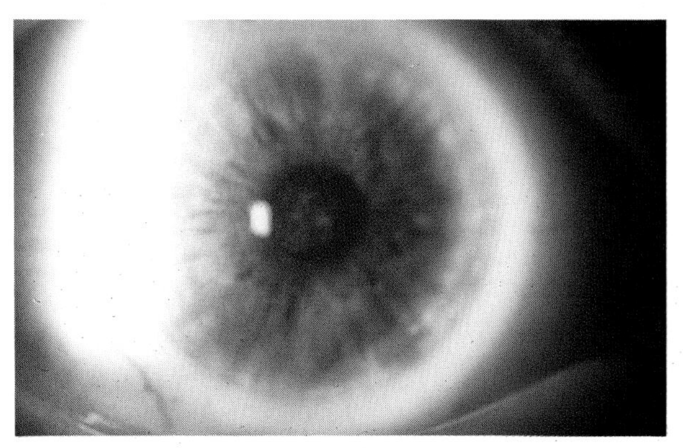

Figure 7.13C.

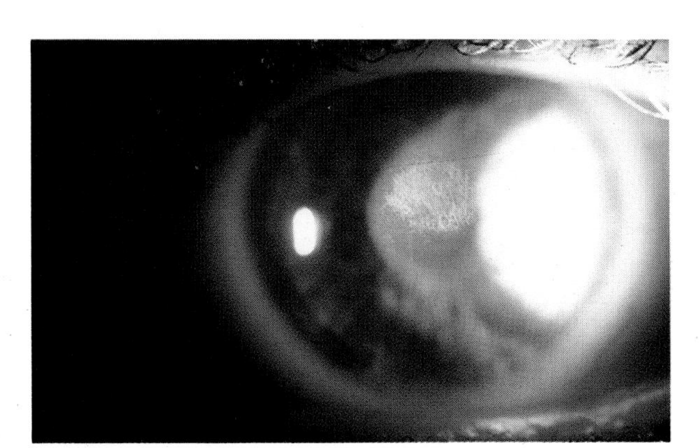

Figure 7.13D.

Figure 7.13: Case with Type III healing. (A) Pre-PRK, (B) 1 month post-PRK, (C) 3 months post-PRK, and (D) 6 months post-PRK.

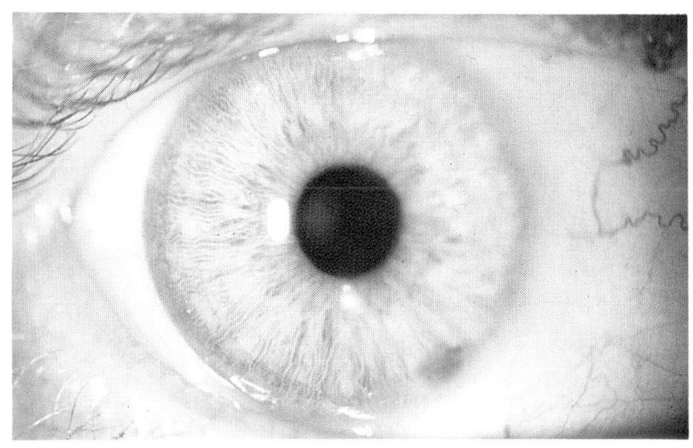

Figure 7.14A.

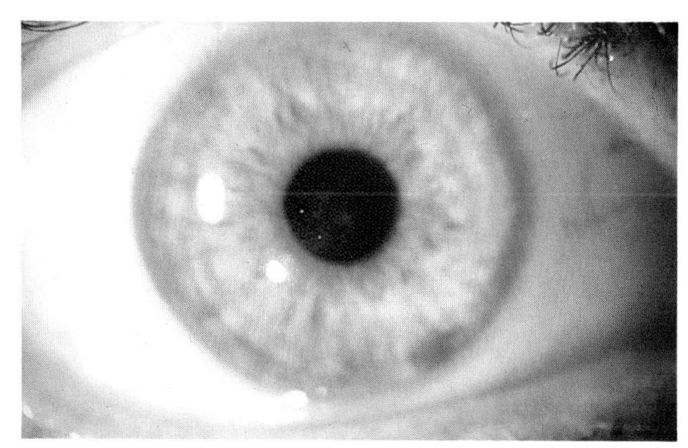

Figure 7.14B.

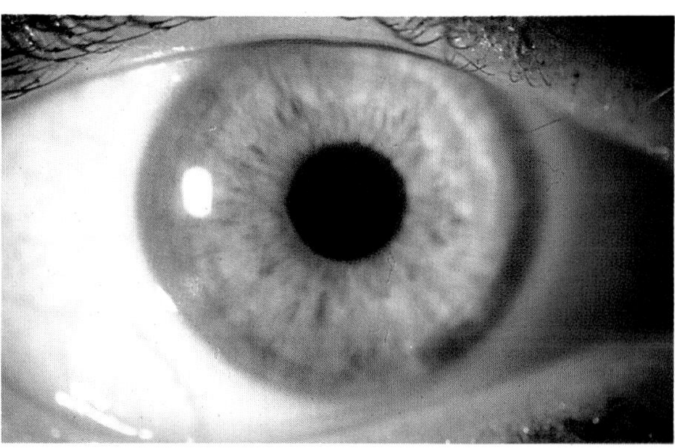

Figure 7.14C.

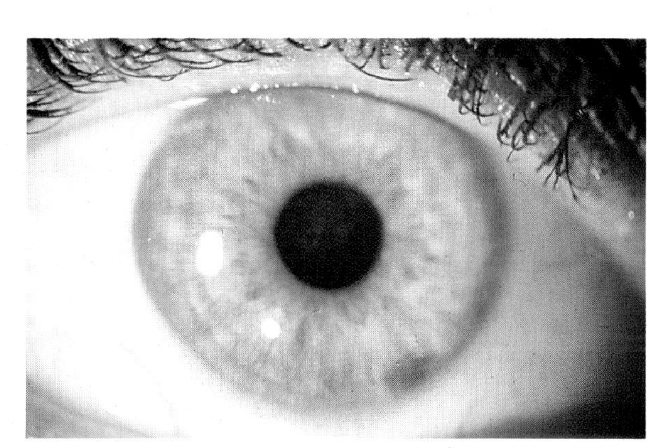

Figure 7.14D.

Figure 7.14: Same case as Figure 7.13 showing how even severe haze can be masked by using direct focal illumination instead of oblique illumination. (A) Pre-PRK, (B) 1 month post-PRK, (C) 3 months post-PRK, and (D) 6 months post-PRK.

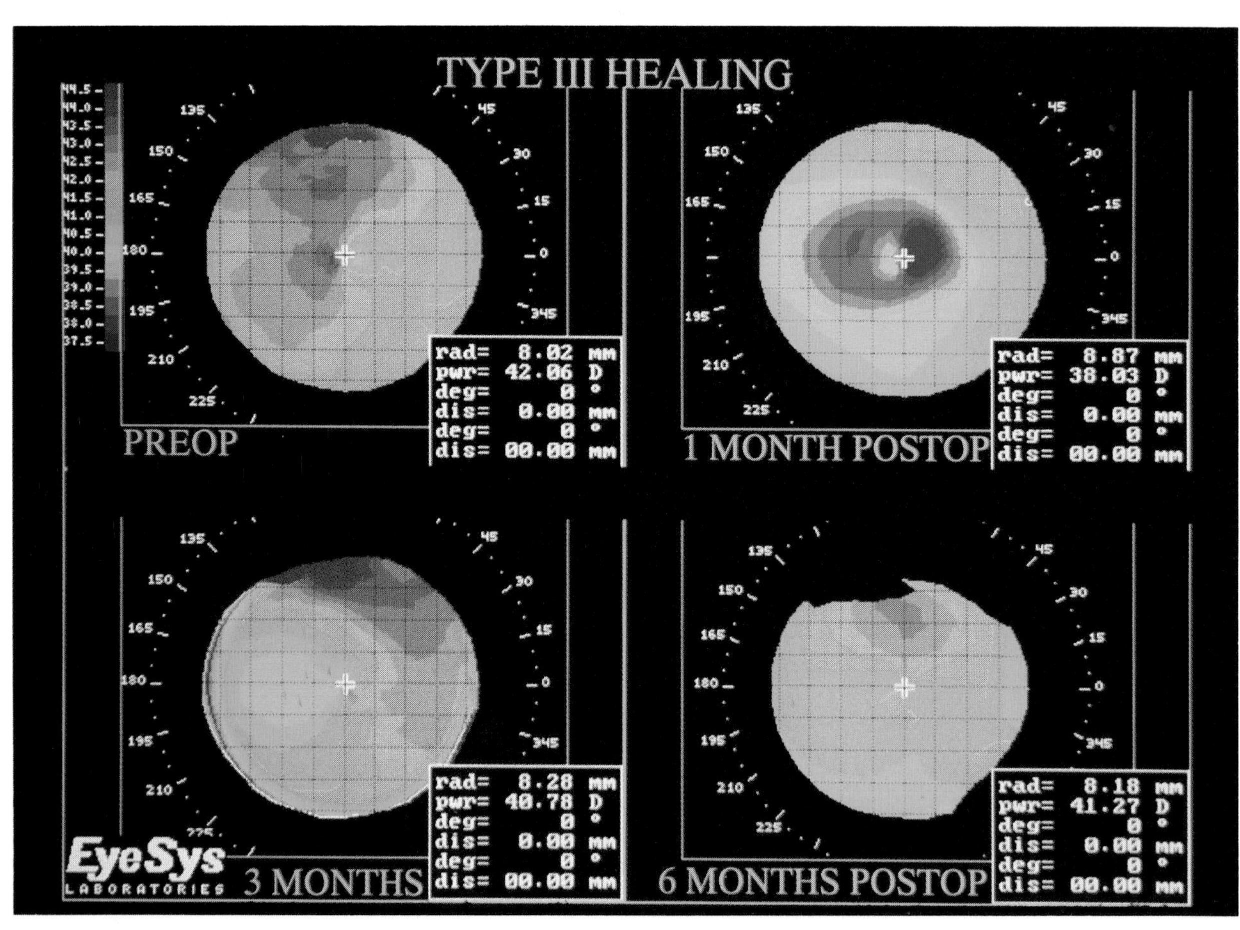

Figure 7.15: Corneal topography of case with Type III corneal healing (same case as Figure 7.13) demonstrating almost complete loss of correction by 6 months post-treatment.

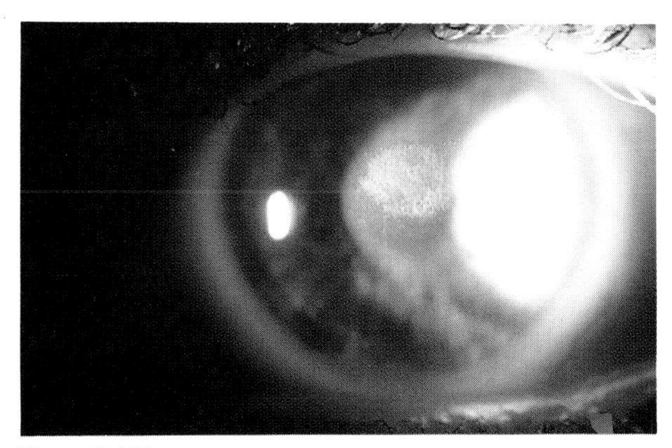

Figure 7.16A.

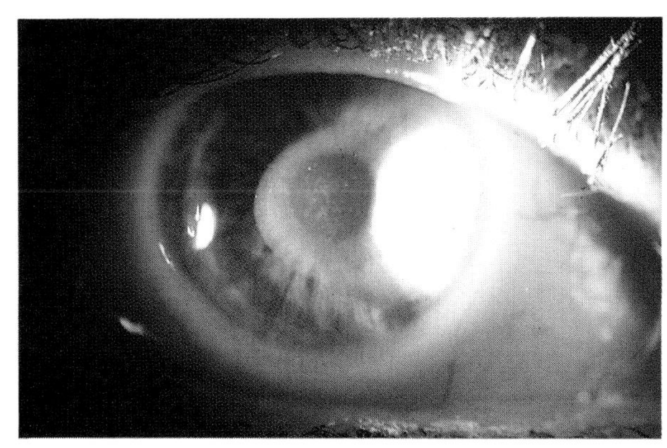

Figure 7.16B.

Figure 7.16: Same case and method of illumination as Figure 7.13. (A) Pre-PRK retreatment (same photo as Figure 7.13D), (B) 1 month post-PRK retreatment, and (C) 3 months post-PRK retreatment.

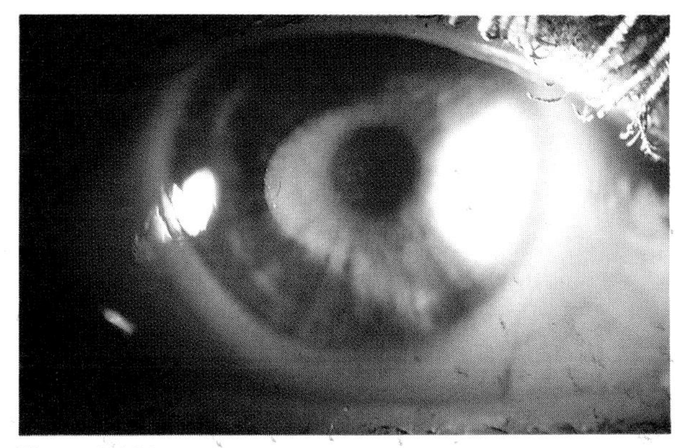

Figure 7.16C.

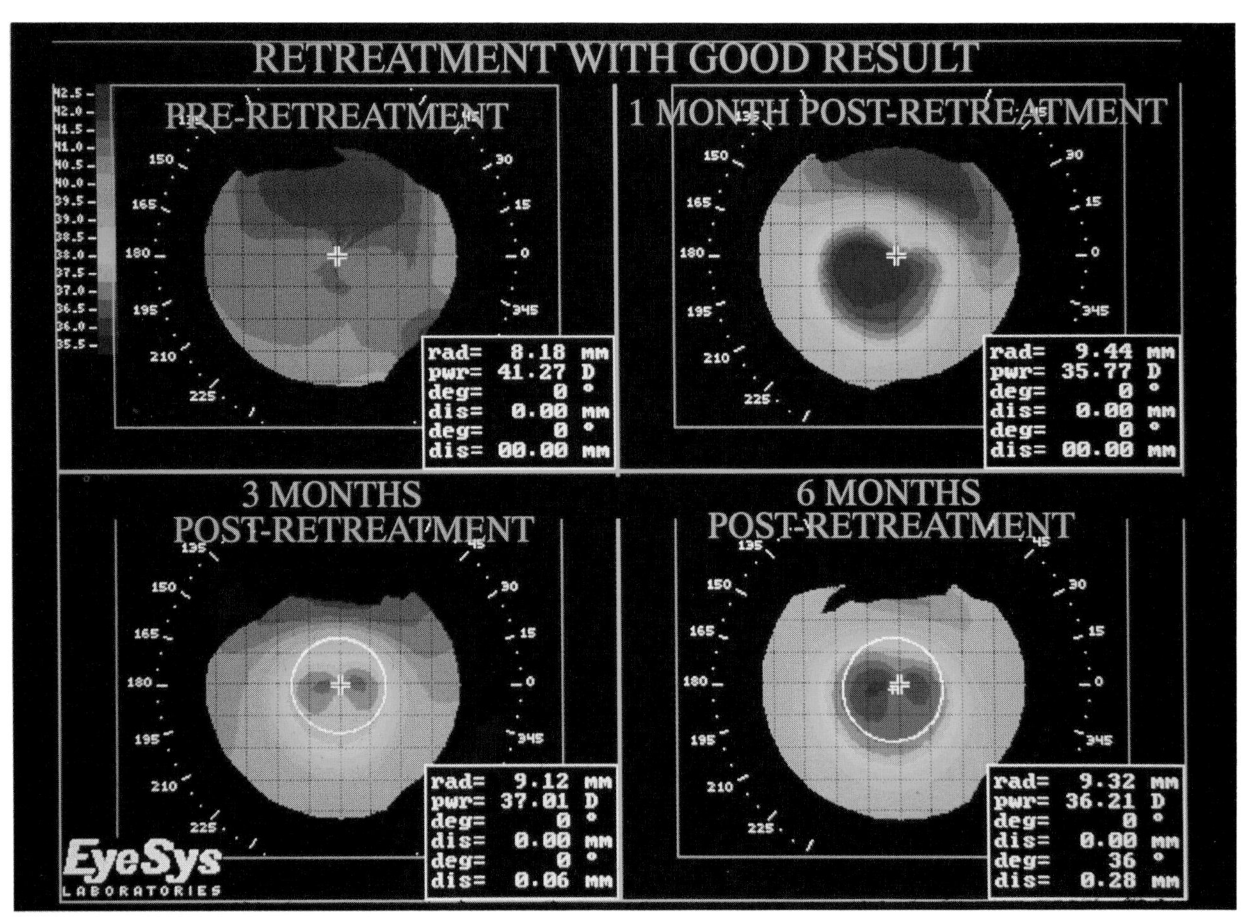

Figure 7.17: Corneal topography of the same case shown in Figure 7.13. Retreatment resulted in significant stable correction.

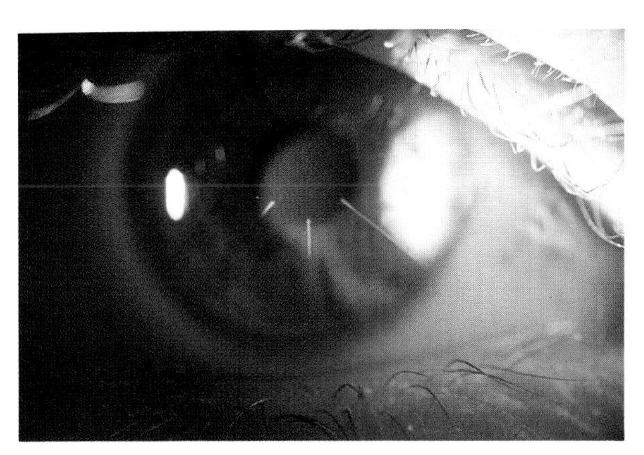

Figure 7.18A.

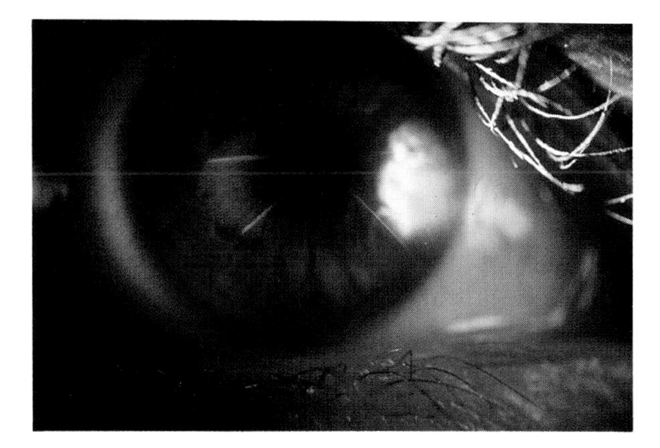

Figure 7.18B.

Figure 7.18: Appearance of undercorrected RK eye treated with PRK. (A) Pre-PRK appearance. (B) One month post-PRK appearance.

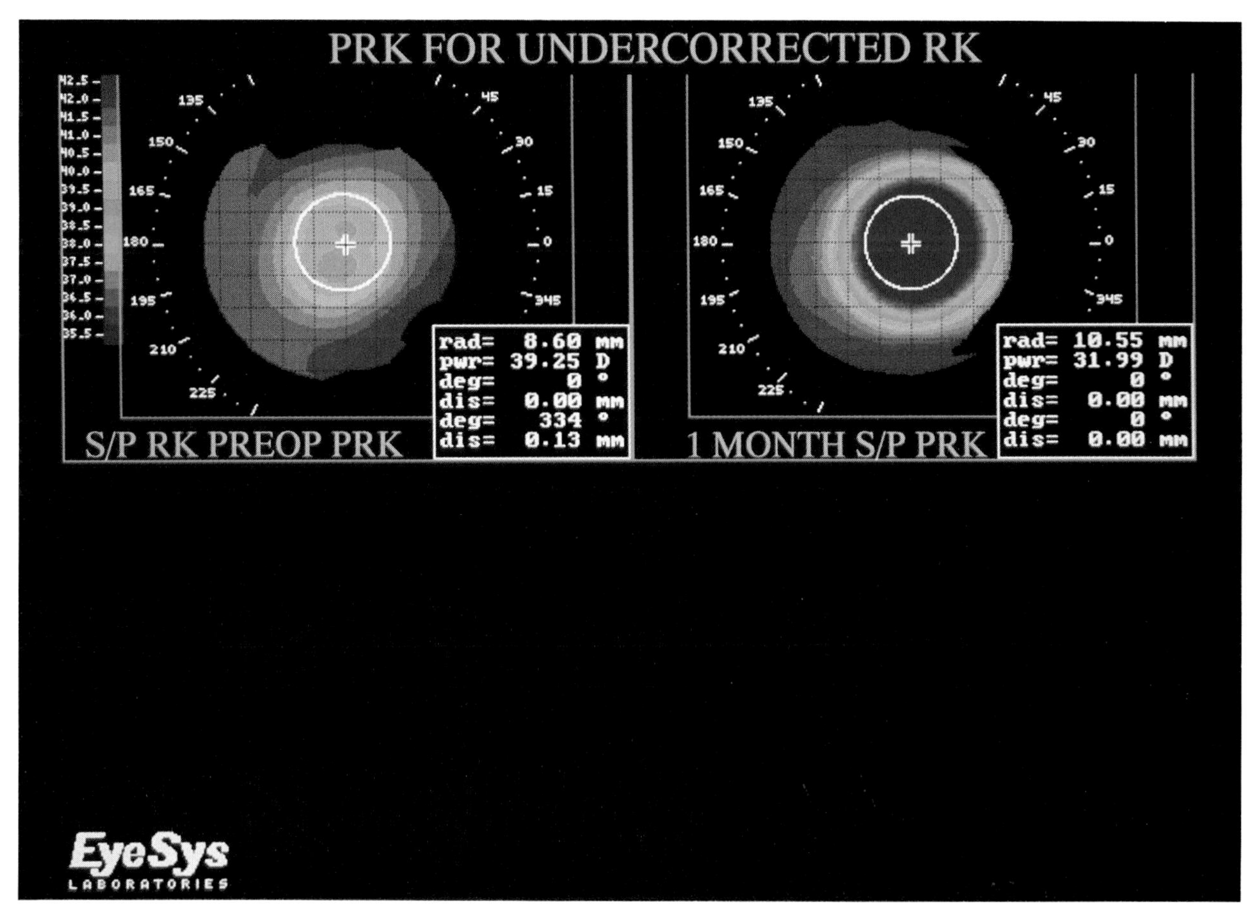

Figure 7.19: Corneal topography of case shown in Figure 7.18.

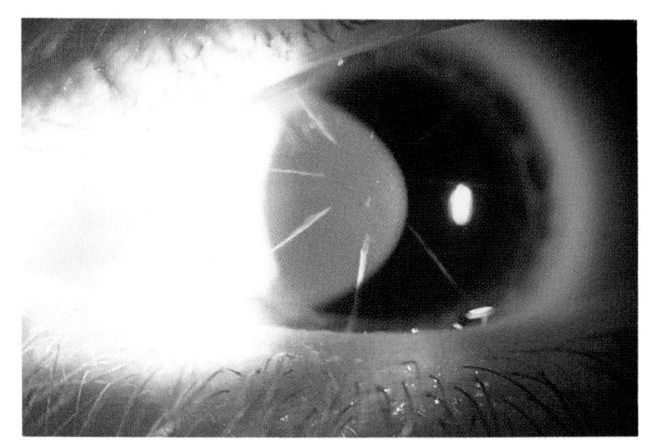

Figure 7.20A.

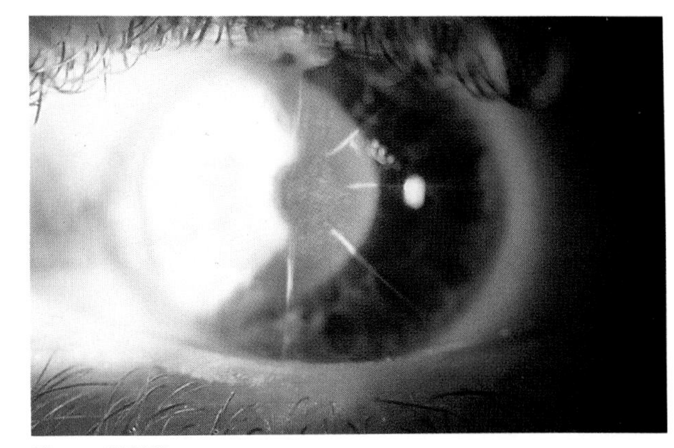

Figure 7.20B.

Figure 7.20: Appearance of undercorrected RK eye treated with PRK. (A) Pre-PRK appearance. (B) One month post-PRK appearance.

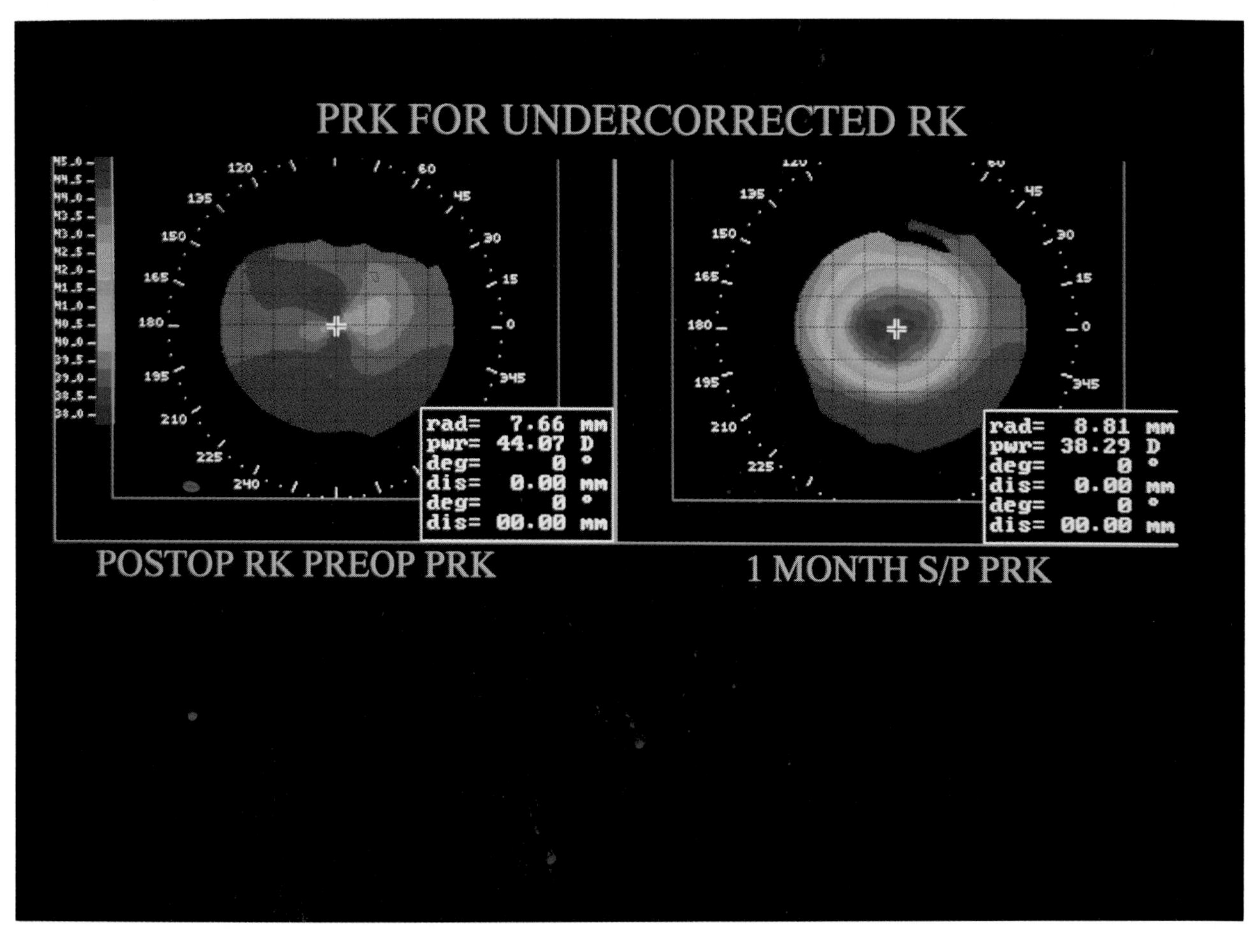

Figure 7.21: Corneal topography of case shown in Figure 7.20.

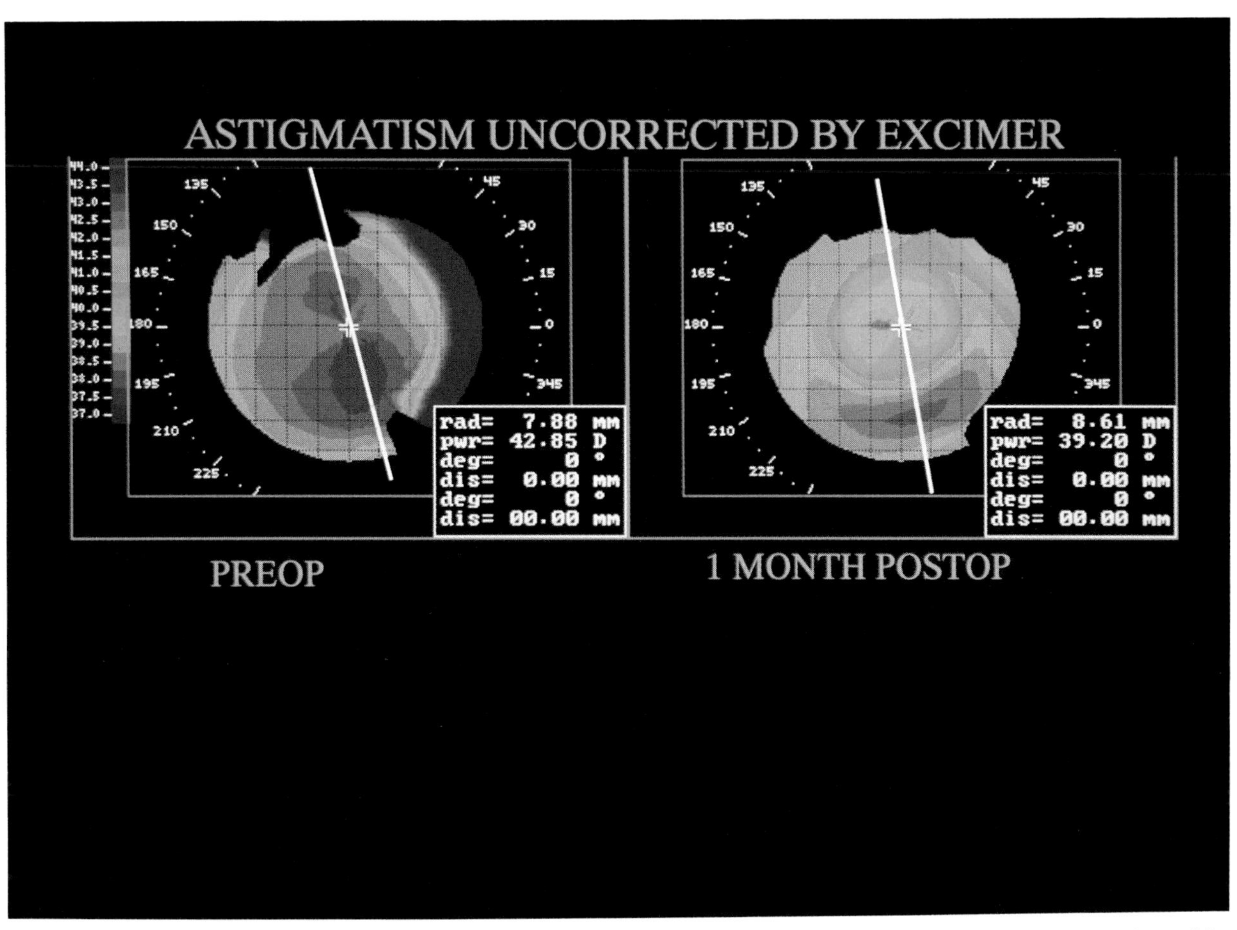

Figure 7.22: Corneal topography with pre-treatment plus cylinder at 100° meridian (left) and also with plus cylinder 100° meridian (right) post-treatment. Large blue crescent in pre-treatment (left) image is an artifact.

rical bow-tie pattern pre-PRK (left image). Although the appearance has changed somewhat post-PRK, the axis of the plus cylinder remains at 100 (right image). We have in other cases performed corneal relaxing incisions after PRK with excellent results.

Conclusions

We have attempted to summarize some of our observations with PRK-related corneal healing and its effect on the refractive and corneal topographic changes. Corneal topography closely parallels refractive change but provides much more clinically relevant information. It has become an indispensable part of our pre-treatment and post-treatment evaluation of the patient.

8

LINDA J. RHODES, FCLSA, NCLE

The Corneal Analysis System Method of Fitting Rigid Contact Lenses

Introduction

It has been over five centuries since Leonardo Da Vinci first considered the effects of corneal aberration and its distorting effect on vision. Since Da Vinci there has been a succession of new ideas which have affected the science of vision. In this last century there have been great strides made by many pioneers who have advanced the concept of contact lenses, developed new and better materials and conceived innovative technologies that have come to serve as the foundation of the contact lens industry.

In this age of computerization, it is only logical that the contact lens industry would take advantage of what computers have to offer, and so it has. With the use of computers and sophisticated image processing, it is now possible for the contact lens fitter to measure corneal topography with extreme accuracy. As a result of this new technology, and the corresponding increase in understanding of the corneal topography, the contact lens fitter now has the tools to design better rigid contact lenses. With the precision that these computer driven imaging processors provide, contact lens manufacturers, who already employ computer driven lathes, will be able to produce lenses tailored to the individual patient's needs that are predictable, consistent, and highly reproducible.

Keratometry

For many years the keratometer was the principal measuring device used for determining the central corneal curvature. Keratometry measurements taken in the flattest and steepest meridians are used to order rigid contact lenses using various fitting techniques. Although the keratometer is an extremely objective instrument with highly repeatable results, there are several shortcomings associated with its use (see also Chapters 1 and 3) that can affect the way in which rigid contact lenses fit and perform. These shortcomings are:

1) Assumes cornea is spherical: The keratometer derives its readings from a direct linear measurement (chord) taken between two pairs of points on a mire approximately 3.2 mm apart that are reflected off the anterior corneal surface. This direct linear measurement is converted to a radius of curvature based on the subtending chord diameter and is reported as if the corneal surface were spherical.
2) Assumes cornea is symmetric: The keratometer assumes that, when the patient is fixating down the center of the instrument and the patient's visual axis is properly aligned with optical axis of the instrument, the true apical cap is being measured.
3) Does not measure corneal topography: The keratometer does not allow the fitter to accurately measure the area inside or outside of the two pairs of points on the reflected mire.

Soper's Topogometer attachment was a valuable addition to the keratometer. It allowed the fitter to determine if there was a steeper "apical reading" outside of the central radius of the curvature, "central reading," and to define the limiting margins of either the central or apical readings in the major and minor meridians. This information was used for determining the diameter of the rigid contact lens and for designing custom rigid contact lenses. Diameter was determined by measuring the distance between the points at which the radius of curvature flattened by 0.5 D in each meridian. The diameter of the lens is calculated by adding 2 mm to the longest of these two readings (LD+2). One millimeter is added for centering and stability, and 1 mm for addition of secondary and peripheral curves. Although Soper's invention was a big step forward in attempting to define corneal topography, it unfortunately is subject to the same basic principles under which the keratometer functions, and thereby is subject to the same shortcomings.

The keratometer has one other limiting factor, its range. The flattest reading possible is 36.00 D and the steepest 52.00 D without the aid of orthogonally corrected lenses for extending the range. It is not possible to perform topographical keratometry to determine the keratometry readings of a displaced apical cap when those readings are beyond the range of the keratometer. This limitation makes it impossible to get accurate readings on patients who have moderate to severe keratoconus or who have had refractive surgery.

Photokeratoscopy

Since the early 1900s, scientists and inventors have been aware that a better method for measuring corneal topography and designing rigid contact lenses was needed. The Placido disc provided the first means for specifying, at least qualitatively, the shape of the corneal surface. Devices for photographing the Placido disc, photokeratoscopes, were developed. Information from the photo was manually compared to theoretical spheres of known radii of curvature and chord diameters to arrive at a base curve for the contact lens. The most notable of the early photokeratoscopes is the Corneascope-Comparator. Although this instrument has been around for many years, it has not been widely used, and the keratometer continued to be the instrument of choice in the fitting of contact lenses.

New high-resolution computer-controlled video-image processing instrumentation can assess data from videokeratographic images to qualitatively and quantitatively measure and plot corneal topography with extreme accuracy. This high-tech instrumentation is perfect for the design and fitting of rigid contact lenses. However, the earliest computerized instruments were not always predictable, and because their cost was prohibitive, few contact lens fitters used them, preferring to stay with the tried-and-true, less expensive keratometer and Topogometer or the Corneascope-Comparator.

With the arrival of second-generation instrumentation, which has proved to be much more precise and more cost effective, most probably all contact lens fitting and manufacturing in the near future will be generated by using information derived from computerized videokeratographs. This advanced technology has enabled the contact lens fitter to measure the shape of the cornea, and in the process it has shown that our concepts of corneal topography and contact lens design must be reassessed.

Shape Factors

The traditional concept of two primary meridians that cross perpendicular to each other to form a central apex no longer holds true, as demonstrated in earlier chapters and in the shape patterns in Figures 8.1 and 8.2. Contrary to the belief that the corneal shape is aspheric and that it flattens as it approaches the periphery in a symmetrical elliptical fashion, video image processing demonstrates that semi-meridians along any given meridian often have clinically important differences in curvature. Video image processing has also shown that the apex of many spherical and/or astigmatic corneas is displaced, and that in general the shape is asymmetric.

Looking at computerized videokeratographic data by semi-meridians, paracentrally and peripherally, is proving invaluable in the initial fitting, refitting, and subsequent follow-up analysis of rigid contact lenses. Topographic asymmetry can have a profound effect on the success of rigid contact lens fitting. If the apical zone is not centrally located, problems with lens positioning, visual acuity, and comfort may result (Figures 8.3 A, B). An understanding of the corneal topography is imperative if success in fitting rigid contact lenses is to be achieved.

Extensive work is in progress with each of the Placido-based videokeratographs to develop programs for contact lens fitting. The author has had the opportunity to work with EyeSys Laboratories, Inc., in developing a software program which includes several universally accepted rigid contact lens fitting techniques. This first-generation rigid contact lens fitting program to be used with the EyeSys Corneal Analysis System (CAS) addresses all of the issues and concerns previously mentioned. This system analyzes data obtained in all semi-meridians, from the center to the periphery of the cornea, in order to design contact lenses that will help maintain normal corneal metabolism and topography and provide optimum comfort for the patient.

EyeSys Corneal Analysis Contact Lens Fitting Program

The first-generation contact lens fitting software allows the contact lens fitter to design rigid lenses using the following fitting philosophies:

- Apical Clearance
- Alignment
- Aspheric

The EyeSys Corneal Analysis System takes into consideration that the experienced or inventive contact lens fitter may wish to make changes to the fitting parameters. In this regard, the fitter has the ability to edit non-protected data which allows the fitter the latitude either to follow the cookbook formula or to adjust the final lens parameters to fit his or her particular fitting

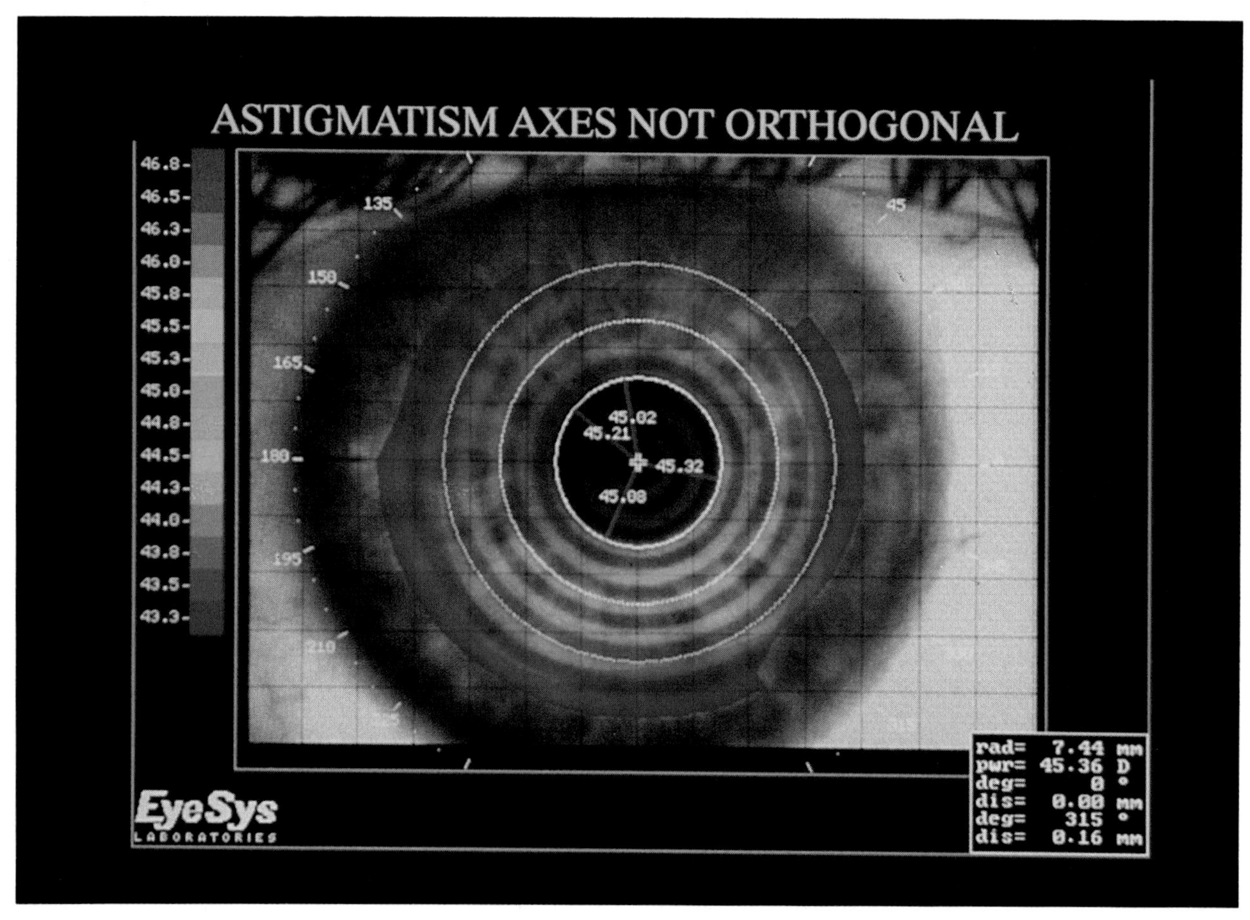

Figure 8.1: Translucent topographic color map superimposed over the eye image demonstrating differences in radii of curvature along semi-meridians at 3 mm. Simulated K's for this cornea are 45.12 × 57/45.37 × 147.

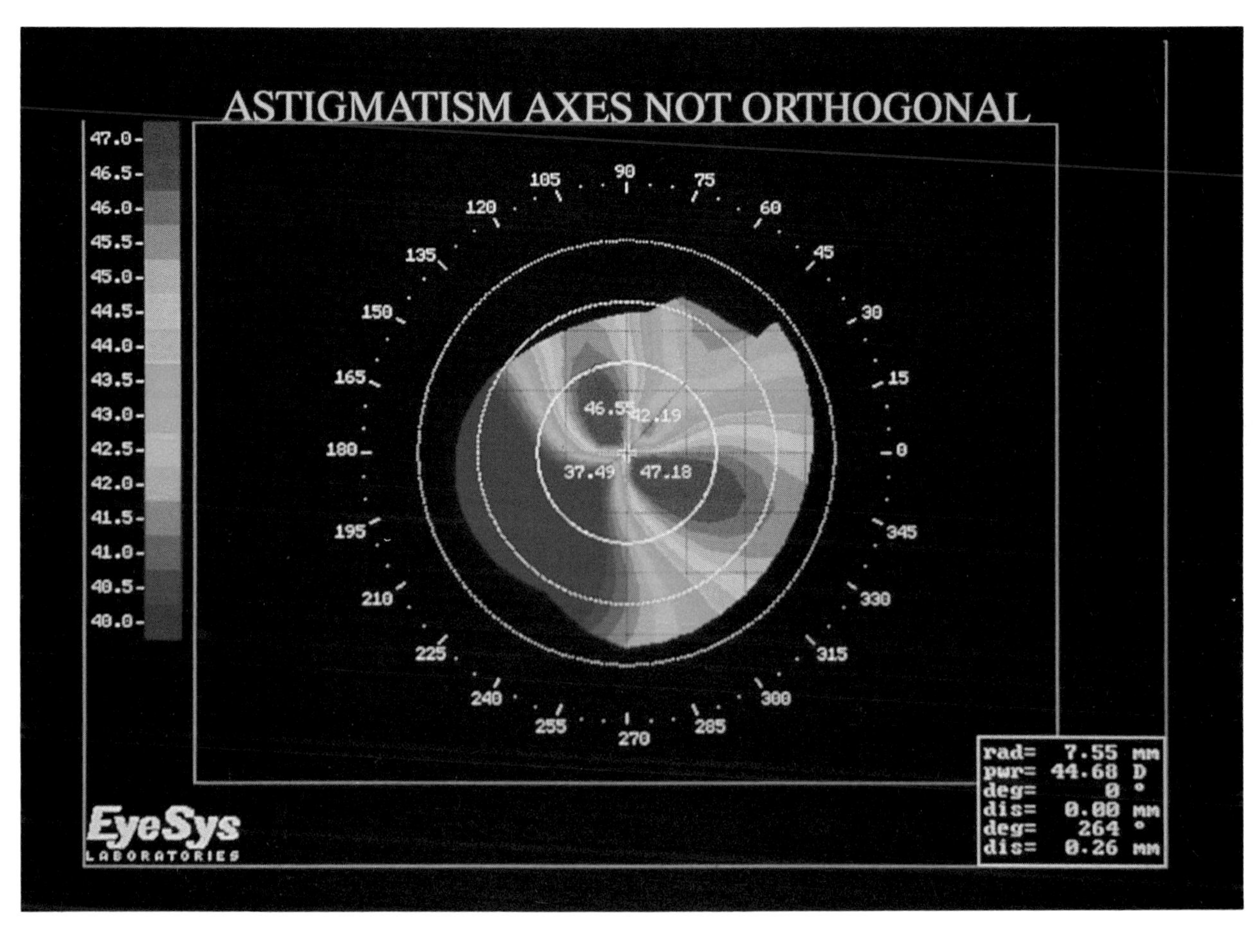

Figure 8.2: Simulated K's for this cornea are 38.87 × 36/46.12 × 126. K's by semi-meridian are 37.49 × 215, 46.55 × 110, 42.19 × 52 and 47.18 × 340.

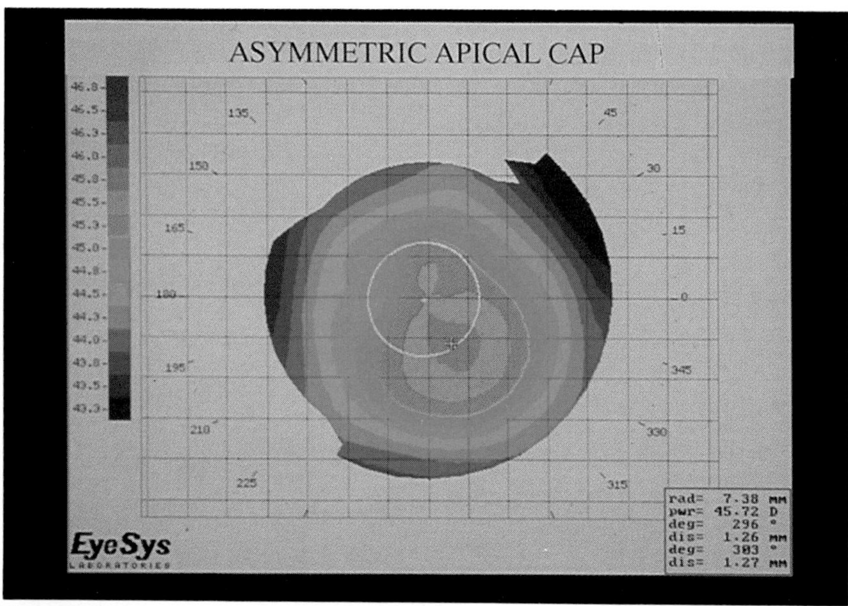

Figure 8.3A.

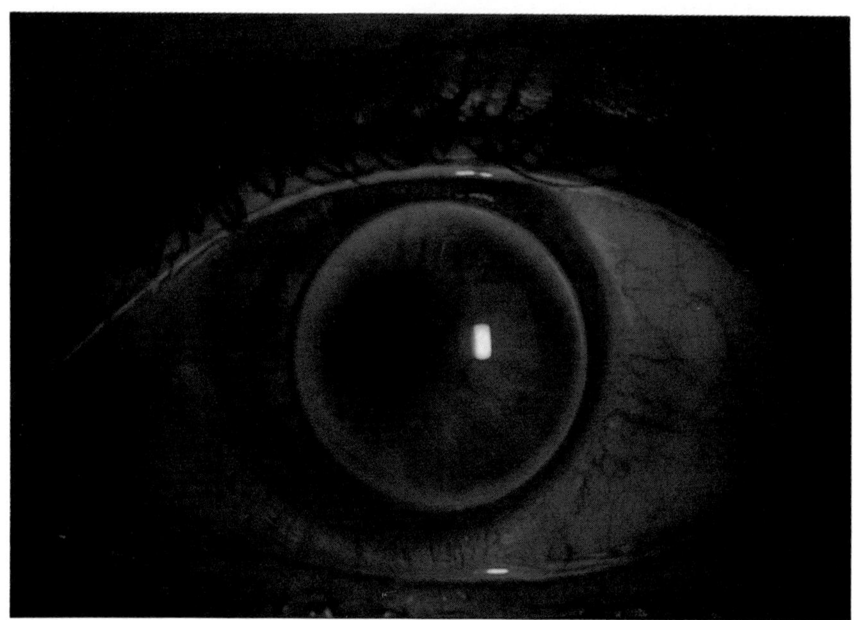

Figure 8.3B.

Figure 8.3: (A) Topographic color map of asymmetric apical cap. Note apical center is positioned inferiorly and temporally 1.13 mm. (B) Slit-lamp photo of a rigid contact lens with a diameter of 8.6 mm positioned over the apical cap. Note lens rides inferiorly and temporally.

philosophy. The ability to compare and evaluate the effects of the lens on the corneal topography in subsequent follow-up visits will allow fitters to test their own fitting techniques as well as provide a stimulus for better designs in the future.

The software is extremely flexible and simple. No prior computer experience and little training is necessary to understand and effectively operate this program. Once the video image of the reflected Placido disc is taken, the computer digitizes the data (information from 5,760 points on the corneal surface compared to four with the keratometer), applies the appropriate formulas, performs the mathematical calculations, displays the information and stores the data to compare with data obtained on subsequent follow-up visits.

The contact lens program has fail-safe measures to help the fitter choose between a spherical or toric lens. For example, if the amounts of refractive cylinder and corneal astigmatism are not reasonably close, a red warning message appears on the screen indicating that there may be residual astigmatism and that a toric lens design may be needed. If the axis of the refractive cylinder and the axis of the corneal astigmatism differ by 10 degrees or more, a warning message to this effect will appear on the screen. The fitter has the ability to override all warnings.

If the fitter unintentionally moves ahead on any screen or menu, pressing the Escape key allows the fitter to move back through the program to the desired screen or back to the main menu. Each screen has a HELP screen (F1) that gives all options for that particular screen. Some screens have the message, "Press C to change." This function allows the fitter to change unprotected parameters, such as the range of the normalized color scale.

For each of the three fitting techniques in this software package the imaging steps are the same. After the video camera captures the image of the reflection of the Placido disc (videokeratograph) off the cornea, the fitter simply follows the prompts on each screen. The Central Processing Unit (CPU) digitizes the data. Once the fitter accepts the image and data, the data is saved by hitting the "S" key on the computer keyboard, which automatically brings up the Patient Information screen. The patient's name, ID number (birth date, or special patient number), address, diagnosis, fitter's initials and who referred the patient, as well as any special comments are entered under New Patient information.

After the patient information has been entered, the fitter has a permanent record of all the data points. The fitter can now call up the patient's record of exams using either the name, ID number, or group classification. Once the record of exams is on the screen, the fitter selects the exam to be viewed. Up to four exams can be viewed with some display formats. Two can be displayed in the contact lens fitting format. After the exams have been selected, the Select Display format screen will appear. The third display option, "Contact Lens Data," provides access to the Contact Lens Data Menu. There are three options on this menu:

1) Numerical Data Map (First exam loaded)
2) Numerical Data Map (Second exam loaded)
3) Contact Lens Fitting

Numerical data map

Options one and two on this screen allow the fitter to view numerical data in topographic color map form and zone averaging (Figure 8.4). In the color map form, the radius of curvature readings along each of the sixteen rings are displayed at fifteen degree increments from 0° to 360°. Radii of curvature values are expressed in dioptric power (D) or in millimeters (M). To toggle

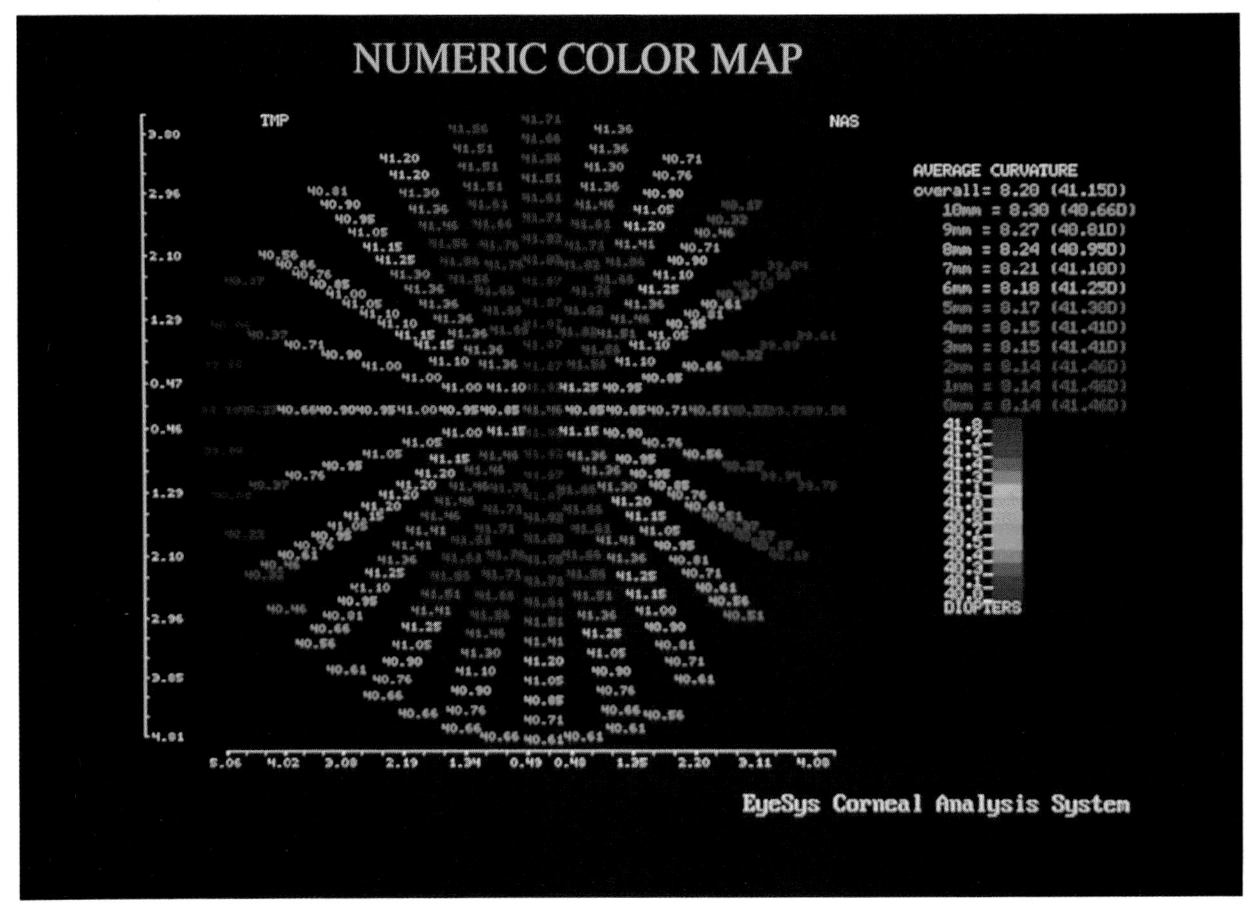

Figure 8.4: Numerical data color map and zone averaging. Can be viewed in millimeters or changed to diopters.

back and forth between the two, the letters "D" and "M" on the keyboard are used. Zone averaging provides information regarding radius of curvature averages within a particular zone of the cornea. All of the values are presented in the corresponding normalized color scale for that particular value. Blue data values correspond to curvatures which are flat and red data values correspond to curvatures which are steep relative to the particular cornea being examined. The color bar in the lower right of the screen defines the normalized color scale for each cornea.

Average curvature along the periphery of different optical zones is displayed above the color scale on the right of the screen. Since these are zone diameters, a 5 mm zone, for instance, would include data points around a 2.5 mm perimeter from the center of the rings. The overall corneal curvature is shown above the zone diameter values.

Applications for the numerical data in the color map and zone averaging include:

- Delineation of the apical cap in the fitting and follow-up analysis of rigid contact lenses.
- Custom designing rigid contact lenses for patients who have keratoconus or who have had corneal refractive surgery or a corneal transplant.
- Designing aspheric contact lenses using paracentral and peripheral data.
- Evaluating the rate of paracentral and peripheral flattening for specifying secondary and peripheral curves.

Data Entry

Selecting option number three, "Contact Lens Fitting," provides access to the three fitting techniques:

1) Apical Clearance
2) Alignment
3) Aspheric

To access any of these three options, press the corresponding number (Figure 8.5A-C).

The data entry screen for each rigid contact lens fitting technique is basically the same. If both the right and left eyes were selected, both will be displayed on the fitting screen which allows the fitter to evaluate and fit both eyes at the same time. Each screen includes a topographic color map for the eyes that were selected. The color map has been included to give the fitter an idea where the contact lens may position relative to the position of the apical cap. The normalized color scale is located next to the color maps and provides a scale for the colors being displayed.

The fitter enters the following information in the data entry section for each eye:

1) Spherical prescription
2) Cylinder in minus form
3) Cylinder axis
4) Vertex distance in millimeters
5) Visible iris diameter in millimeters
6) Pupil diameter in millimeters
7) *Lens diameter will be automatically calculated*
8) *Lens base curve (CPC) will be automatically calculated*
9) Base curve (CPC) of diagnostic lens in diopters
10) Power of diagnostic lens
11) Over-refraction over diagnostic lens

As the data is entered into the data entry section, the software automatically calculates the Base Curve, Power, Diameter, Optical Zone, Peripheral, and Secondary Curves or eccentricity value of the lens to be ordered. On the Aspheric fitting screens, the eccentricity value "E" is reported. There are no secondary curve values on the Aspheric fitting screen. Parameters for ordering the contact lens for all fitting screens are displayed on the prescription line at the bottom of the screen.

Although it is possible to edit all parameters on the prescription line, the K values, Lens Diameter, and Lens Base Curve

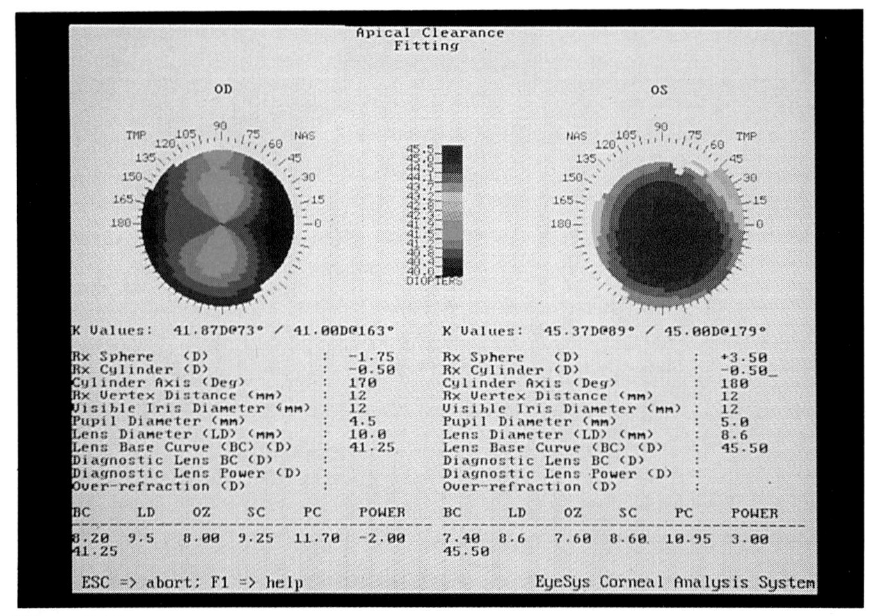

Figure 8.5A.

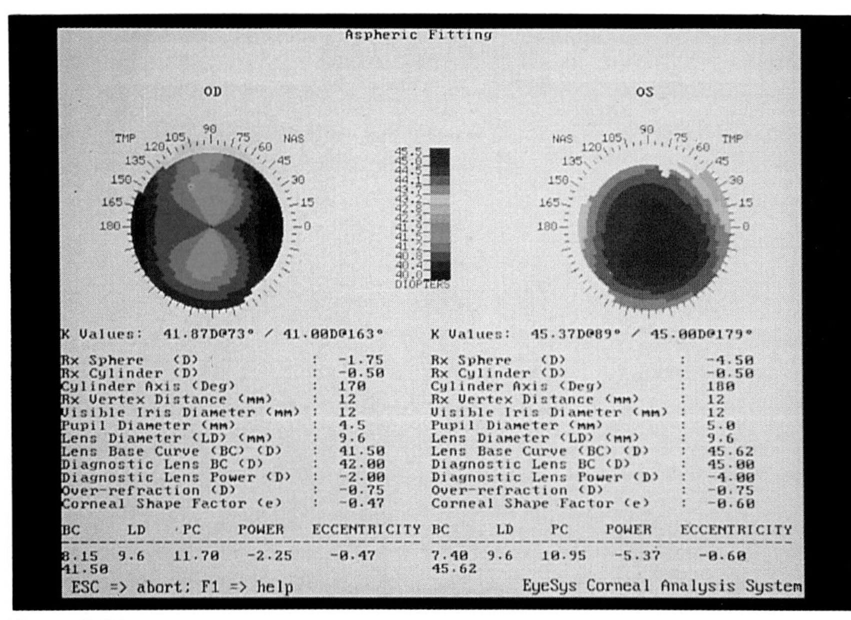

Figure 8.5B.

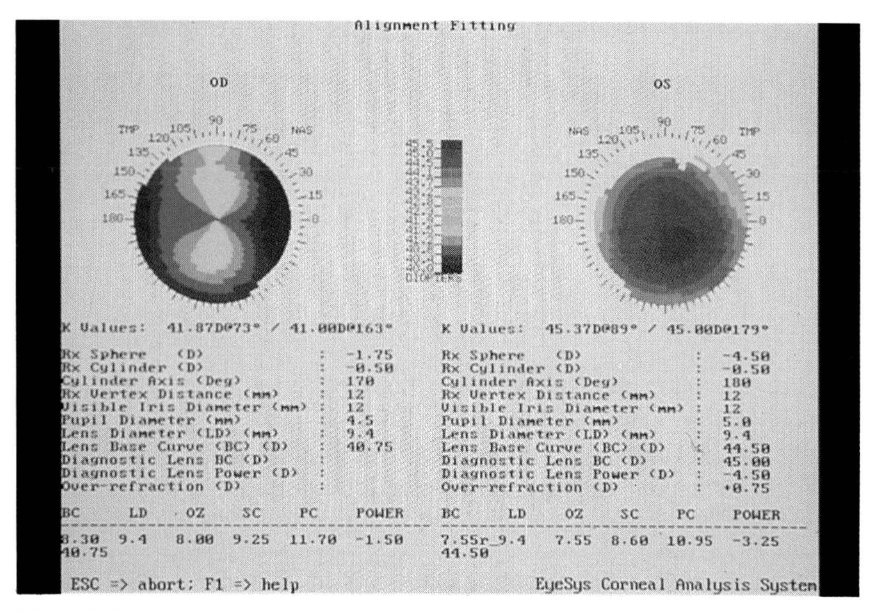

Figure 8.5C.

Figure 8.5: Contact lens fitting screens. (A) Apical Clearance contact lens fitting screen. Power calculated using manifest refraction. Note diameter of right lens changed to 9.5 mm on prescription line. (B) Alignment contact lens fitting screen. Power of left contact lens calculated using diagnostic lens and over-refraction data. (C) Aspheric contact lens fitting screen. Power for both eyes calculated using diagnostic lenses and over-refractions. Note eccentricity value for each eye.

are protected in the data entry section displayed on the upper part of the screen. The program automatically recalculates any parameter which is dependent on another parameter. For example, if the base curve (CPC) on the prescription line is altered, the program will automatically recalculate the power. If the diameter is altered, the program will recalculate the optical zone.

Data entry is repeated for the second eye. Once all the data has been entered for both eyes, hitting the "Enter" key on the computer keyboard "fixes" the data. A printout of the information on any screen can be made to be used as a permanent record for the patient's chart and to order lenses. This information is stored in the main drive of the CPU for comparison with data obtained on the subsequent follow-up visits. Topographical data can be stored on a floppy disc.

Rigid contact lens fitting techniques

Apical clearance. The Apical Clearance or "Steeper than K" fitting philosophy ideally requires the rigid contact lens to center within the interpalpebral fissure and vault the apical zone.

This first-generation software uses a variation in the Soper LD+2 method for determining the overall diameter needed in the Apical Clearance technique. Once the diameter of the lens has been determined, the following rules are applied to calculate the base curve (CPC):

- If the diameter is less than 9.0 mm, one-half of the corneal astigmatism or 0.5 D, whichever is the greatest, is added to the flat "K."
- If the diameter is 9.0 mm or greater,

> one-quarter of the corneal astigmatism or 0.25 D, whichever is the greatest, is added to the flat "K."

It is not necessary to measure the visible iris diameter or pupil diameter if the Apical Clearance method is used. The Apical Clearance formula for diameter will always override data entered on pupil and visible iris diameter.

Power of the lens is calculated using either a manifest refraction (sphere, cylinder, axis) in minus cylinder form and vertex distance, or a diagnostic lens (base curve, power) and over-refraction. This information is entered in the data entry section. If a manifest refraction is used, the software calculates the vaulting effect of the base curve to be ordered, adjusts for the resultant tear power and takes into consideration the vertex distance measurement entered by the fitter. If the manifest refraction is over + or − 4.00 D, it is suggested that power be determined by using a diagnostic contact lens plus over-refraction. When a diagnostic lens is used, the fitter enters the base curve of the diagnostic lens in diopters, the power of the diagnostic lens, and the over-refraction in the data entry section. The computer program then calculates the power of the lens to be ordered in terms of total need of the eye, adjusting for the difference between the base curve of the diagnostic lens and the base curve of the lens to be ordered. The resultant power will appear in the prescription line at the bottom of the screen. Diagnostic lens and over-refraction data will always override manifest refraction and vertex distance data that may have been entered previously.

Optical zone diameter is determined by the overall diameter less 2 mm. For example, if the overall diameter of the final lens is 8.8 mm, the optical zone would be 6.8 mm. Allowances are made for 1 mm of peripheral and secondary curves, 0.5 mm on each side. Peripheral and secondary radii are displayed in the lower prescription line. It is possible to edit parameters in the lower prescription line without affecting the protected data in the upper data entry section.

Alignment fitting. In the Alignment fitting technique, the diameter and optical zone are dependent on the diameter of the visible iris diameter in relationship to pupil size. A hand-held PD ruler can be used to measure both the pupil size and the visible iris diameter. The millimeter grid in the Data Fusion display with an eye image can also be used to determine the visible iris diameter. Visible iris diameter is measured using the horizontal meridian. Pupil size is determined in dim lighting to ensure that the optical zone of the lens will adequately cover the pupil under all lighting conditions. Table 8.1 was used for determining the base curve (CPC) in the Alignment fitting technique.

Optical zone diameter is calculated as 1.4 mm less than the overall diameter. For example, if the overall diameter is 8.8 mm, the optical zone would be 7.4 mm. The maximum optical zone in this fitting technique is equal to the radius of curvature of the base curve. For example, if the base curve of the lens in millimeters is 7.60, the largest optical zone allowable would be 7.6 mm. However, the fitter does not have to worry about this calculation; the software automatically makes the necessary adjustments.

To determine the peripheral curve of the contact lens, the program analyzes and averages peripheral ring data obtained from a 22° section along the flat meridian. Two millimeters are then added to the averaged reading. The resultant radius of curvature is the suggested peripheral curve.

The secondary curve is based upon the average reading of data obtained from a 22° section just outside the optical zone along the flat meridian. The program adds 0.75 mm to this value to calculate the sug-

Table 8.1
Determining the base curve (CPC) in the Alignment fitting technique.

Degree of Corneal Astigmatism	Base Curve (CPC) Determined By
0 to 0.50 (D) diopter flat	"K" (D) -0.50 (D) diopter
0.50 to 1.00 (D)	flat "K" (D) -0.25 (D)
1.00 to 1.50 (D)	on flat "K" (D)
1.50 to 2.00 (D)	flat "K" (D) +0.25 (D)
2.00 to 3.00 (D)	flat "K" (D) +0.50 (D)
Greater than 3.00 (D)*	Delta "K"/4

* If the corneal astigmatism is greater than 3 D, a warning message appears that recommends consideration of a toric lens design.

gested secondary curve.

The EyeSys system takes into consideration the importance of edge clearance based on the patient's corneal topography as opposed to edge lift as determined by the base curve of the lens. This program allows the fitter to custom design the finish of a rigid contact lens according to the patient's own corneal topography.

The power of the lens to be ordered is calculated in exactly the same manner as with the Apical Clearance technique, taking into consideration the vaulting effect in each fitting situation.

Aspheric. The EyeSys Corneal Analysis System is the first videokeratographic program that allows the fitter to achieve some control over the fitting aspects of aspheric lenses. It does this by providing all the information on the eccentricity value obtained from the patient's corneal topography data. Using a section of the flat meridian, the radius of curvature information is converted to sagittal depth data. A basic conic equation for converting sagittal depth data to an eccentricity value is applied. The resulting value equals the best eccentricity value for the patient's corneal topography. Table 8.2 is used to determine

Table 8.2
Determining the central radius of curvature in the aspheric lens design.

Degree of Corneal Astigmatism	Base Curve (CPC) Determined By
0 to 1.00 (D)	flat "K" (mm) -0.10mm
1.00 to 2.00 (D)	average "K" (mm) -0.10mm
2.00 to 3.00 (D)	average "K" (mm) -0.15mm
Greater than 3.00 (D)*	average "K" (mm) -0.15mm

* If the corneal astigmatism is greater than 3 D, a warning message appears that recommends consideration of a toric lens design.

the central radius of curvature of the aspheric lens design:

Diameter is calculated by measuring the visible iris diameter less 2.4 mm. For example, if the visible iris diameter is 12.0 mm, then 12.0 mm less 2.4 mm gives an overall diameter of 9.6 mm. In an aspheric design, consideration for pupil size, optical zone, and calculation of secondary curves is not needed. Peripheral curves are determined in the same manner as they are in the Alignment fitting technique.

Although the power can be calculated using a manifest refraction, the use of a diagnostic lens and over-refraction is the preferred method for determining the power needed in the final lens.

Post-fitting Analysis

The Corneal Analysis System allows the fitter to qualitatively and quantitatively evaluate the effect of fitting techniques on the patient's corneal topography. On each follow-up visit, a computerized videokeratograph is taken and compared to the prefitting data or any previous data the fitter may wish to compare. Data can be compared on several different screens. Data Fusion allows the fitter to compare up to four exams using several different display modes (Figure 8.6). Each of the four screens in the Data Fusion display can be tailored to suit the fitter's needs. For example, the fitter can compare the right and left eyes using pre-fit data with the right and left eye data obtained in subsequent follow-up visits. As modifications are made to the fit, changes in the data can be assessed for consideration for further changes to the fit (Figures 8.7A-C and 8.8A and B).

Refitting the Previous Wearer

Computerized videokeratographs can play a vital role in refitting rigid contact lens wearers who have developed corneal warpage from poorly fitting rigid contact lenses. One key function is to demonstrate when a cornea is stable and therefore ready to be refit. Once the patient has been refit, videokeratography allows the fitter to maintain a stable fit by following the changes in corneal topography.

Other Applications

Fitting keratoconus and post-surgical cases

Art and science go hand in hand when it comes to fitting keratoconus, corneal transplants, and patients who have had corneal refractive surgery. Although the Corneal Analysis System currently does not have a contact lens fitting software program to design rigid contact lenses for these typically very difficult cases, the system does make it possible to decrease the amount of time needed and the number of diagnostic contact lenses necessary to achieve a good fit for these patients. Numerical data in topographic color map form and zone averaging information found in the contact lens menu will aid the fitter in determining the best fit possible (Figures 8.9A and B and 8.10A-C). Simulated fluorescein patterns calculated from sagittal depth data also aid the fitter in determining the ideal lens-cornea relationship.

Fluorescein patterns

Sagittal depth measurements between the back surface of the proposed rigid contact lens and the anterior surface of the cornea provide a mechanism for illustrating fluorescein patterns which the Corneal Analysis System presents in a static format. The fluorescein patterns allow the fitter to look at several fitting techniques superimposed on the same corneal topography. The manner in which each fitting technique aligns with corneal topography provides the fitter

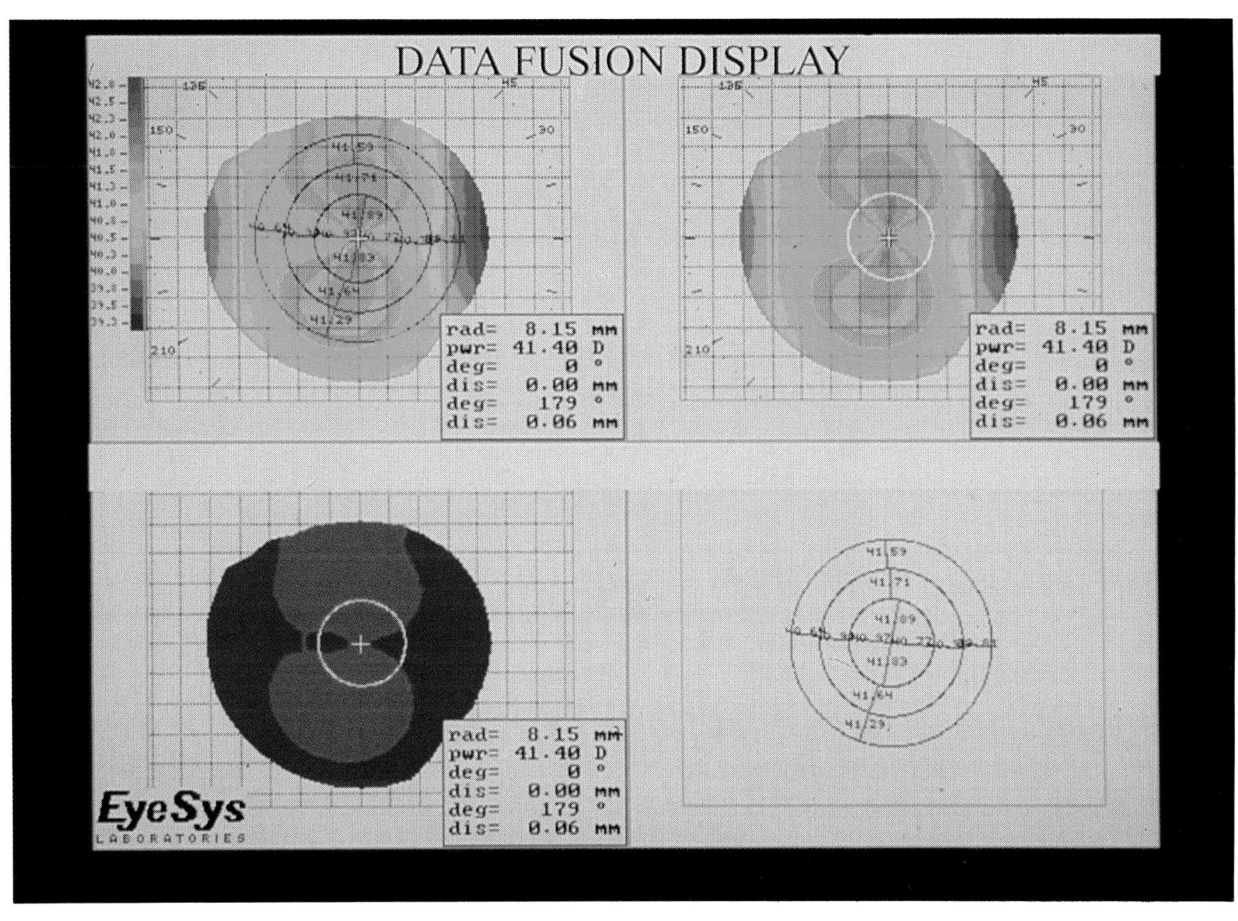

Figure 8.6: Data fusion display of right cornea using four different views of same data. All displays in data fusion can be tailored to individual user's requirements.

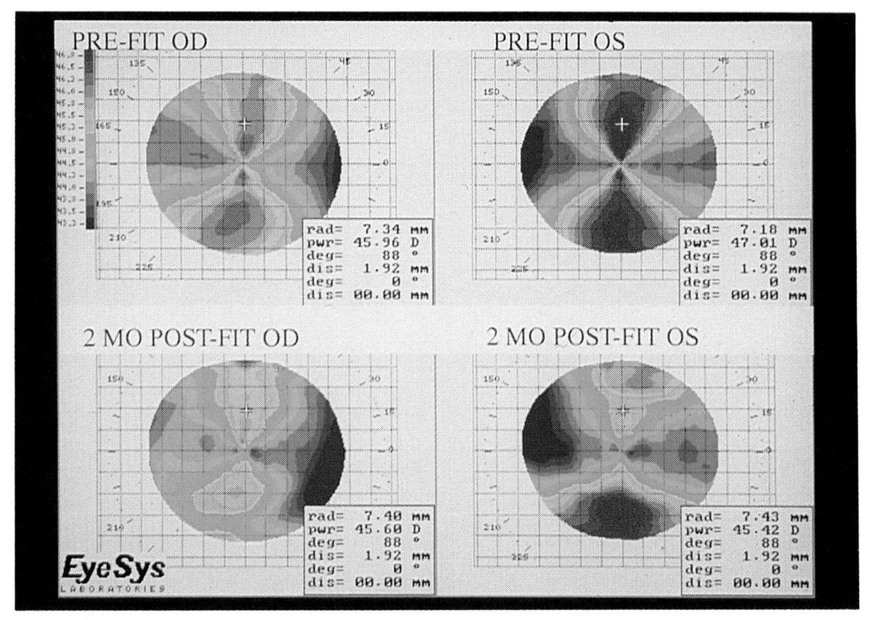

Figure 8.7A.

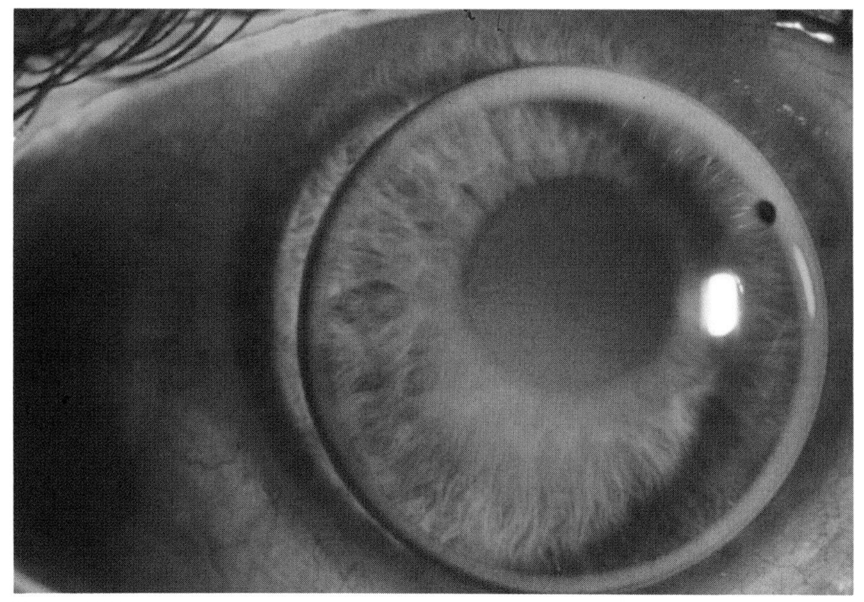

Figure 8.7B.

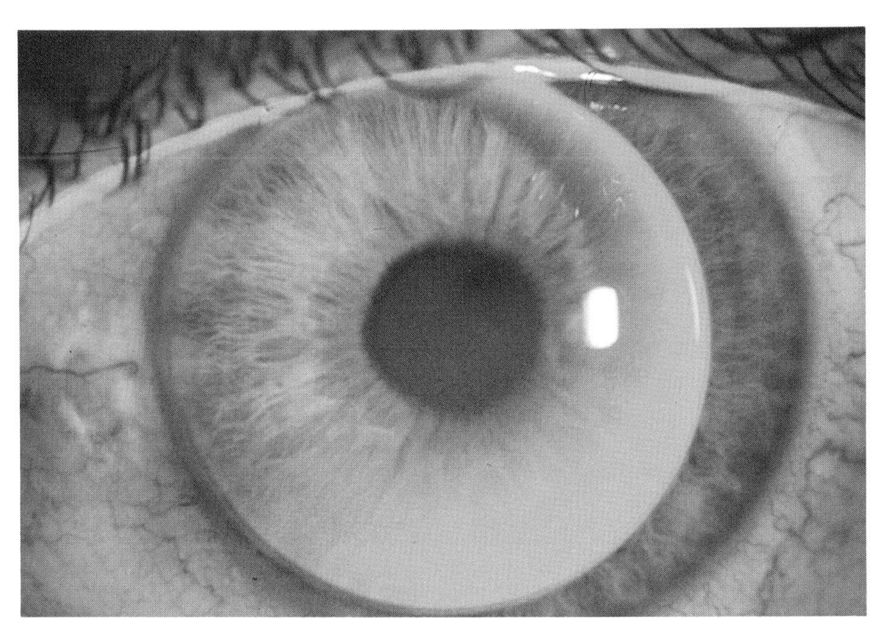

Figure 8.7C.

Figure 8.7: (A) Pre-fitting topographical color maps of right and left cornea (top figures) are compared to two month follow-up data (bottom figures). Right eye fit with Apical clearance technique and left eye fit with Alignment technique. Note displaced apex on left cornea. (B) Slit-lamp photo of Apical clearance lens-cornea relationship. Note central pooling of fluorescein. (C) Slit-lamp photo of Alignment lens-cornea relationship. Note superior bearing and inferior edge stand off.

with the information needed to determine which of the contact lens fitting techniques will be best for the individual patient.

Assessment of rigid contact lens parameters

The anterior and posterior surface of a rigid contact lens can be read by mounting the lens on the system's calibration stand (Figures 8.11A-C). It is also possible to determine the optical quality of the anterior and posterior surface of the rigid contact lens using the Corneal Analysis System.

Establishment of fitting criteria

Computerized videokeratographs have created a new era for contact lenses. With increased use of these instruments for the fitting and follow-up analysis of rigid contact lenses, new standards for qualitative and quantitative fitting criteria are sure to follow. Information and insights gained from these systems will have tremendous effects on the way contact lenses will be fit in the future.

Contact lens manufacturing interface

More and more contact lens manufacturers are turning to highly sophisticated computer-driven contact lens manufacturing lathes to make rigid contact lenses. These double and triple axial lathes have air-bearing spindles that are capable of cutting such ultra-smooth surfaces that the finished lenses need minimal surface polishing. This highly precise instrumentation is a must for cutting aspheric surfaces. These lathes can be programmed to cut the base curve (CPC),

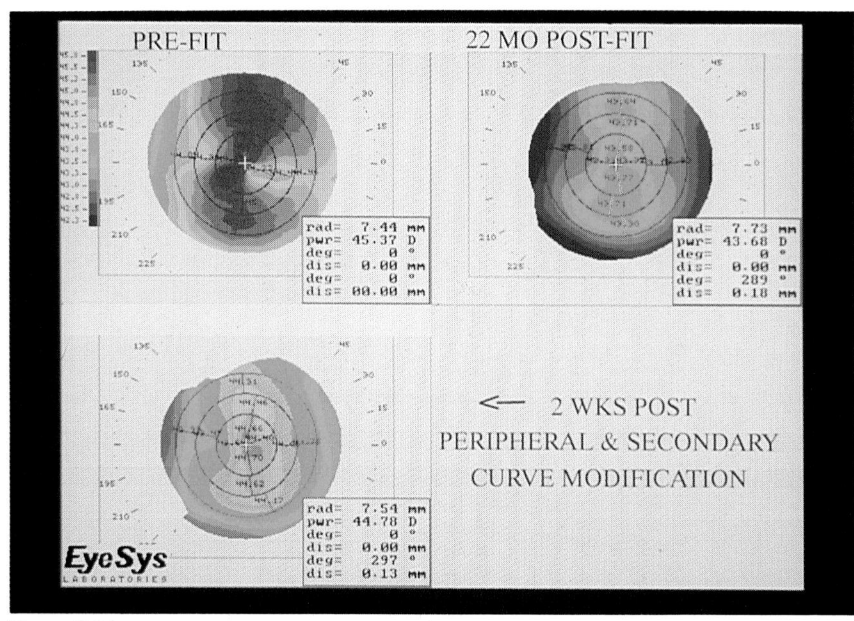

Figure 8.8A.

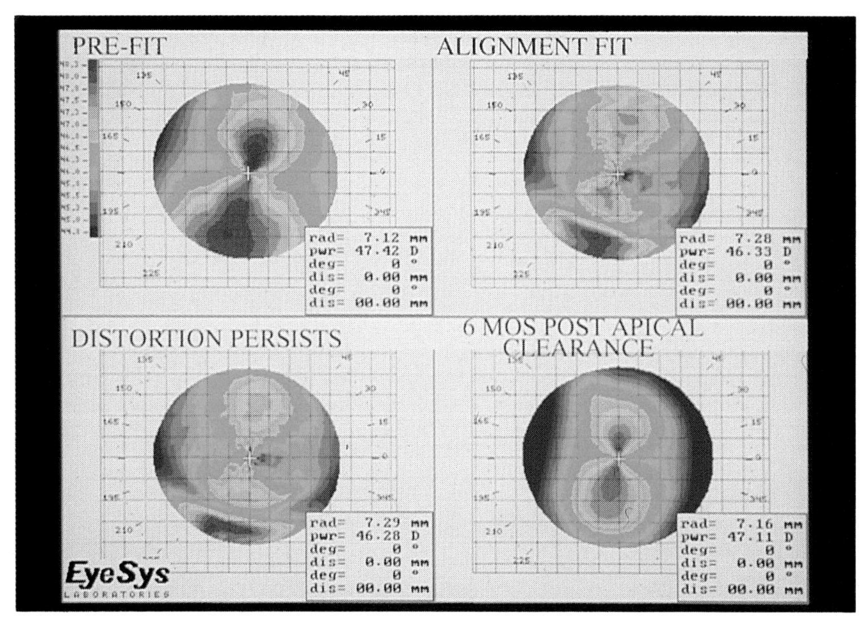

Figure 8.8B.

Figure 8.8: (A) Data fusion display. Upper left, pre-fit rigid contact lens; upper right, 22 month follow-up (note cornea over 1.5 D flatter); and lower left, 2 weeks after modification to peripheral and secondary curves. Readings are returning to normal. (B) Data fusion display. Upper left, pre-fit rigid contact lens using Alignment technique; upper right, lens positioned under upper lid causing gross distortion; lower left, 3 weeks later distortion persists and fit changed to Apical clearance lens; and lower right, six months later cornea now stable.

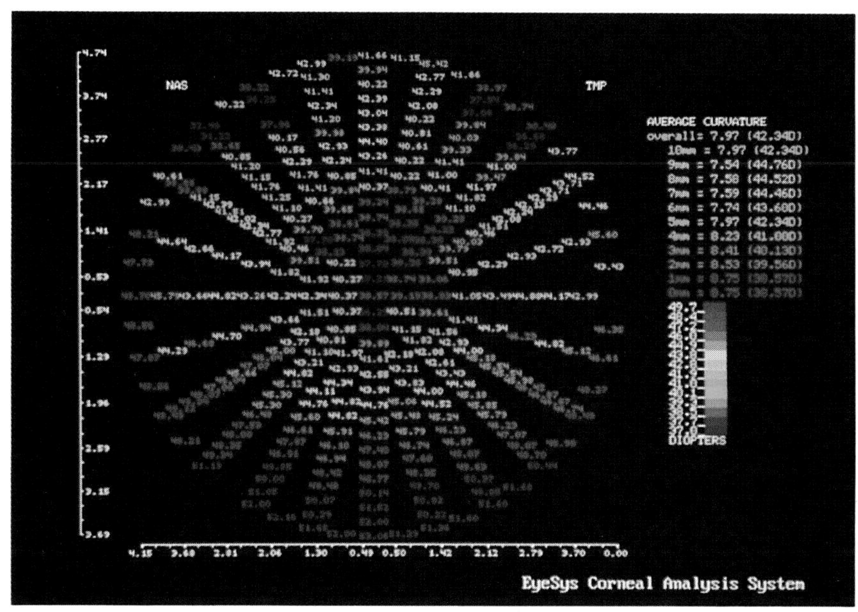

Figure 8.9A.

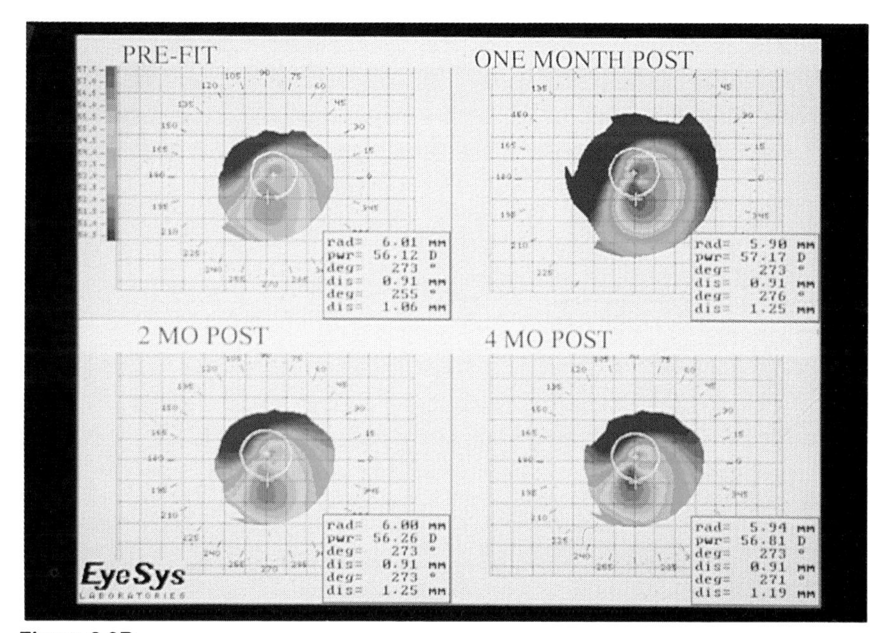

Figure 8.9B.

Figure 8.9: Keratoconus case. (A) Numerical data map and zone averaging display. Information from zone four was used to determine base curve of rigid contact lens. Best fit was 54.00 D base curve with a diameter of 8.0 mm. (B) Data fusion display of pre-fit and 1, 2 and 4 month follow-ups. Cone has remained relatively stable.

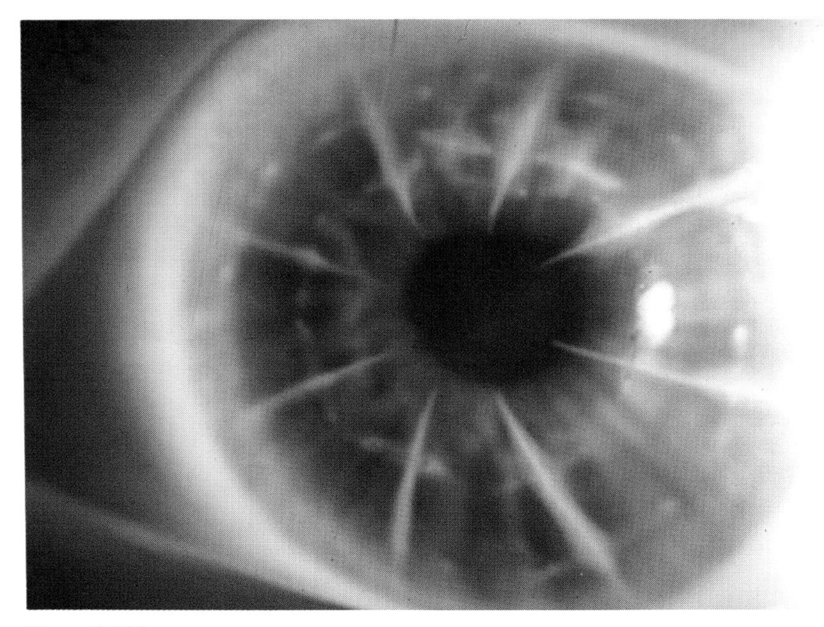

Figure 8.10A.

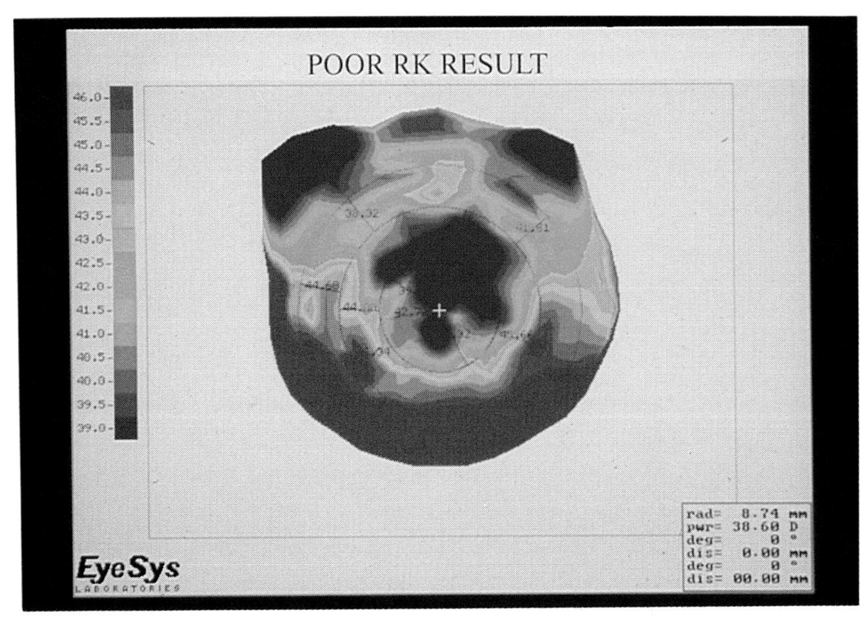

Figure 8.10B.

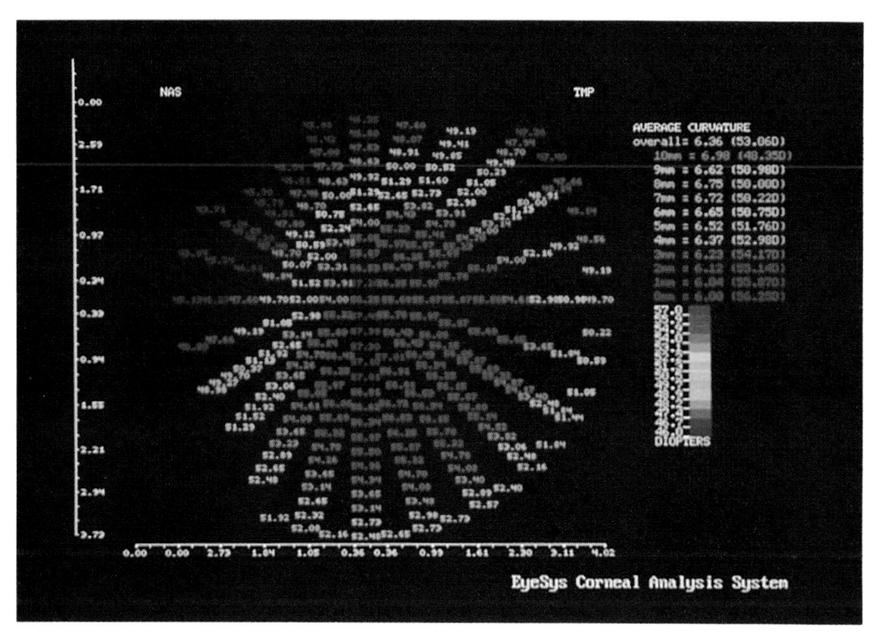

Figure 8.10C.

Figure 8.10: (A) Slit-lamp photo of RK cornea with poor result. (B) Topographical color map of same case. (C) Numerical data map and zone averaging data is used to determine base curve of rigid contact lens. Zones five through seven gave best fit. Base curve ordered was 43.50 D with 10.0 mm diameter.

peripheral, and secondary curves in one continuous process, thereby eliminating the necessity of manually finishing the edge. Inconsistent edge designs are eliminated by avoiding human error in the manual finishing process.

By interfacing computer videokeratographic systems with computer-driven lathes and linking them via modem, lens parameters can be sent directly from the fitter's computer to the manufacturer's computerized lathe. This link-up would reduce handling of contact lens orders and reduce errors in manually filling out forms. The ability to interface and link-up by modem would allow the fitter to maintain complete control of all of the patient's contact lens fitting parameters and the manufacturing of the lenses, including the generation of the peripheral and secondary curves. Once the patient has been fit satisfactorily, duplicates of the fit can be ordered with the assurance that each and every subsequent lens will be exactly the same as the original.

Use of computer videokeratographs to design rigid contact lenses and the potential for linking these instruments with computer-driven lathes will promote many new and innovative rigid contact lens designs and fitting techniques. The same is true for improvements in peripheral and secondary curve finishing techniques. A contact lens fitting program based on computer videokeratographs enables the fitter to order rigid

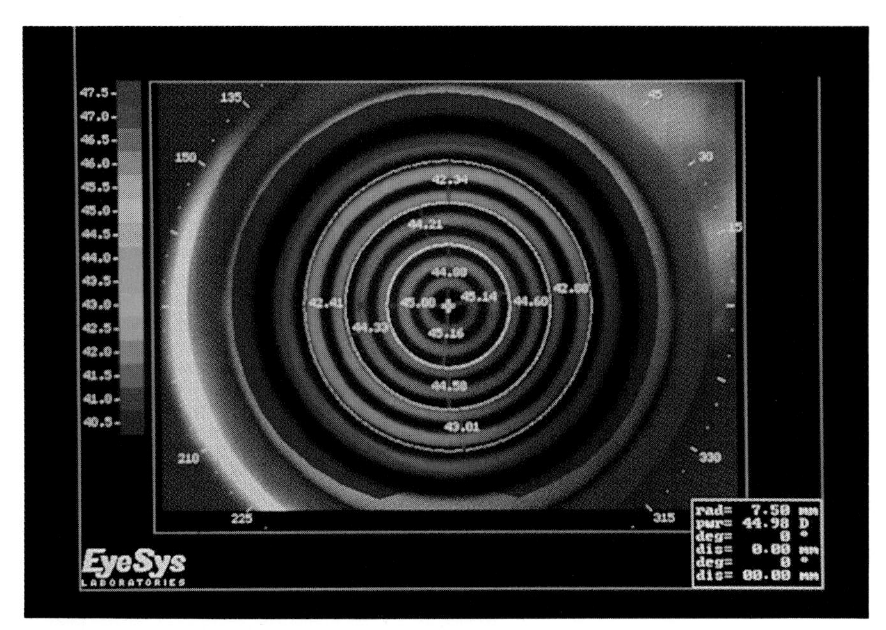

Figure 8.11A.

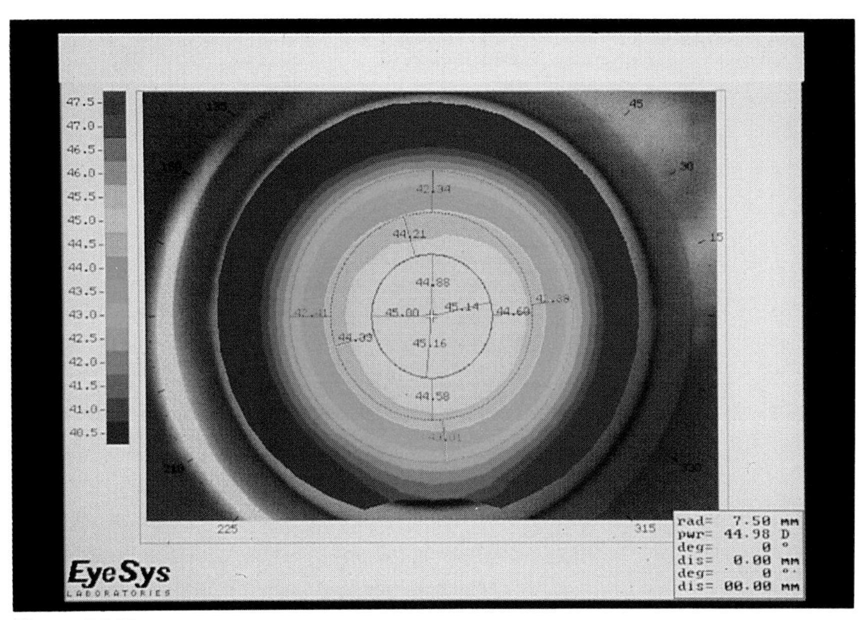

Figure 8.11B.

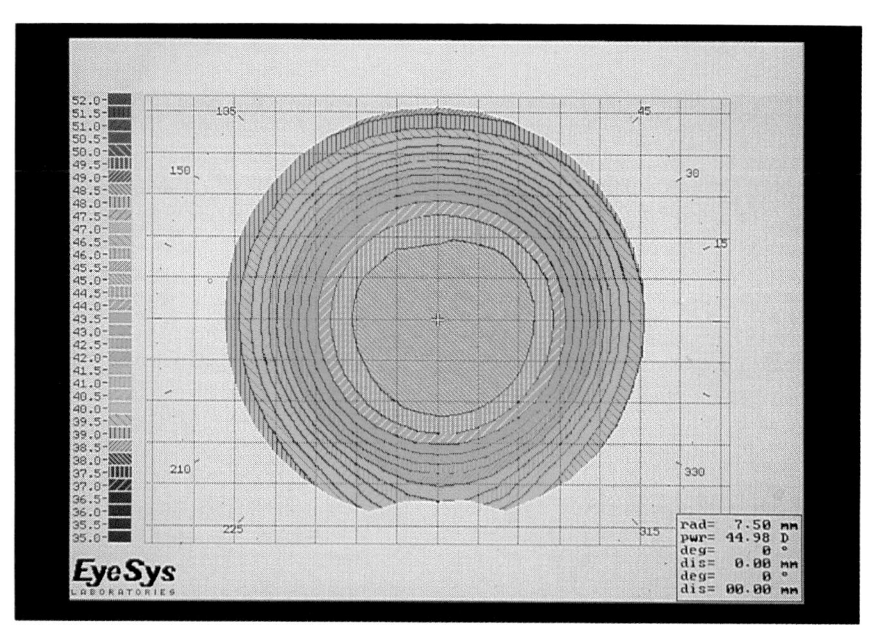

Figure 8.11C.

Figure 8.11: (A) Keratograph of aspheric rigid contact lens with translucent topographic color map. (B) Opaque topographic color map with radii of curvature data by semi-meridian at 3, 5, and 7 mm. (C) Absolute scale demonstrating 4.25 mm optical zone, smooth surface, and 0.5 D changes in radii of curvature from the optical zone to periphery of the lens.

contact lenses with predictable, consistent, and reproducible results. The system enhances the fitter's subjective judgement and ability to objectively evaluate any patient's needs. Best of all, today's technology will enable manufacturers to produce a superior product that will help maintain normal metabolism and corneal topography while providing the patient with a precisely fitting, comfortable lens.

Bibliography

1. Arffa RC: Clinical applications of corneal topographic analysis. *Seminars in Ophthalmology* 6(3):122-132, Sept. 1991.
2. Benjamin WJ, Rosenblum WM: Radii of curvature and sagittal depths of conic sections. *ICLC* 9:76-82, March/April 1992.
3. Bogan SJ, Waring III GO, Ibrahim O, et al: Classification of normal corneal topography based on computer-assisted videokeratography. *Arch Ophthalmol*108, July 1990.
4. Davis LJ, Dresner MS: A Comparison of the EH-270 corneal topographer with conventional keratometry. *CLAO Journal* 17:191-196, July 1991.
5. Dingeldein SA, Klyce SD: Imaging the cornea. *Cornea* 7(3):170-183, 1988.
6. Girard LJ, Sampson WJ, Soper JW: *Corneal Contact Lenses* CV Mosby, St. Louis, 1966.
7. Gormley DJ, Gertsen M, Koplin RS, Lubkin V: Corneal modeling. *Cornea* 7:30-35, 1988.
8. Hamano H, et al: Fundamental and clinical studies of corneal physiology and contact lenses, G. Peter Halberg Lecture. *Asia-Pacific J Ophthalmol* 3(2):77-83, April 1991.
9. Hannush SB, Crawford SL, Waring III GO, et al: Accuracy and precision of keratometry and corneal modeling on calibrated steel balls. *Arch Ophthalmol* 107:1235-1230, Aug 1989.
10. Hannush SB, Crawford SL, Waring III GO, et al.: Reproducibility of normal corneal power measurements with a keratometer, photokeratoscope and video imaging system. *Arch Ophthalmol* 108:539-544, April 1990.

11. Johnson LA: Calculating corneal curvatures. *Contact Lens Forum* 19-25, April 1985.
12. Kastl PR: 'Unbelievable' corneal flattening caused by RGP lenses. *Contact Lens Forum* 71, July 1987.
13. Klyce SD: Color-coded maps enhance corneal topography analysis. *Ophthalmol Times* 15, April 1992.
14. Koch DD, Foulks GN, Moran T, Wakil JS: The corneal EyeSys system: accuracy analysis and reproducibility of first generation prototype. *Refract Corneal Surg* 5:424-429, Nov/Dec 1989.
15. Manabe R, Matsuda M, Suda T: Photokeratoscopy in fitting contact lenses after penetrating keratoplasty. *Brit J Ophthalmol* 70:55-59, 1986.
16. Mandell RB: *Contact Lens Practice, Fourth Edition,* Charles C. Thomas Publisher, Springfield, IL, 1988.
17. McGuire LJ, Singer DE, Klyce SD: Graphic presentation of computer-analyzed keratoscope photographs. *Arch Ophthalmol* 105:223-230, Feb 1987.
18. Rabinowitz KS, Mc Donnell PJ: Computer-assisted corneal topography in keratoconus. *Refract Corneal Surg* 5:400-408, Nov/Dec 1989.
19. Rowsey JJ, Reynolds AE, Brown R: Corneal topography: corneascope. *Arch Ophthalmol* 99:1093-1100, June 1981.
20. Schanzlin DJ, Robin JB: *Corneal Topography, Measuring and Modifying the Cornea,* Springer-Verlag, New York, 1991.
21. Siegel IM, Cohen ML: Post-RK contact lens fitting. *Contact Lens Spectrum* 41-43, April 1992.
22. Soper JW: Follow-up keratometry. *Transactions of The World Congress,* 1966.
23. Soper JW, Sampson WG, Girard LJ: Corneal topography, keratometry and contact lenses. *Arch Ophthalmol* 67:753, 1962.
24. Stein HA, Slatt BJ, Stein RM: *Fitting Guide for Rigid and Soft Contact Lenses, A Practical Approach, Third Edition,* CV Mosby, St. Louis, 1990.
25. Tate Jr. GW, Safir A, Mills CZ, et al: Accuracy and reproducibility of keratometer readings. *CLAO Journal* 13(1):50-58, Jan 1987.
26. Weinstock FJ: *Contact Lens Fitting, A Clinical Text Atlas,* Gower Medical Publishing, New York, 1989.
27. Wilson SE, Lin DTC, Klyce SD, et al: Topographic changes in contact lens-induced corneal warpage. *Ophthalmology* 97(6):734-744, June 1990.
28. Winkler TD: Correct equation for calculating the sagittal depth of a hyperboloidal lens surface. *ICLC* 9:68-70, March-April 1992.

9

ROGER F. STEINERT, MD
ELLEN KELLEY McHALE, COT

Evaluating the Corneal Transplant Patient

Corneal topography is valuable in evaluating the corneal curvature changes induced by corneal transplantation (Figure 9.1). However, as the rate of corneal transplants remaining clear in the long term has improved, increasing attention has been directed at control of postoperative astigmatism. An anatomically clear graft with poor optical function is a functional failure. Over the past decade many surgeons changed suturing techniques to improve their results with postoperative astigmatism, including different styles of single and double running sutures and different suture materials. In the mid 1980s, surgeons began using combined interrupted and running sutures.

Selective Suture Removal

Selective suture removal of tight interrupted sutures in the steep meridian helped to reduce suture-in astigmatism. With the advent of computer-assisted topographic analysis as a clinical tool, discrimination of the precise etiology of the astigmatism improved further. The most immediately obvious application was to identify the exact location of the tight interrupted suture(s) causing the astigmatism (Figure 9.2) and to evaluate the immediate effects on the cornea of the suture removal (Figures 9.3, 9.4).

Not only can one evaluate the effects of removing interrupted sutures, but also the effects of removing the running suture (Figure 9.5), or the combined effects of removing running and interrupted sutures (Figure 9.6), or even the effect of removing interrupted sutures and rotation of the remaining running suture (Figure 9.7).

These illustrations demonstrate how keratometry may be misleading since clearly the corneal power changes are neither orthogonal nor symmetrical across a given meridian (i.e., 0° to 180° axis or 90° to 270° axis).

Suture Rotation

Van Meter et al[1] introduced a further refinement in postoperative suture adjustment by utilizing a 24 bite running suture as the sole closure. Tension on the suture is then adjusted postoperatively, guided by the computer-assisted topographic analysis. In a prospective randomized study, we have shown both more rapid recovery and less final astigmatism with the 24 bite running suture adjustment technique compared to a technique utilizing 8 interrupted sutures combined with a 16 bite running suture.[2]

Figures 9.8 to 9.12 represent detailed case reports documenting the value of this technique and powerfully demonstrate the use of corneal topography in postoperative suture adjustment.

Relaxing Incisions

Obviously none of the dramatic effects outlined in the cases above are useful once all the sutures have been removed. At this point, corneal relaxing incisions provide a useful alternative. Figures 9.13 and 9.14 not only demonstrate the value of these incisions but document the necessity to perform asymmetric surgery for the asymmetric astigmatism frequently present.

Summary

As the above described examples amply demonstrate, corneal topography has dramatically improved the post-surgical management of astigmatism in the corneal transplant case.

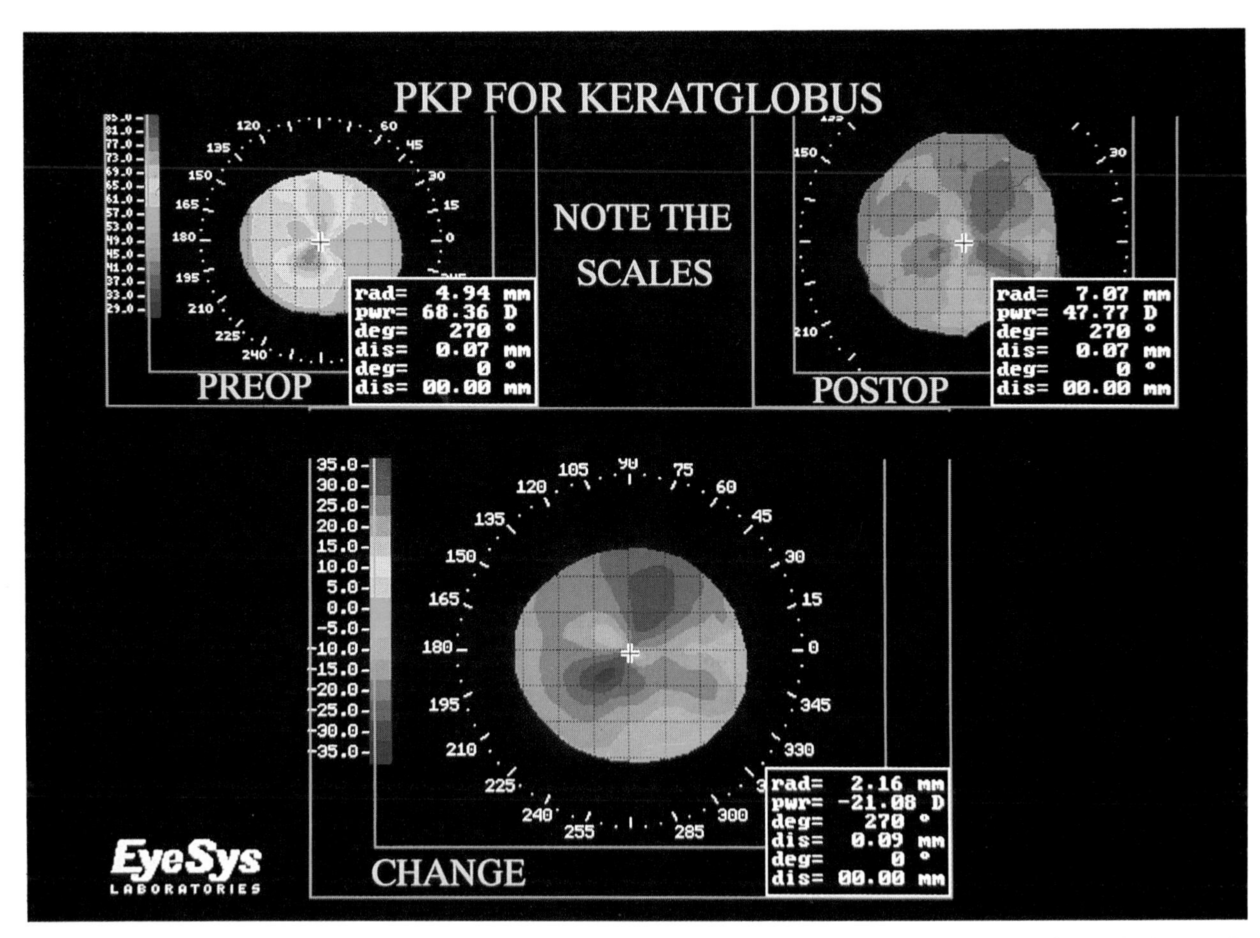

Figure 9.1: Penetrating keratoplasty for keratoglobus one day preoperatively (left) and one day postoperatively (right). Note the marked conversion of central steepness to relative central flatness. Bottom, subtraction, or change, map shows the dramatic postoperative flattening in excess of 20 D (courtesy of Douglas Koch, MD).

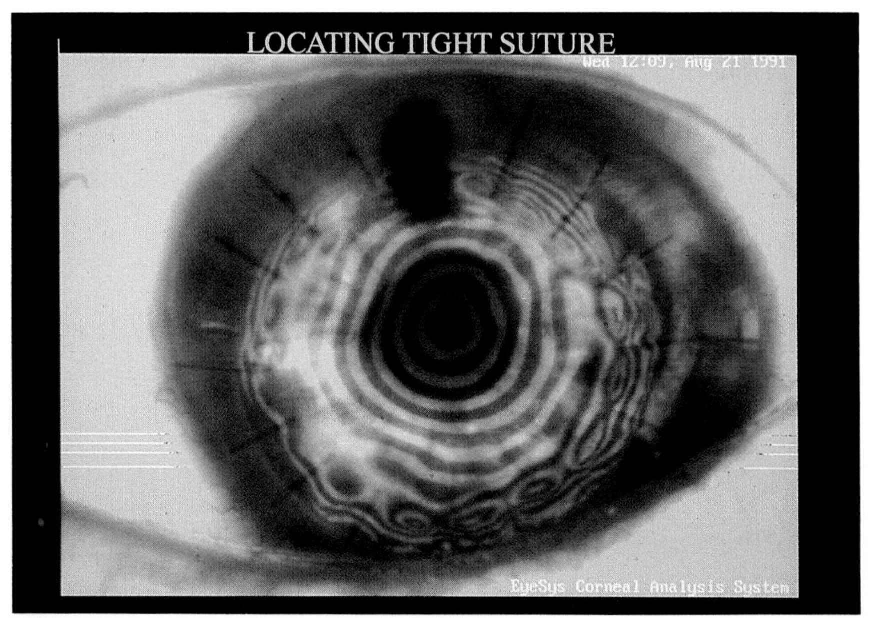

Figure 9.2A.

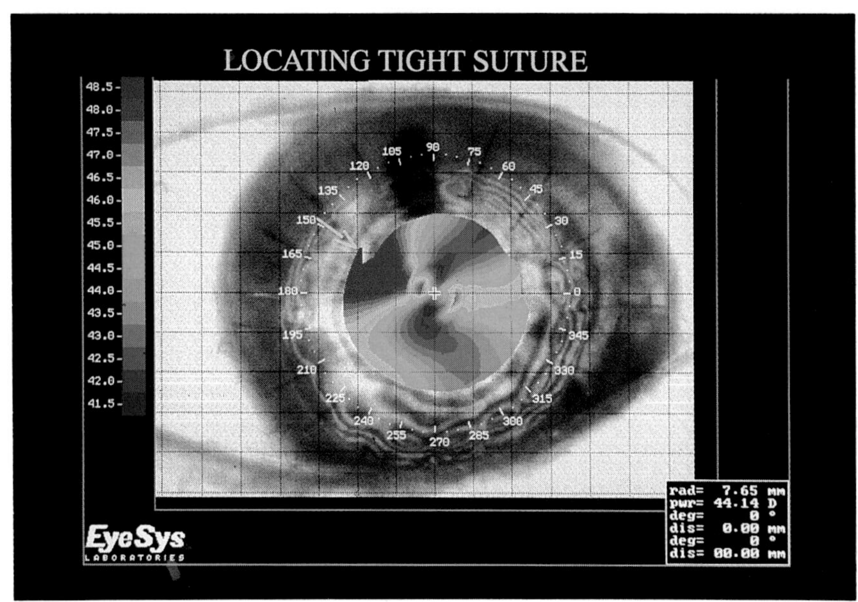

Figure 9.2B.

Figure 9.2: Localization of tight interrupted suture. (A) Placido image: location of tight suture not obvious. (B) Overlay corneal map: marked area of steepening (arrow) localizes the suture(s) that needs removal.

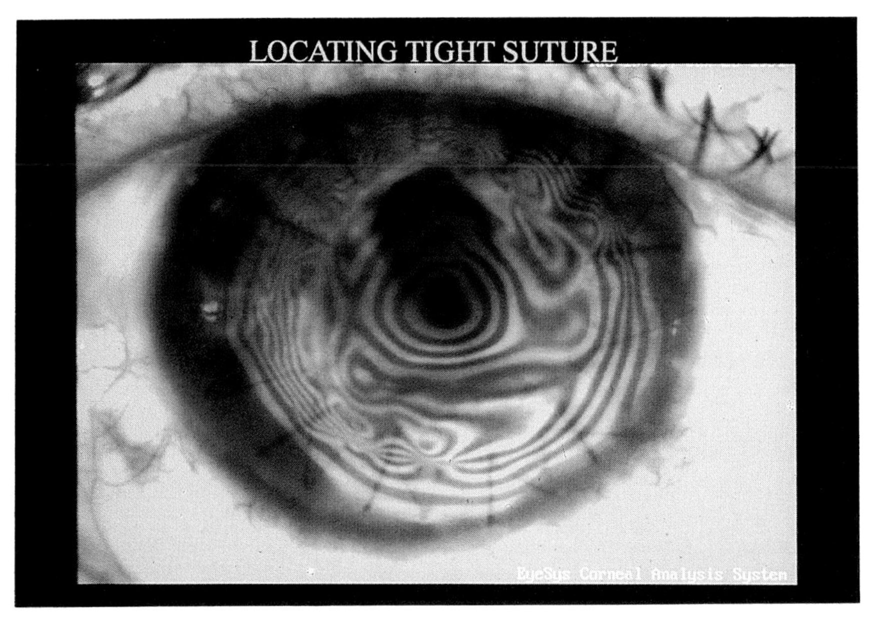

Figure 9.3A.

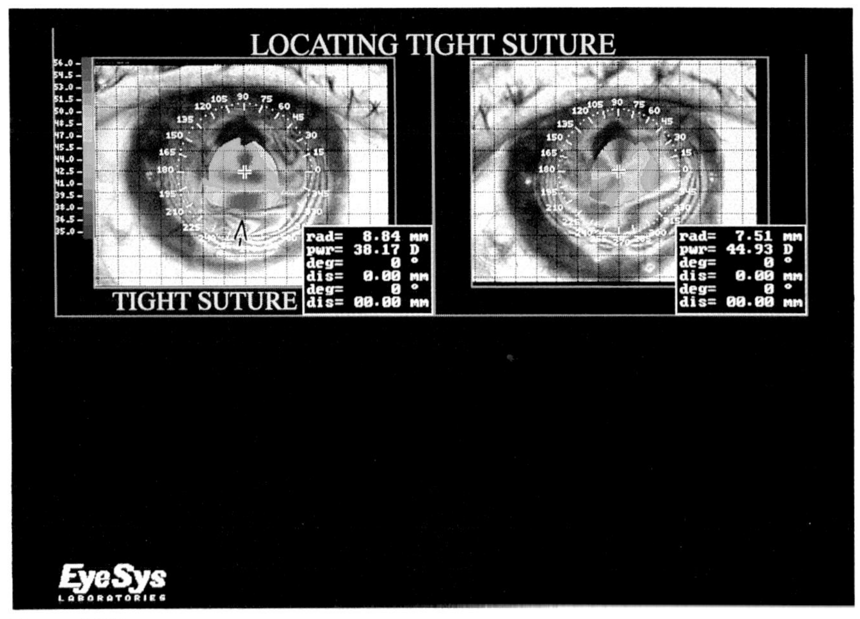

Figure 9.3B.

Figure 9.3: Localization and removal of tight interrupted suture. (A) Placido image difficult to interpret. (B) Overlay corneal map. Left, inferior area of steepening due to tight suture (arrow) is obvious. Right, 20 months following suture removal the central topography assumes a more regular astigmatic pattern (courtesy of Douglas Koch, MD).

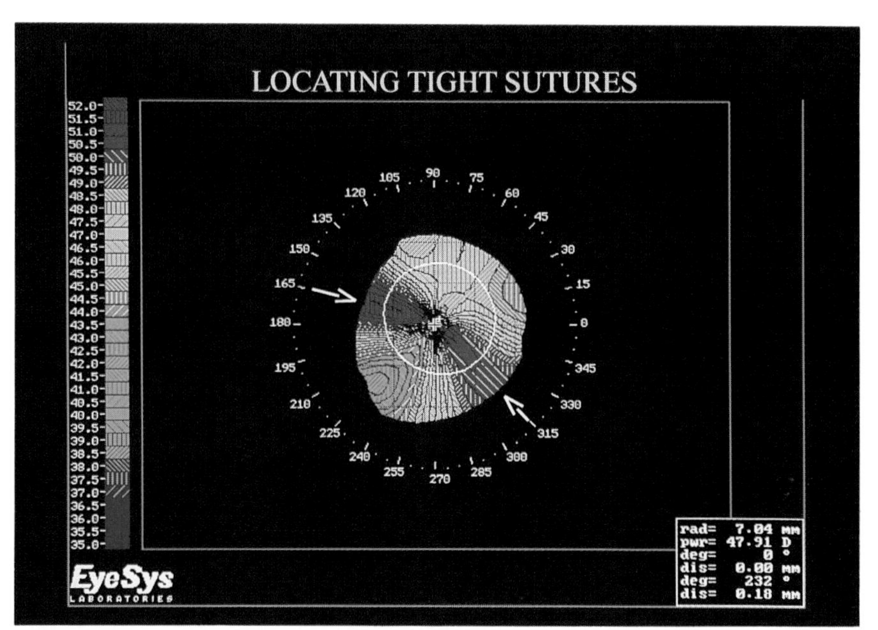

Figure 9.4A.

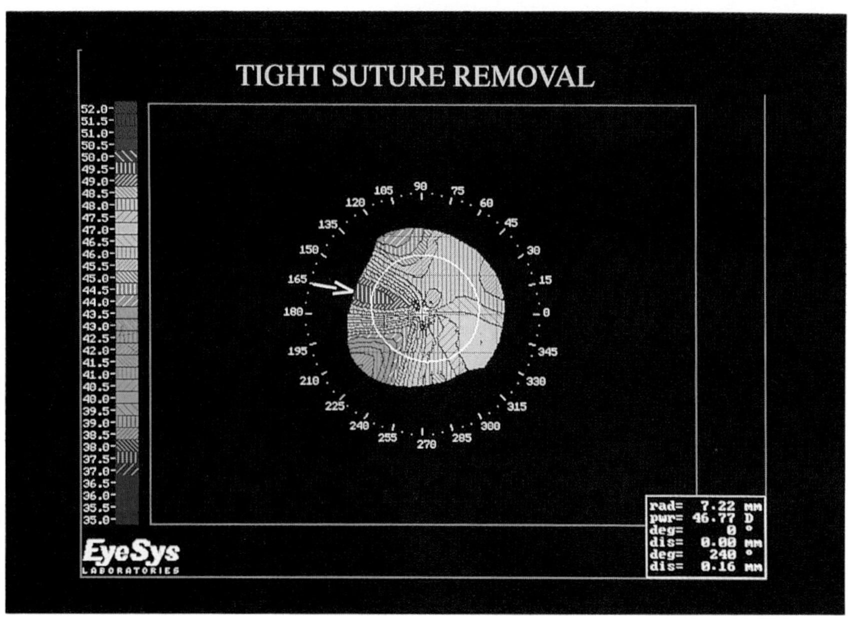

Figure 9.4B.

Figure 9.4: Localization and removal of tight interrupted suture. (A) Corneal topography reveals steep hemi-meridians at 165° and 315° (arrows, 150° apart) corresponding to areas with tight sutures. (B) Corneal topography 30 minutes after suture at 315° removed, with dramatic decrease in the astigmatism. The examiner advised the patient to wait until the next visit to consider suture removal at 165° (arrow) (courtesy of Daniel Durrie, MD).

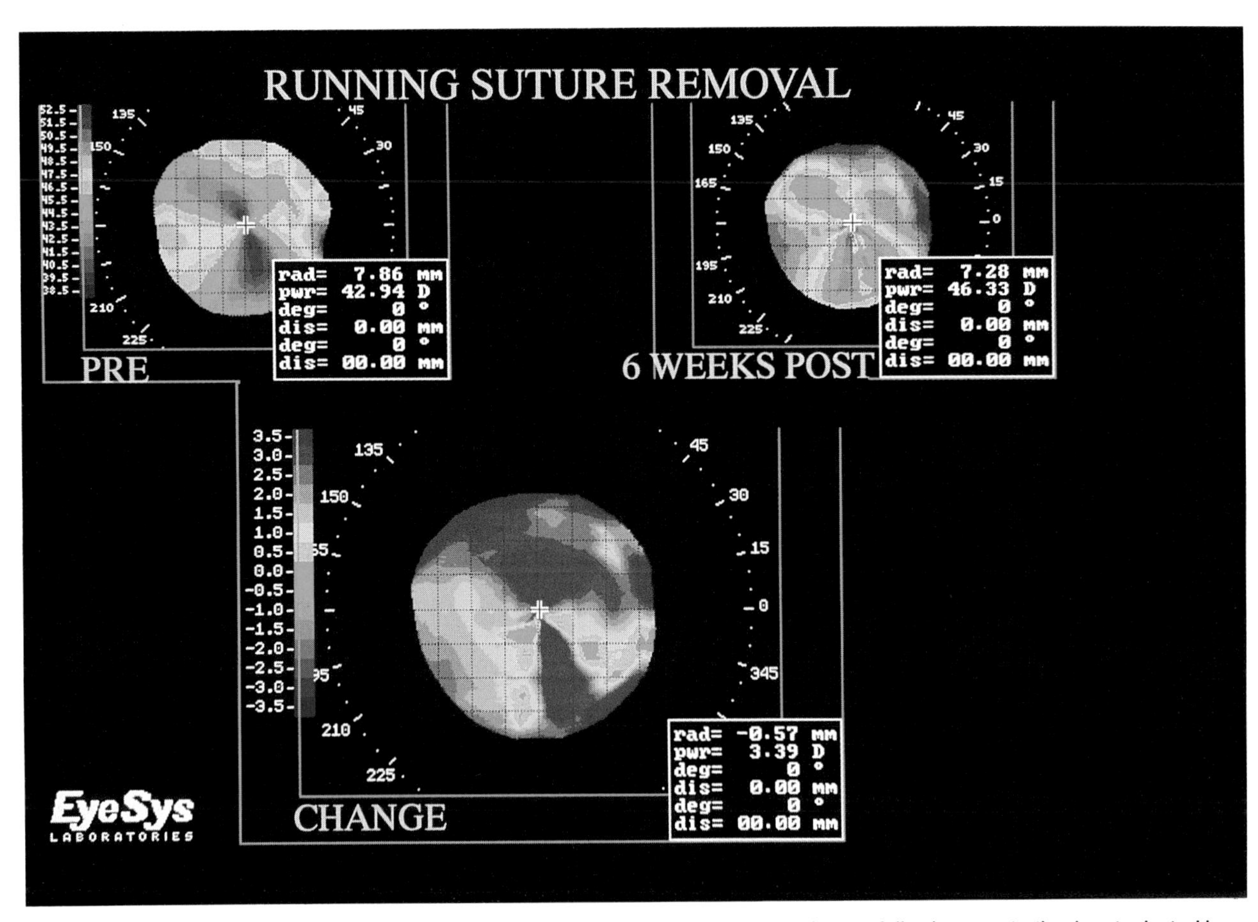

Figure 9.5: Topographic maps of the right cornea of an 85 year old, one-eyed male, 4 years following penetrating keratoplasty. Upper left, 16-bite running suture is still in place. Upper right, 6 weeks following removal of the running suture, the cornea has steepened with a reduction of astigmatism. Bottom, subtraction, or change, map showing greater steepening vertically than horizontally, reducing astigmatism by 1 D.

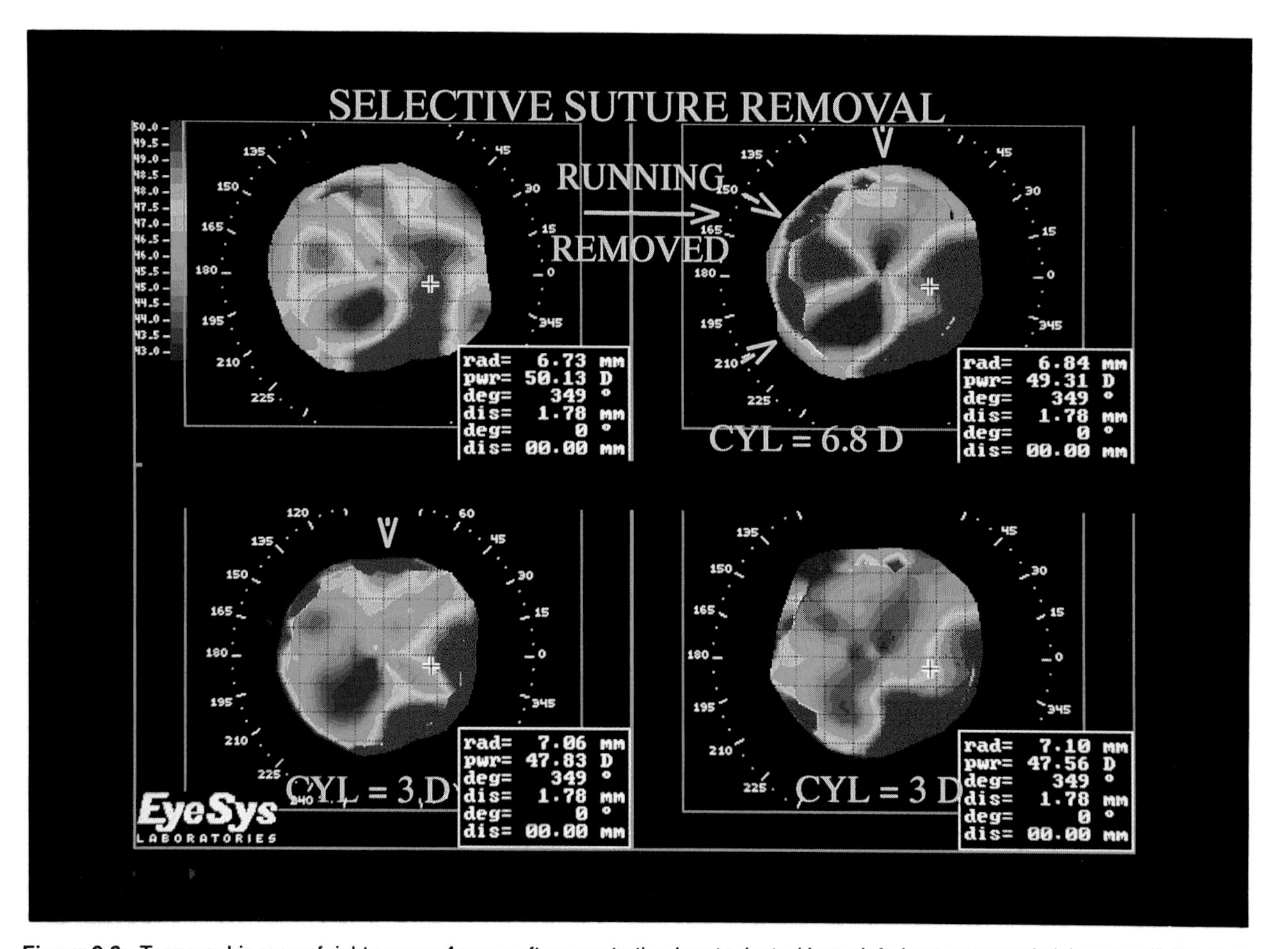

Figure 9.6: Topographic map of right cornea 4 years after penetrating keratoplasty. Upper left, best-corrected vision was 20/70. Note irregular astigmatism. Upper right, following removal of the running suture, the corneal topography is more regular. Interrupted sutures remain at the 8:00, 10:00 and 12:00 positions (arrows). Lower left, following removal of the 8:00 and 10:00 sutures, astigmatism has been reduced from 6.83 D to 3.00 D, although some irregularity is present. The 12:00 suture is still in place (arrow). Lower right, following removal of the 12:00 suture, astigmatism is still 3.00 D, but the cornea is more regular. Best-corrected vision is 20/30. Note the persistent steep zone inferonasally.

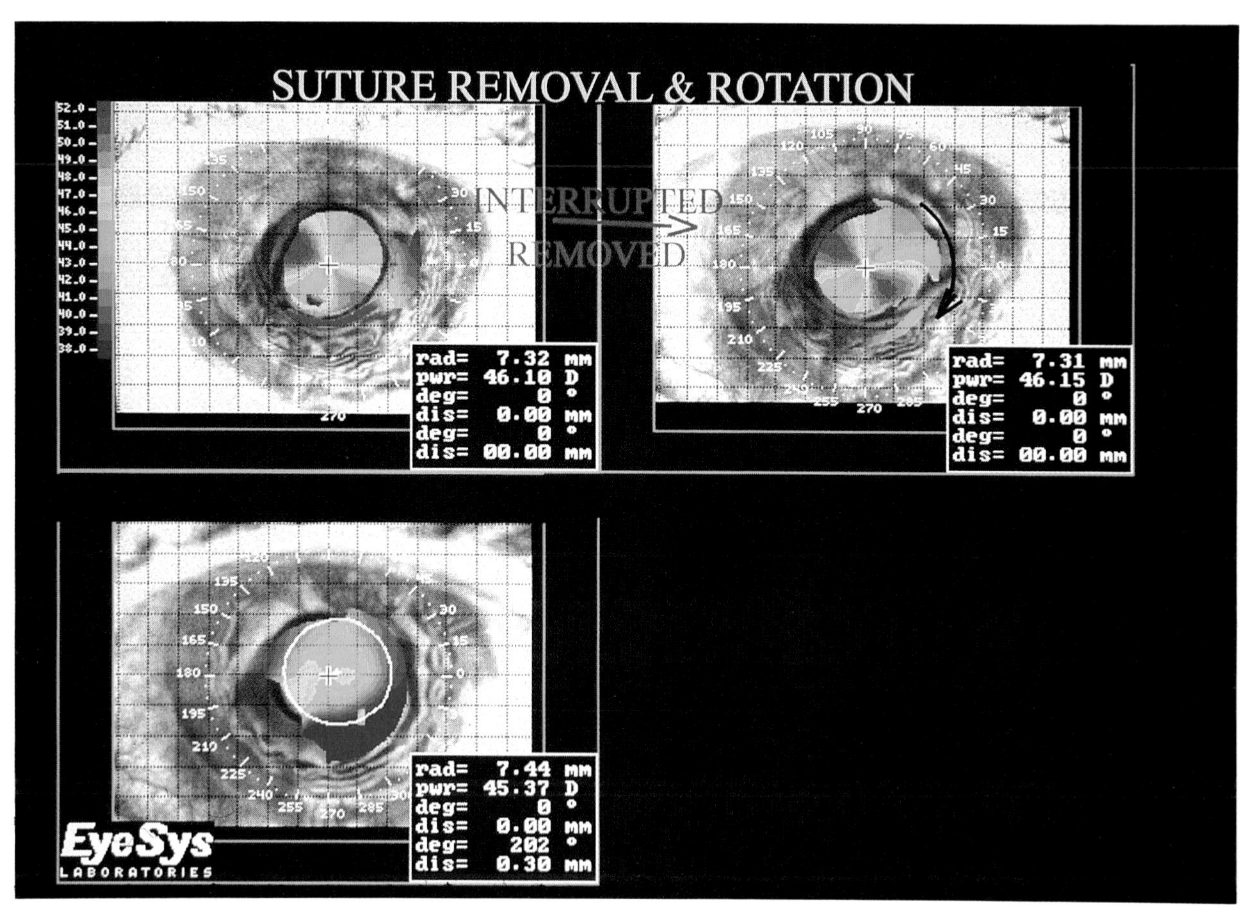

Figure 9.7: One-eyed 73 year old male with severe open-angle glaucoma. Fellow eye is blind secondary to glaucoma. He is 4 months status post penetrating keratoplasty and eager for improved vision. He describes his acuity of 20/400- as "very faint" with poor edge definition. Initial topography (upper left) shows the explanation for this problem, with a very high degree of semi-regular, asymmetric astigmatism. This patient had undergone suturing of the transplant with eight interrupted 10-0 nylon sutures in addition to a 16-bite running 10-0 nylon suture for added security in view of his one-eyed status. Upper right, all of the interrupted sutures were removed, which resulted in some improvement of the regularity, but with persistence of the same orientation of astigmatism. The 16-bite suture was therefore adjusted. Suture material from the flattest hemi-meridian centered at 50° was shifted inferotemporally toward 315° (shift from 1:00 to 4:00, arrow). Lower left, repeat topography shows marked improvement in the overall astigmatism. There is still some component of irregular astigmatism but markedly improved. The patient's acuity improved slightly to 20/200, but he reported markedly improved vision qualitatively, with much better edge definition to objects. The suture in the wound will be allowed to settle for approximately 1 month and the patient will return for re-measurement and refraction with further suture adjustment if needed.

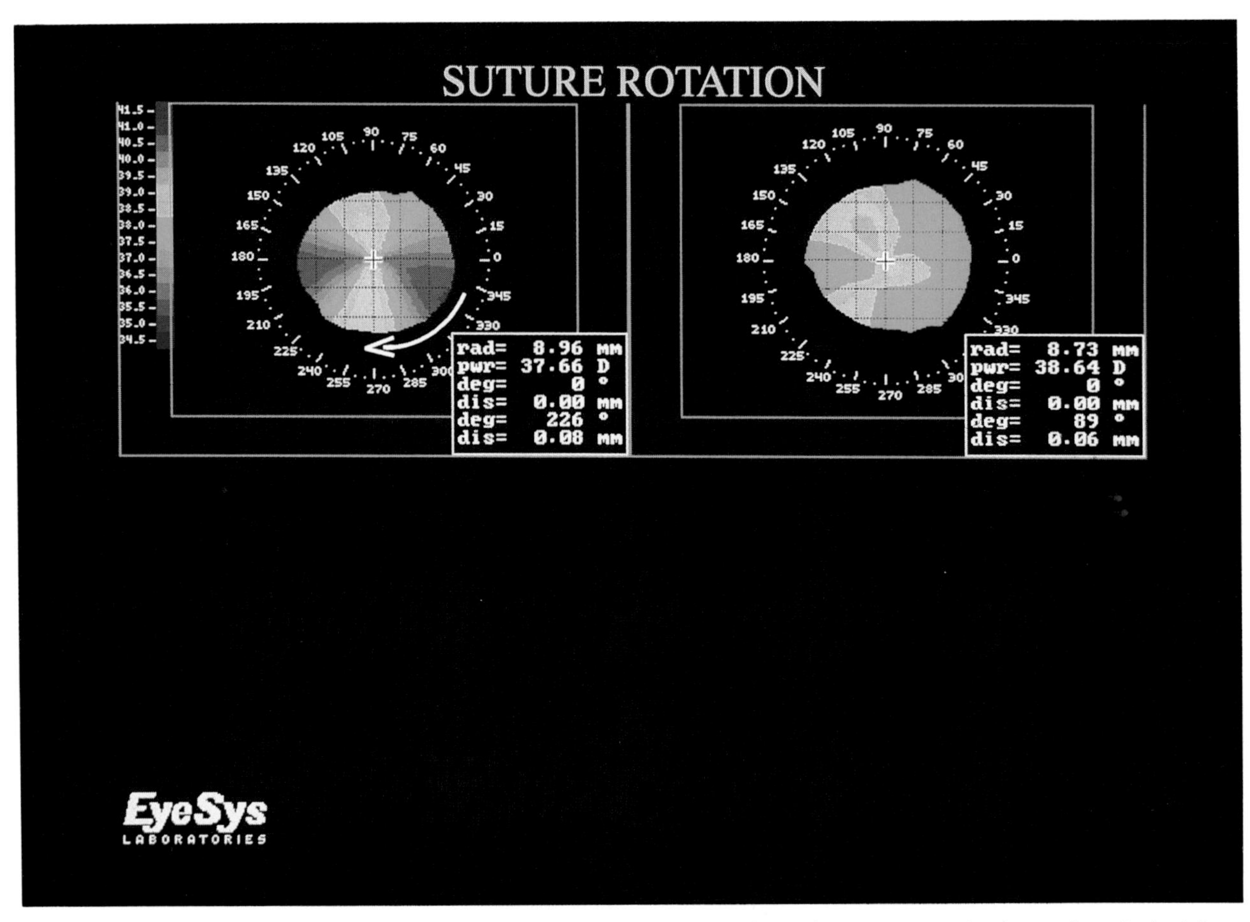

Figure 9.8: Case M.P. The patient is a 27 year old female with keratoconus who underwent penetrating keratoplasty in the left eye utilizing the 24-bite 10-0 nylon running suture technique. The first topographic image, 1 month postoperatively (left), shows fairly regular astigmatism. Both keratometrically and refractively, she had 4 D of astigmatism with the steep orientation vertically. The suture was adjusted by moving suture material from the flattest hemi-meridian as indicated by the peripheral blue coloration at 4:00, or the hemi-meridian centered at 330°. Suture material was moved from this flat hemi-meridian inferiorly toward the 6:00 position at 270° (arrow). Repeat topography approximately 35 minutes later (right) shows marked improvement in overall sphericity with reduction in cylinder. There is still some component of irregular astigmatism. At this point the wound is left to settle down and re-evaluation will be performed in 1 month. The patient notes qualitatively marked improvement in uncorrected vision.

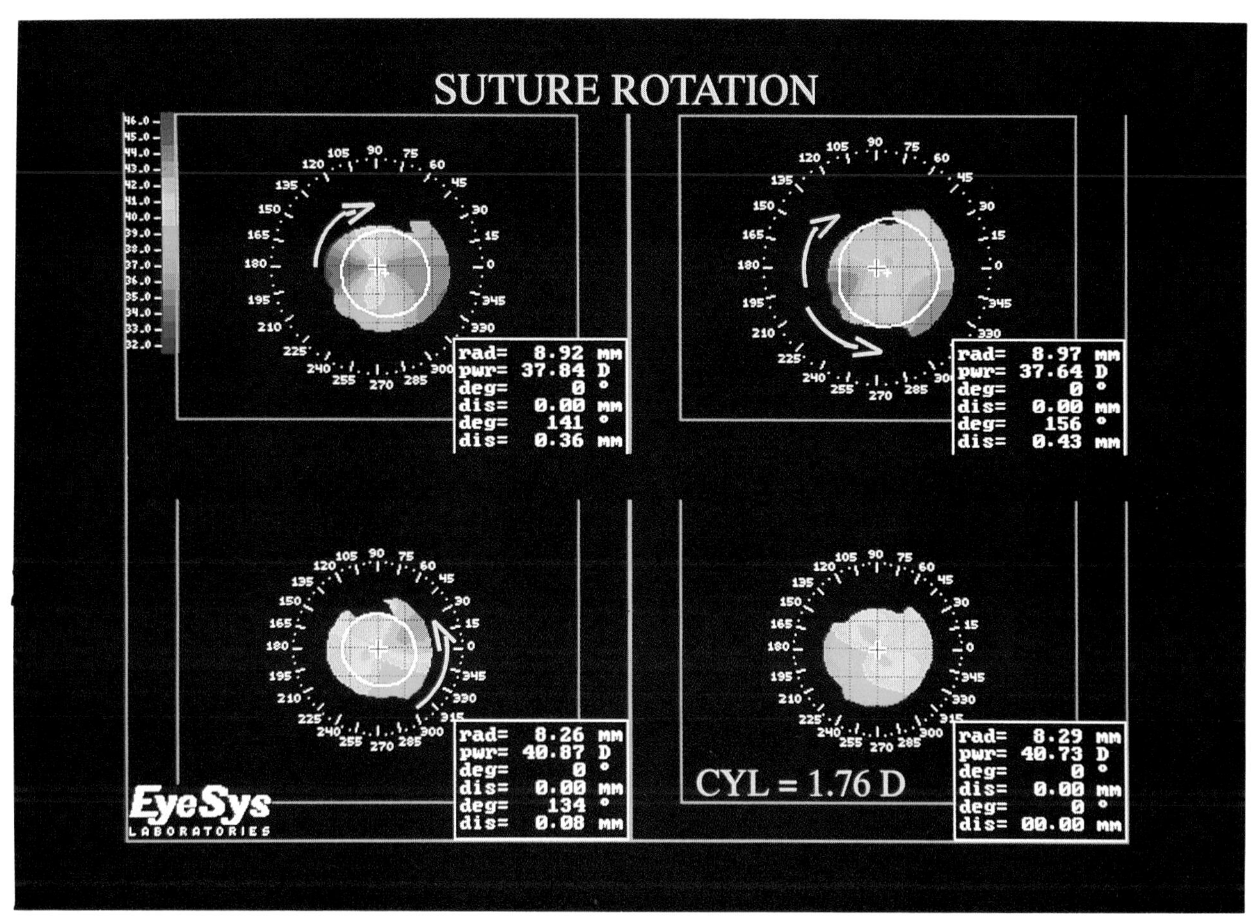

Figure 9.9: Case A.A. The patient is a 30 year old male with keratoconus. Five weeks earlier he had undergone penetrating keratoplasty in his left eye. The baseline topography (upper left) shows steepening vertically and flattening horizontally, with more prominent steepening at the 90° hemi-meridian. The tension on the running suture was adjusted by tightening suture loops from 180° (9:00) and moving the suture material toward 90° (12:00, arrow). Upper right, re-evaluation one hour later shows dramatic reduction in total astigmatism but a shift toward some irregular astigmatism with maximal steepening at the 125° hemi-meridian and maximal flattening at 195°. This astigmatism was then adjusted on a second immediate revision by tightening suture loops centered at 195° and moving tension both toward 140° and toward 270° as indicated by the topographic analysis (suture shifted from 8:00 toward 10:30 and toward 6:00, arrows). Lower left, re-evaluation 30 minutes later shows further reduction in net astigmatism but marked asymmetry with a maximally steep hemi-meridian at 30° and a maximally flat meridian at 290°. Accordingly a third revision was performed, tightening loops at 290° and moving them toward 30° (5:00 toward 2:00, arrows) Lower right, the final keratograph 30 minutes later shows a return to relatively regular astigmatism with a net keratometric astigmatism of 1.76 D. This series of adjustments and consecutive topographic analyses were performed to demonstrate the power of the computer-assisted corneal topography to follow and direct the suture adjustment. Our more typical procedure is to begin suture adjustment 1 month postoperatively, as soon as the surface is smooth enough to permit it, but rarely do we perform more than one adjustment at a given session. Some realignment of the suture occurs in the weeks following the adjustment, and we will typically allow 2 to 4 weeks to pass before bringing the patient back for reanalysis with refraction, repeat topographic analysis, and further adjustment if needed.

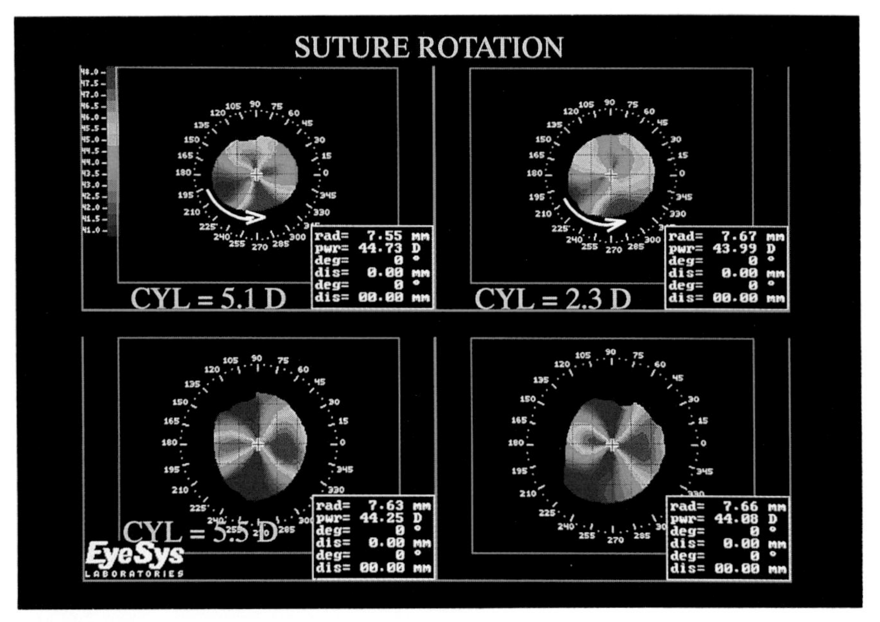

Figure 9.10A.

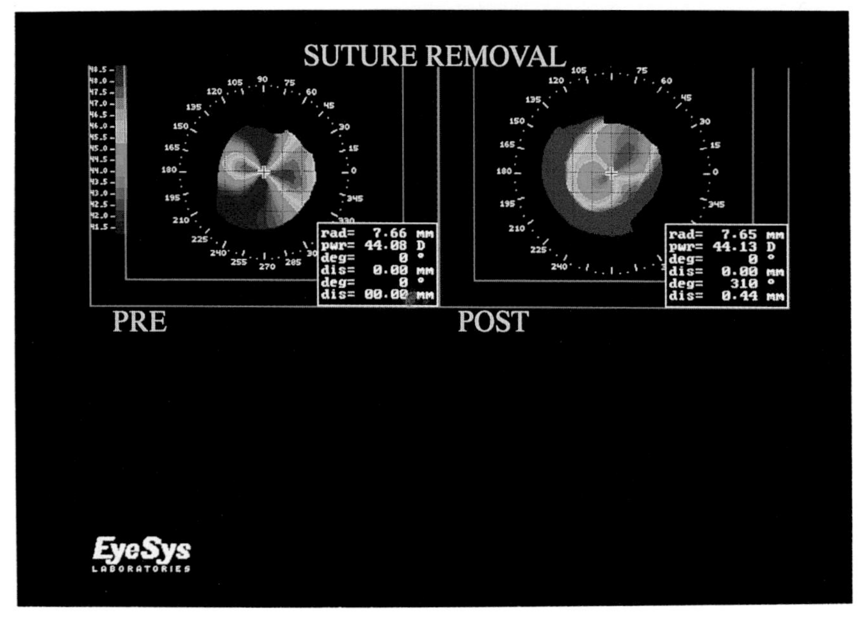

Figure 9.10B.

Figure 9.10: Case T.T. (A) This 21 year old female underwent penetrating keratoplasty due to central corneal scarring from a *Pseudomonas* ulcer acquired during extended wear soft contact lens use. Suturing utilized the 24-bite 10-0 nylon running suture technique. Upper left, 1 month postoperatively the topography exhibited 5 D of central astigmatism with mild asymmetry of the hemi-meridians but good orthogonality. Guided by the topography, suture material was tightened in the flattest hemi-meridian at 195° and passed to the steepest hemi-meridian centered at 285° (8:00 to 5:00, arrow). Upper right, by the third postoperative month repeat topography showed less central astigmatism by conventional keratometry (5 D had been reduced to 2.3 D), but the residual astigmatism was asymmetric, limiting best spectacle correction to 20/40. A second suture manipulation was therefore performed, shifting more suture material from the flattest hemi-meridian centered at 200° to the steepest hemi-meridian centered at 290° (arrow). Lower left, 90 minutes later repeat topography showed marked improvement in the regularity of the astigmatism with return of orthogonality but with a net increase in conventional keratometric cylinder (2.3 D increased to 5.5 D). Lower right, by the fifth postoperative month, no spontaneous improvement in the residual astigmatism had occurred. (B) After a graft rejection episode successfully reversed with intense topical steroids, the suture spontaneously loosened and was removed. The wound appeared anatomically stable. Topographic analysis (right) 1 year postoperatively showed mildly asymmetric astigmatism with conventional keratometric cylinder of 3 D. Compare this image to topography with suture-in 8 months earlier (left). This case dramatically illustrates the power of suture adjustment on astigmatism, both regular and irregular. Also clearly illustrated by the suture-out topography 1 year postoperatively is the appearance of an entirely different topographic pattern, which is consistent with the literature suggesting that, based on historical controls, there is no evidence yet that suture manipulation affects the ultimate astigmatism after full suture removal. Until a suture manipulation technique does demonstrate such an effect, the working hypothesis is that postoperative suture manipulation has the goal of improving suture-in astigmatism. Depending upon the patient's age and underlying pathology, as well as the surgeon's own technique, nylon sutures are typically retained between 1 and 5 years. Restoration of good acuity during this period is therefore an important goal.

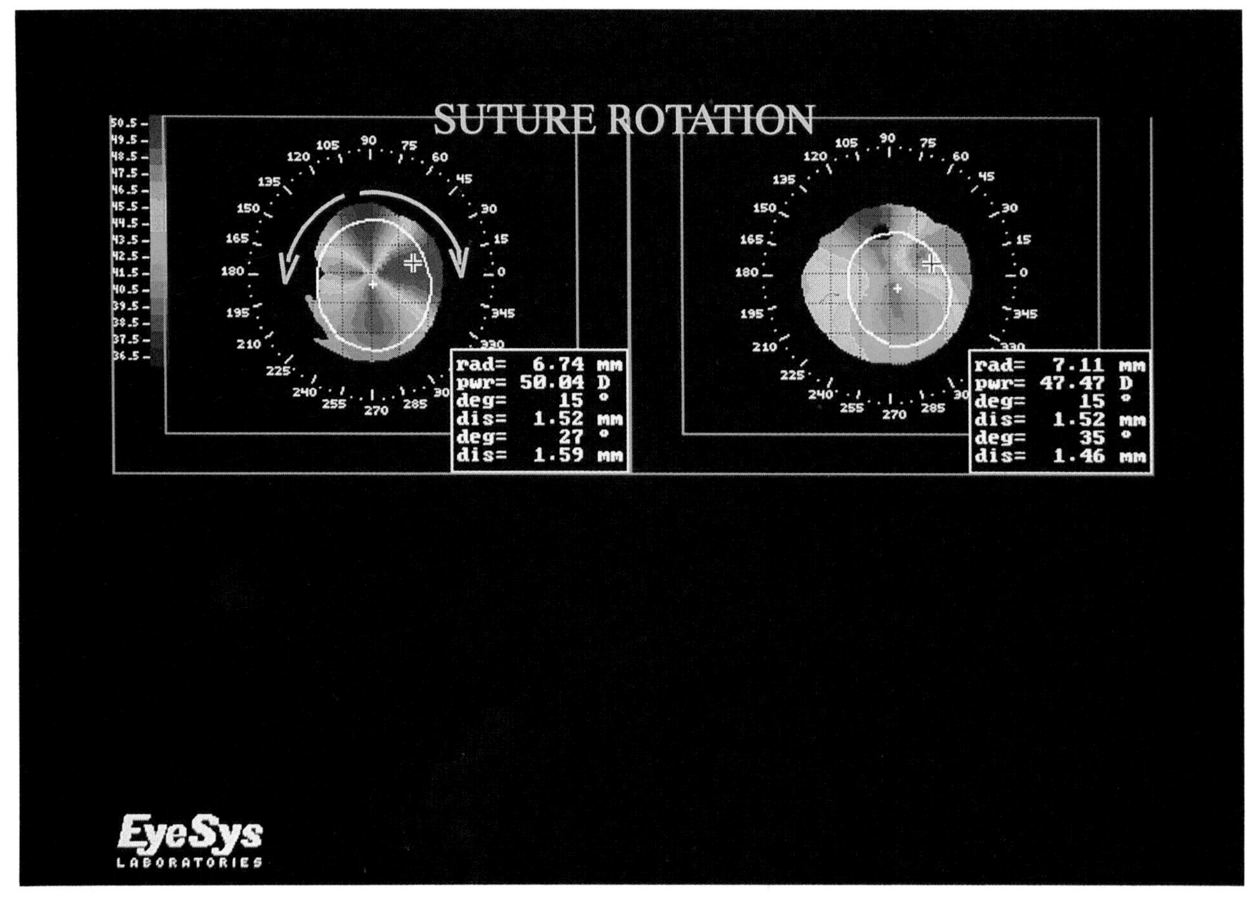

Figure 9.11: Case C.T. This 40 year old male is status post repeat penetrating keratoplasty for corneal decompensation secondary to congenital glaucoma and multiple ocular surgeries. His most recent transplant in the eye was 7 weeks prior to this examination. Upper left, right eye topography shows fairly symmetrical vertical flattening but asymmetrical steepening horizontally with the steepest hemi-meridian at 0°. His 24-bite running suture was adjusted based on the topography. The knot was located precisely at 95°, in the middle of the flat superior hemi-meridian. Beginning at the knot, the superior suture was tightened and the generated slack suture moved toward both 0° and 180° (arrows), which resulted in the improvement illustrated at the upper right. The cursor shows reduction in the steepest hemi-meridian from 50.04 D to 47.47 D. Acuity was markedly improved by the procedure. Uncorrected acuity had improved from 20/400 to 20/100. Best-corrected acuity improved further to 20/80.

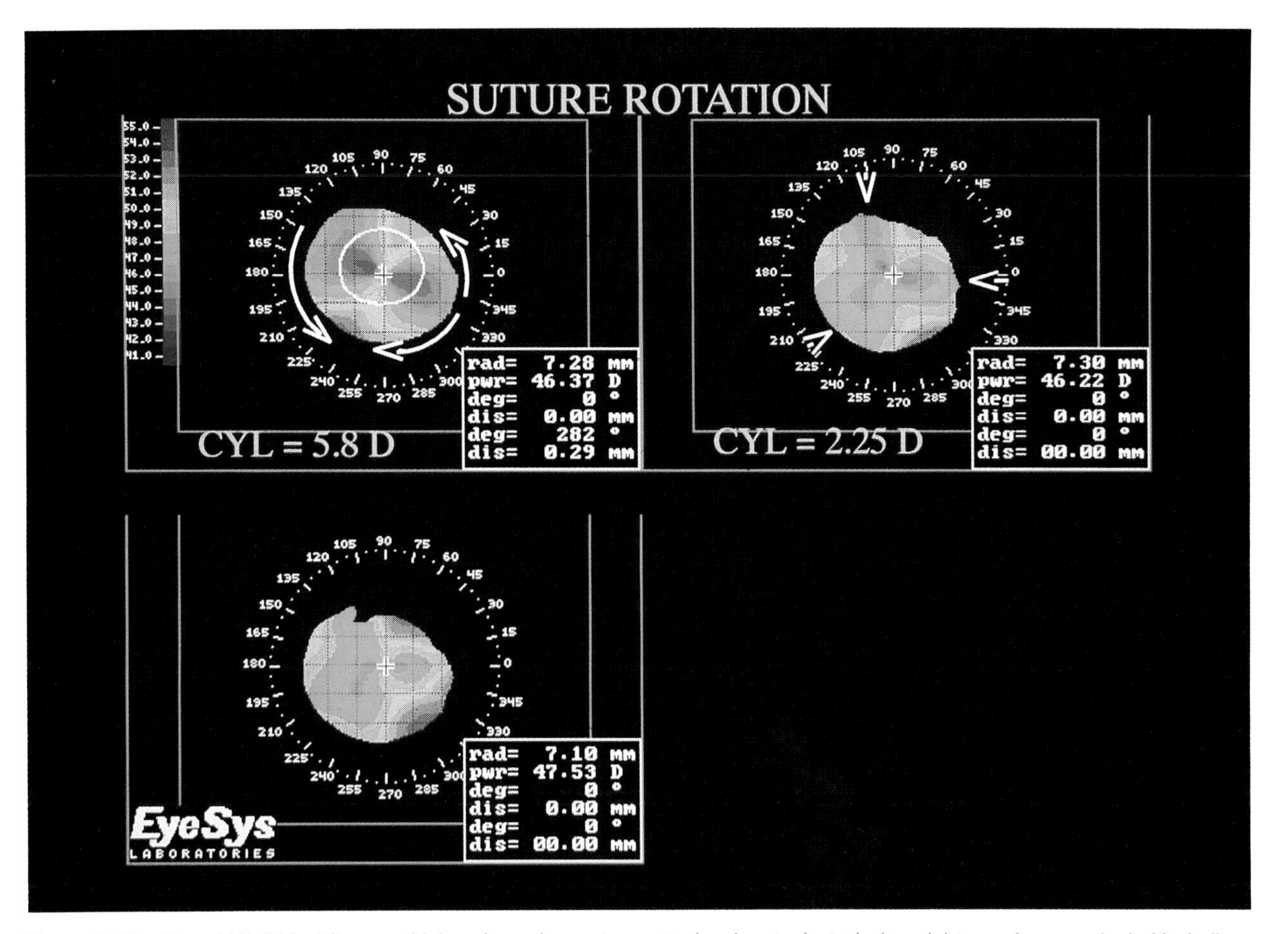

Figure 9.12: Case H.T. This 83 year old female underwent penetrating keratoplasty in her right eye for pseudophakic bullous keratopathy. The 24-bite running 10-0 nylon suture technique was used. Early postoperative filamentary keratitis gradually cleared and topographic analysis became possible 10 weeks postoperatively. Upper left, initial astigmatism disclosed regular astigmatism with 5.8 D of keratometric cylinder. Suture tension was adjusted moving suture material from the flat hemi-meridian at 345° both toward 60° and 240° and from the opposite flat hemi-meridian at 150° toward the steep hemi-meridian at 240° (arrows). Upper right, 5 months postoperatively a marked reduction in total astigmatism had occurred, but with development of an interesting pattern of three flat hemi-meridians (arrows). Nevertheless, refractive astigmatism dropped from 5.5 D prior to the manipulation to 2.25 D. No further suture manipulations were undertaken. The irregular astigmatic component diminished by 7 months postoperatively (lower left).

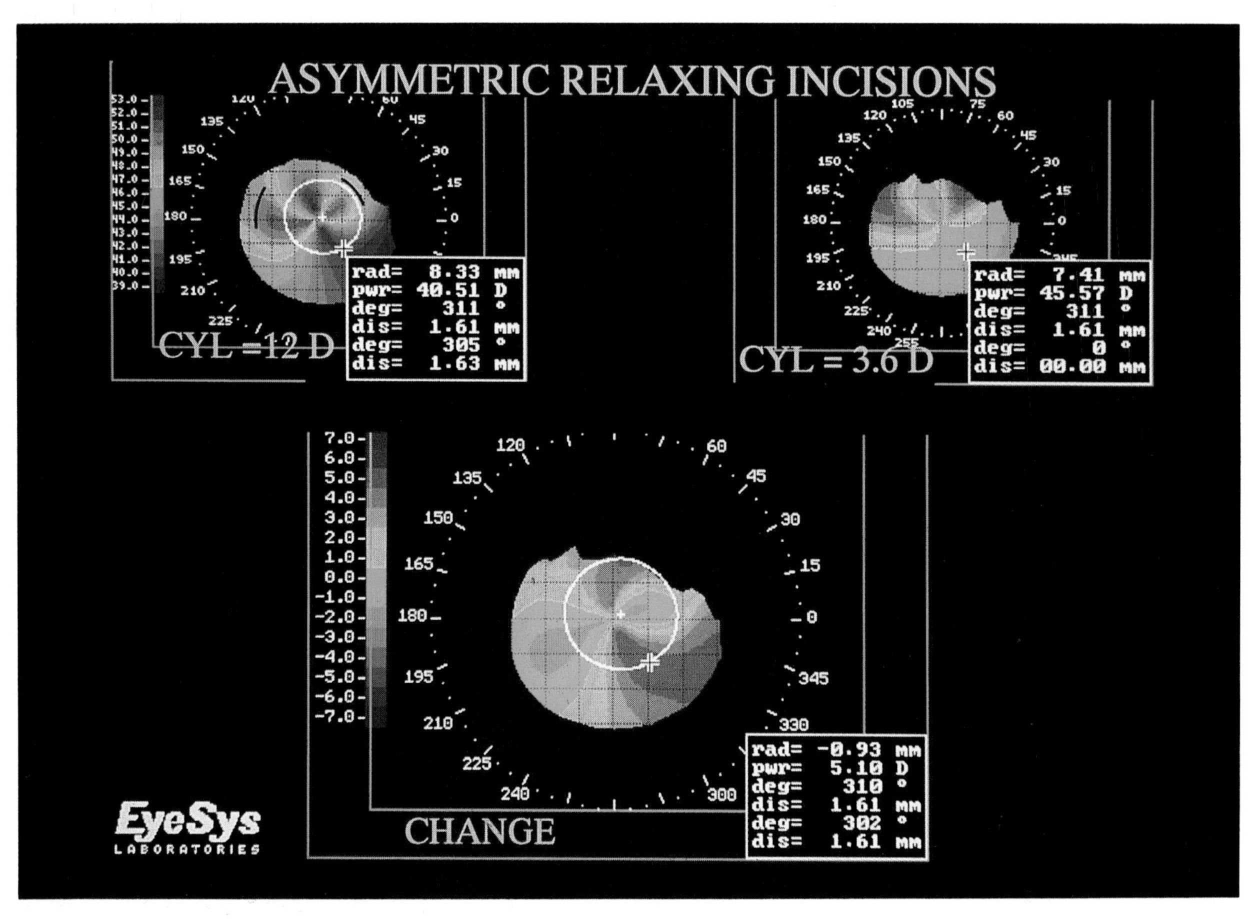

Figure 9.13: Case P.M. Upper left, topographic map of right cornea of a 52 year old male with 12 D of astigmatism 10 years following penetrating keratoplasty. Contact lens fitting was unsuccessful due to lens decentration. Relaxing incisions in the graft-host junction along the 30° and 190° semi-meridians were placed (curved lines). Upper right, 3 month postoperative appearance. Keratometric cylinder is now 3.6 D at 32°. Bottom, difference map shows that the greatest change consisted of steepening of the flat zones approximately 90° from the sites of the incisions.

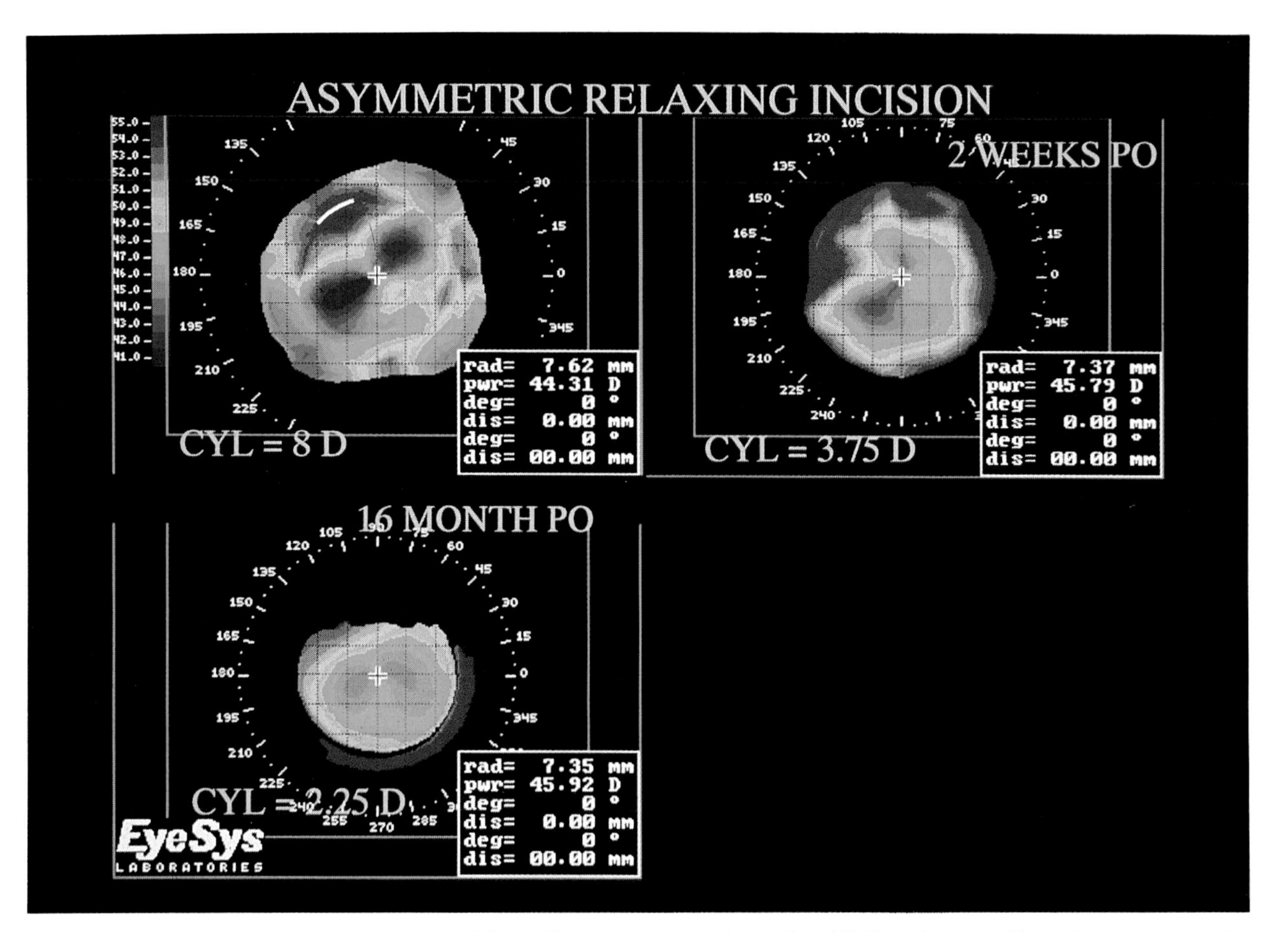

Figure 9.14: Case H.M. 65 year old male physician with keratoconus and pseudoexfoliation glaucoma. He underwent penetrating keratoplasty in the left eye due to contact lens intolerance in April, 1989. Upper left, after full suture removal, he was left with an unacceptable degree of astigmatism. Examination of the topography showed a relatively symmetrical flat meridian at 50° but asymmetry of the steep hemi-meridians, with most of the steep meridian concentrated at the superonasal quadrant centered at 125° A relaxing incision (curved line) was placed in the wound down to approximately 95% depth as guided by computer topography. His refraction prior to the relaxing incisions was -1.50 -8.00 X 55, yielding 20/30^{-2} vision. The cornea could not retain a stable hard contact lens. Upper right, re-evaluation 2 weeks later showed dramatic improvement. Much less residual astigmatism is present. A refraction of - 1.75 - 3.75 X 75 yielded the same 20/30 acuity. Lower left, ongoing wound healing improved the situation further. In follow-up more than 1 year later, the computer topography shows more regularity in the optical zone. A spectacle correction was now - 2.00 - 2.25 X 150, yielding 20/30. This case illustrates the utility of the topographer in designing astigmatic keratotomies for postoperative astigmatism. A symmetrical keratotomy as indicated by keratometry readings and refraction would have resulted in an inappropriate incision in the inferotemporal quadrant.

References

1. Van Meter WS, Gussler JR, Soloman KD, Wood TO: Postkeratoplasty astigmatism control: single continuous suture adjustments versus selective interrupted suture removal. *Ophthalmology* 98:177-183, 1991.
2. Filatov V, Talamo J, Steinert RF. Postkeratoplasty astigmatism: Single running suture adjustment versus selective removal of interrupted sutures—a prospective randomized study. *Arch Ophthalmol* (in press).

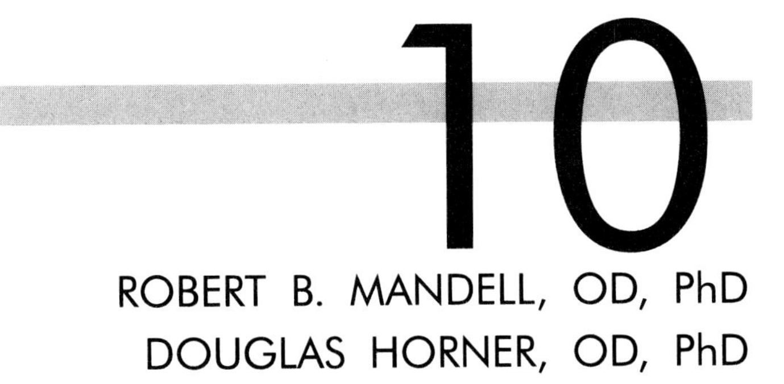

ROBERT B. MANDELL, OD, PhD
DOUGLAS HORNER, OD, PhD

Alignment of Videokeratoscopes

What may first appear to be a trivial problem of aligning a videokeratoscope appropriately with the cornea has proven to be a challenging task. The same problem is shared by the alignment of a photorefractive system and hence is of critical importance.

Understanding the alignment of videokeratoscopes is made complex by the confusion surrounding the various reference points and axes of the eye, which require clarification.

Entrance Pupil

The primary reference point of the eye for refractive procedures is the center of the entrance pupil. The entrance pupil is the image of the real pupil formed by the optics in front of it. Since we can never actually see the real pupil of a patient when the eye is intact, we have only its image available to us, which fortunately serves quite well. Basic optics dictate that any ray directed towards a point on the entrance pupil will, after refraction, pass through the corresponding point on the real pupil (Figure 10.1).

Line of Sight

The line of sight is the most appropriate reference axis of the eye to be used in videokeratoscopy because it can be accurately determined clinically and it relates closely to the optical properties of the ocular system. It is also unaffected by most of the irregularities commonly encountered in the real eye. The line of sight is defined as the straight line from the fixation point to the center of the entrance pupil. This definition is deceptively simple. If a light ray traveled from the fixation point along the line of sight, it would actually be deviated from the line of sight at the tear layer where refraction would begin. It would then be refracted

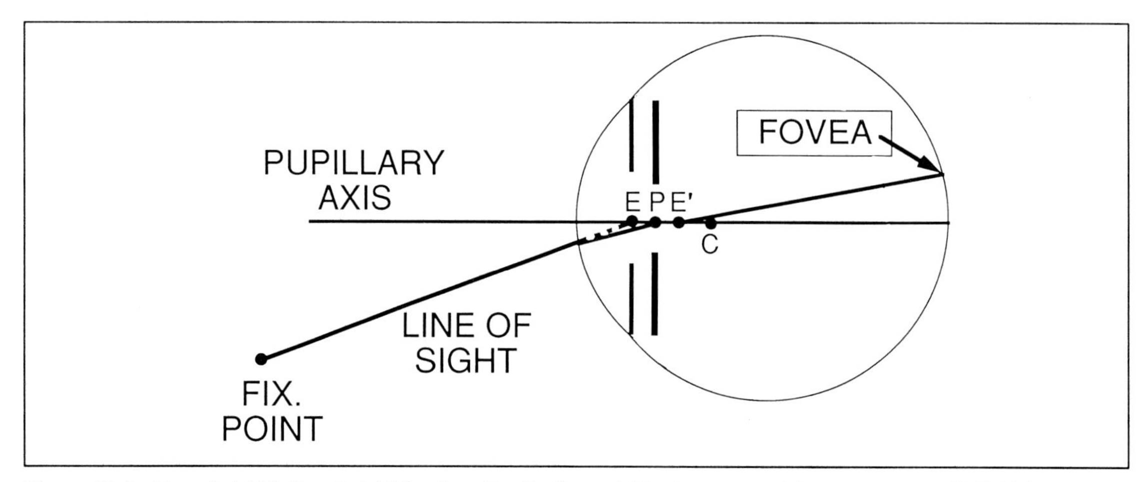

Figure 10.1: Line of sight is the straight line from the fixation point to the center of the entrance pupil, E. Light traveling along the line of sight is refracted at the cornea and passes through the center of the real pupil, P. Light leaving the crystalline lens passes to the retina as though coming from the exit pupil, E′.

by the cornea, pass through the real pupil and be refracted by all the remaining optical elements of the eye until it eventually reached the retina at the foveal position. It must ultimately strike the fovea because by definition the subject is looking at the fixation point.

When a patient looks at an object point all the rays from that point which are directed towards the entrance pupil will, after refraction, pass through the real pupil after refraction and come to a focus at the fovea, assuming emmetropia (Figure 10.2). These rays form a cone of light that is centered on the line of sight, which makes the line of sight the primary reference axis. For an ammetropic eye the blur circle would be symmetrical with respect to the same axis.

Two points in space must be located in order to identify a patient's line of sight, of which one must be the fixation point (Figure 10.3). The second point may be located by the patient as in using a gunsight or may be found objectively by directing the optic axis

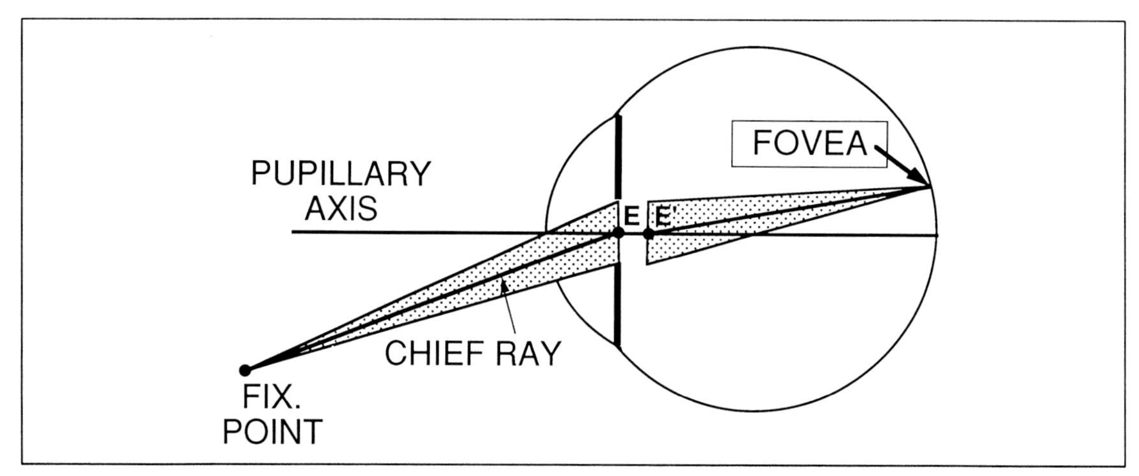

Figure 10.2: Line of sight is the chief (central) ray for the bundle of light that actually passes through the eye to the fovea, as though from the exit pupil, E′.

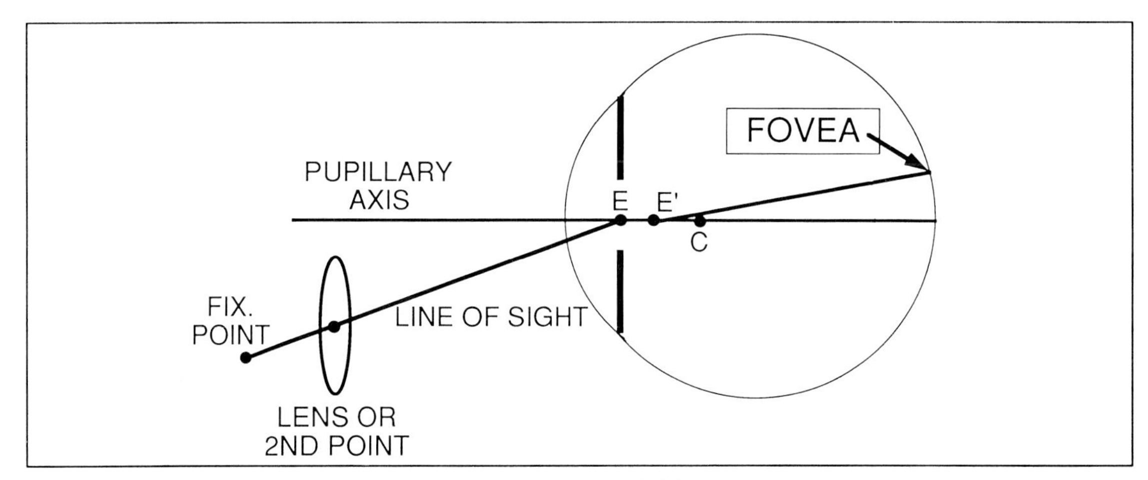

Figure 10.3: Two points in space are required to locate the line of sight.

of a microscope at the center of the patient's entrance pupil. Additionally, the patient must fixate an object point on the optic axis of the microscope.

Visual Axis

The commonly used reference line known as the visual axis should not be used with respect to videokeratoscopy because it cannot be found using clinical testing methods. The visual axis is defined in the visual science literature as the line from the fixation point which passes undeviated through the nodal point (or points) of the eye to the fovea. The visual axis is a useful construct when calculating the relationship between object and image sizes and primarily has theoretical applications. Since the nodal points cannot be found in a real eye without measuring every ocular component, they cannot be used to define the bundle of light which passes through the eye. Indeed, a ray which passes through the nodal point may in some circumstances miss the pupil entirely and by striking the iris never continue to the fovea (Figure 10.4).

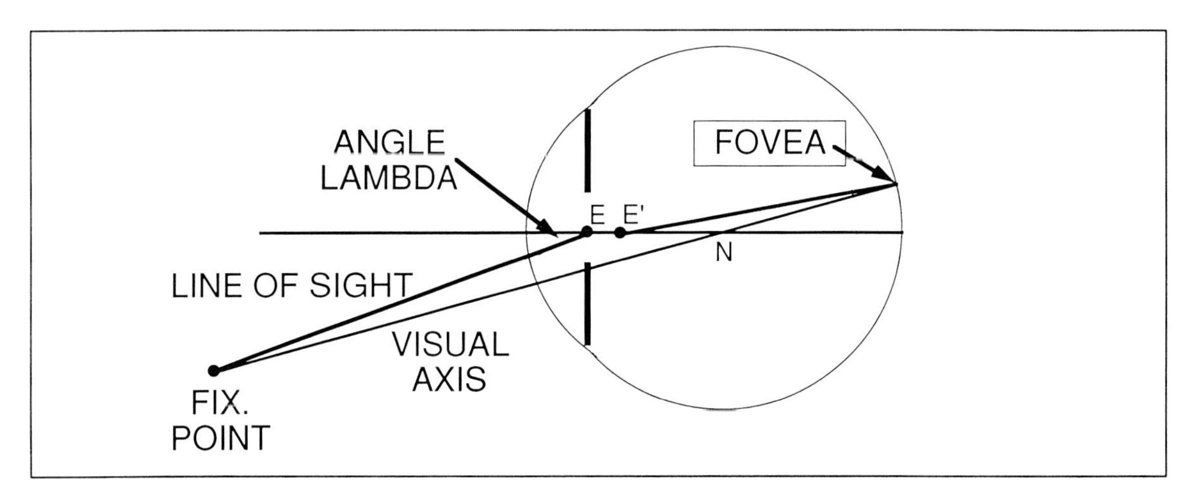

Figure 10.4: Visual axis, defined as the fixation point through the nodal points N and N to the fovea, relates object to image characteristics but does not show actual path of light passing through the eye.

Pupillary Axis

Another very useful axis in videokeratoscopy and other clinical applications is the pupillary axis. Unfortunately, the pupillary axis has been defined in several ways by various investigators. We shall adopt the definition that the pupillary axis is the line from the center of the real pupil that is perpendicular to the cornea (Figure 10.1). It matters not whether the cornea is considered as a simple sphere or is aspherical; the pupillary axis would also pass through the center of curvature of the cornea and would be unique. As with the line of sight, the pupillary axis can be located using clinical test methods.

Asymmetric Eyes

Since the human eye is by no means a perfect optical system, we cannot neglect its imperfections, including the misalignment of the various optical components. We must also take into account that the fovea is usually decentered in a temporal and inferior position from what would be the symmetrical pole. Hence, even for an idealized eye with a symmetrical optical system, the line of sight is usually angled with respect to the pupillary axis, forming angle lambda. Angle lambda should be distinguished from the more commonly used angle kappa, which is defined with respect to the visual axis. Thus, in a clinical setting it is angle lambda that is measured rather than angle kappa as described.

The pupil is not generally a perfect circle and is often found in an eccentric position. With this in mind, it has become common to adopt the use of the centroid rather than the center of pupil as the primary reference point. While the use of the centroid is a useful concept and is likely the best choice for this application, it is not necessarily the optical centroid about which the light bundle is distributed. It would appear to be the most practical solution, however, to the problem of handling asymmetric pupils until more sophisticated techniques are developed. The centroid of the entrance pupil will also be the centroid of the real pupil.

The fact that the line of sight does not coincide with the optic axis would by itself make the entrance pupil appear asymmetric if one were viewing along the line of sight. In most cases it would be more like a slightly asymmetric ellipse than a circle.

For the pupillary axis, finding a unique line to fit the definition becomes more difficult. If the pupil is decentered then the pupillary axis can be deviated significantly. Nevertheless, the pupillary axis is an experimentally definable reference and even in extremely asymmetrical eyes is found to be reproducible. Hence, the pupillary axis has merit simply as a reliably measurable axis for all eyes. It thus serves as a second reference line together with the line of sight in order to describe certain properties of the eye.

Apex Normal

This line defined as the normal to the corneal vertex is confusing because the vertex may be defined in several ways, such as the point of maximum height from the pupil or the point of maximum curvature.

Videokeratoscope Alignment

Currently videokeratoscopes are aligned along the axis which is neither the line of sight nor the visual axis. The videokeratoscope axis is aligned perpendicular to the cornea and hence it is directed towards the center of curvature of the cornea for some unknown peripheral corneal position (Figure 10.5). Redirecting the videokeratoscope so that it is aligned on the line of sight could be accomplished by simply centering the system with respect to the subject's entrance pupil as viewed through the instrument (Figure 10.6). With this adjustment, however, the videokeratoscope would not be aligned perpendicular to the cornea and hence the algorithm would be no longer valid. A proper alignment along the line of sight would require that the subject view an eccentric fixation point in the videokeratoscope adjusted as shown in Figure 10.7. In this way, the videokeratoscope would be aligned at the point on the cornea through which the line of sight passes and would accomplish the desired result. The alignment error would depend on the application desired and is more relevant to problems relating to vision than for studies of the geometry of the cornea.

Reliability of Videokeratoscopy

How well are current videokeratoscopes able to repeat measurements (reliability or precision) and do the measurements really measure what they are supposed to measure (validity or accuracy)? The reliability of commercially available videokeratoscopes has been measured by several investigators who determined the repeatability of a number of measures under one of various sets of conditions, carried out on either test spheres or human eyes. All of the instruments got high marks for repeatability when the test conditions were held constant. Most of the repeatability error came from variations in focusing each time a videokeratogram was taken.

My colleagues and I approached the reliability problem in a somewhat different way. We determined the error from defocusing the instrument by known distances in order to predict what might be expected to occur in a clinical setting for the two most popular commercial instruments, the TMS (Computed Anatomy) and EyeSys videokeratoscopes. These error magnitudes were obtained by mounting a calibrated test sphere on a micromanipulator positioned in front of the videokeratoscope so that the test sphere could be moved a known amount out of focus in 0.1 mm steps away and towards the videokeratoscope. The results are presented in Figure 10.8A,B and they are distinctly different for the two instruments. The TMS

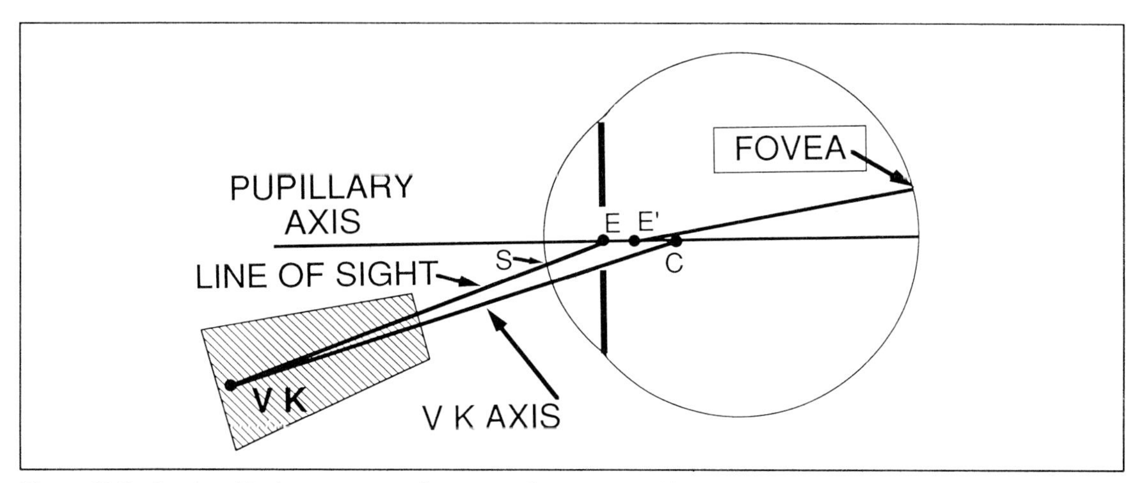

Figure 10.5: Current videokeratoscopes align on a reflected corneal image of a target that is symmetrical with the VK optic axis, which is thus detected towards the center of curvature C for the corneal position measured. VK axis deviates from S where line of sight crosses the cornea.

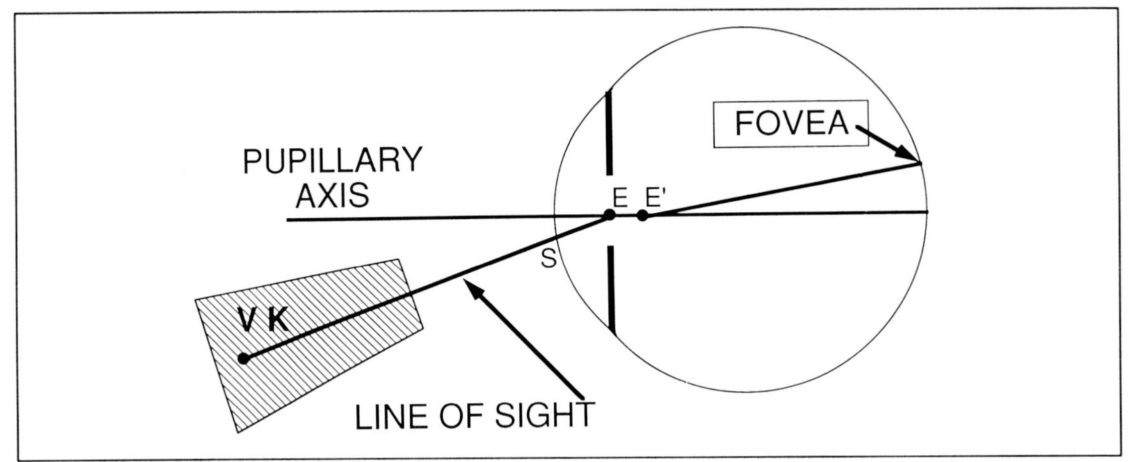

Figure 10.6: Alignment of videokeratoscope so that its optic axis is on the line of sight but not perpendicular to the cornea. Subject views fixation point located on the optic axis of the instrument.

system produced a significant focusing error that was greatest in the periphery of the test ball. The EyeSys system, on the other hand, had less overall error and that was actually less in the periphery. Although informative for finding the nature of the focusing error, these results only have practical significance when viewed in the clinical domain. The significant question is how much out-of-focus can a given operator be expected to be in a clinical situation. The answer may be found from our observations of a number of operators carrying out the focusing task for these two instruments.

With the TMS instrument there was considerable variation from operator to operator in the effort expended to achieve a perfect focus. The poorer operators tended to have errors which correspond to as much as 0.03 mm out of focus and commonly had errors of 0.2 mm out of focus. This produced a final error of approximately ±0.37 D in the central region and up to ±1.00 D in the most peripheral region of the test ball. What can be learned from these test results is that it is imperative that the operator devote maxi-

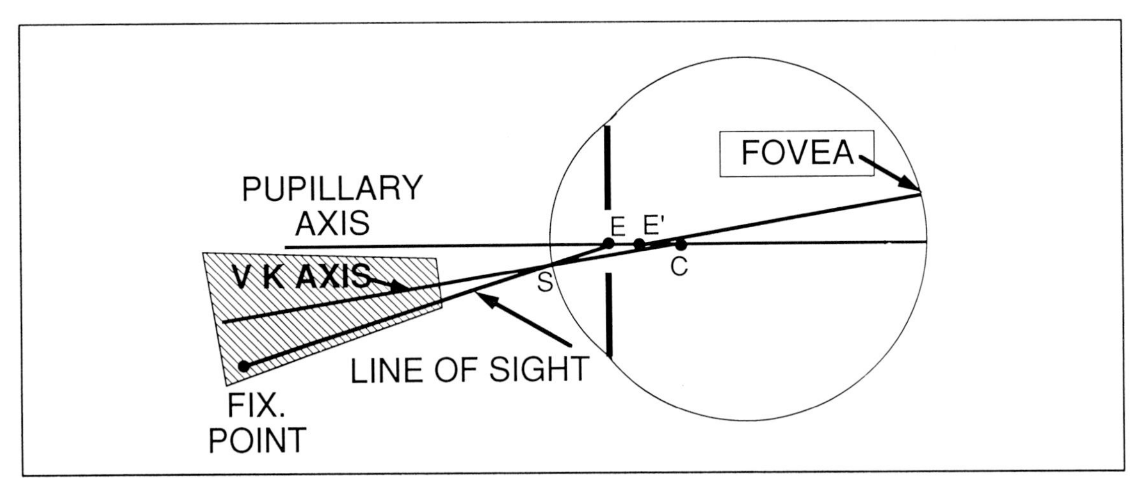

Figure 10.7: Alignment of videokeratoscope so that its optic axis is on the line of sight and also perpendicular to the cornea. Subject views fixation point located at angle from the optic axis of the instrument.

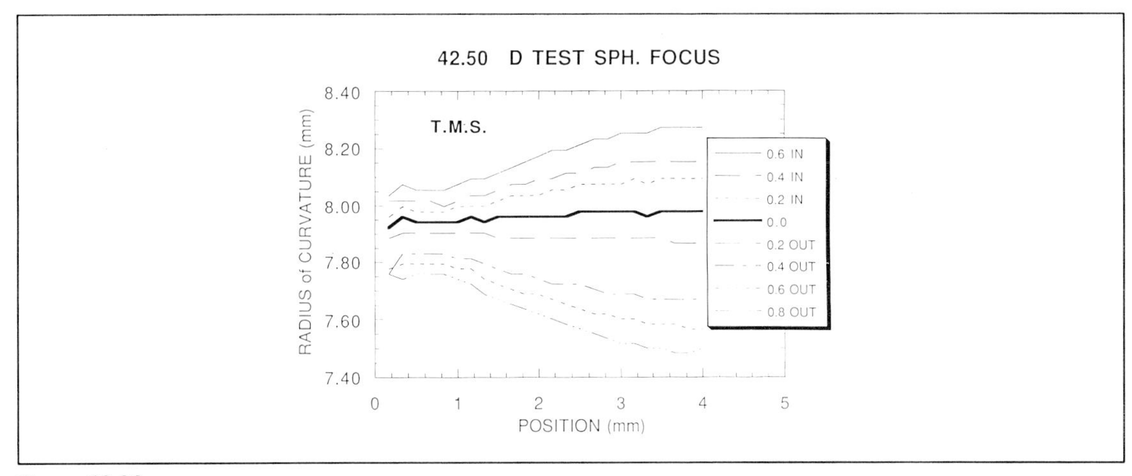

Figure 10.8A.

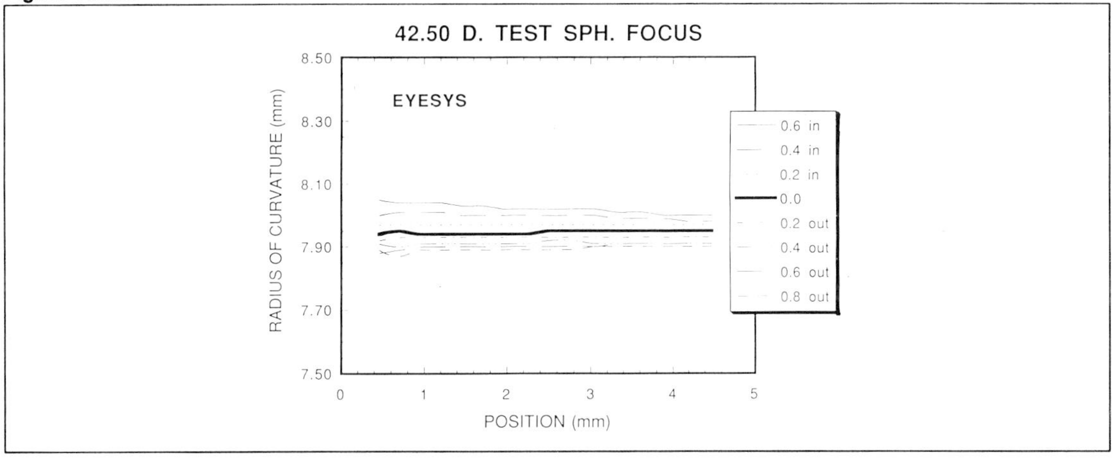

42.50 D. TEST SPH. FOCUS
EYESYS
RADIUS OF CURVATURE (mm)
8.50
8.30
8.10
7.90
7.70
7.50
0
1
2
3
4
5
POSITION (mm)
0.6 in
0.4 in
0.2 in
0.0
0.2 out
0.4 out
0.6 out
0.8 out

Figure 10.8B.

Figure 10.8: Power values found from the videokeratoscope when a test sphere is measured in focus and out of focus by steps of 0.1 mm. (A) TMS Computed Anatomy system. (B) EyeSys system.

mum effort towards obtaining the best focus of the TMS system. The EyeSys system has a less-critical focusing problem primarily because of the large object distance from the instrument target. With a larger object distance, a small shift in focus produces less change in the corneal image size which results in a smaller error.

Lateral decentration of the TMS system also produces greater errors than for the EyeSys system, which has implications for the accuracy of the instruments when measuring aspherical surfaces, which brings up the question of the accuracy for the instrument or how well the instrument is able to measure the curvature of any small area, regardless of its corneal location. The result will depend largely on the instrument algorithm, which is the series of calculations involved in converting the videokeratoscope image sizes into radius of curvature values for the cornea. Several procedures for accomplishing this conversion have been published but we do not know exactly what method is used for each of the commercial instruments, as this information is proprietary.

Nevertheless, by some reverse engineering it is possible to find out how successfully the instrument does measure aspherical surfaces. A discussion of this topic is beyond the scope of this chapter and I can only say that both instruments fall short in this area. However, it would appear that at least from a clinical standpoint the errors occurring from an inaccurate algorithm are less important than the errors produced by improper focusing or misalignment of the system. The latter problem has been generally ignored and needs further attention. There is also a serious problem from the confusion created by the lack of standardization of terminology.

In spite of these problems as the clinical examples demonstrate, currently available videokeratoscopes provide a tremendous amount of clinically useful information not presently obtainable by any other means.

Index